the women's fitness book

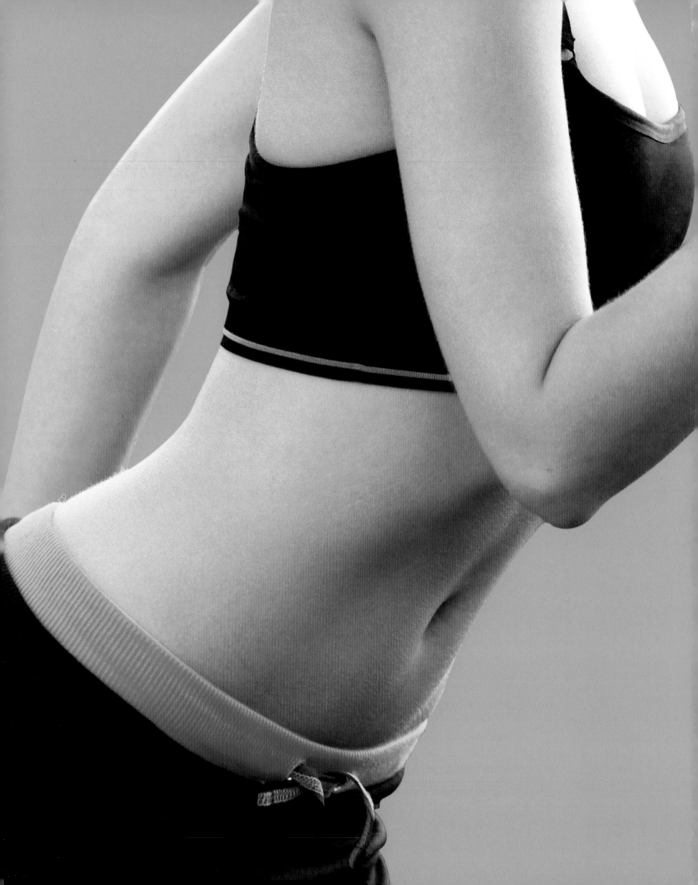

the women's
fitness
book

LONDON, NEW YORK, MUNICH,
MELBOURNE, and DELHI

Principal writer Kelly Thompson

Additional writing Becky Alexander, Fiona Bugler
Senior Editors Andrea Bagg, Corinne Masciocchi, Helen Murray
US Senior Editor Shannon Beatty
Senior Art Editor Wendy Bartlet
Senior Production Editor Jennifer Murray
Senior Production Controller Seyhan Esen
Design Assistant Charlotte Johnson
Creative Technical Support Sonia Charbonnier
Managing Editor Penny Smith
Managing Art Editor Marianne Markham
Art Director Peter Luff
Publisher Peggy Vance

Consultants Lucy Wyndham-Read, Graham Stones, Elisa Withers

DK INDIA
Editors Mahima Barrow, Kokila Manchanda
Assistant Editor Tina Jindal
Senior Art Editor Anchal Kaushal
Assistant Art Editors Zaurin Thoidingjam, Pooja Verma, Neetika Vilash
CTS Manager Sunil Sharma
Production Manager Pankaj Sharma
DTP Designers Dheeraj Arora, Sourabh Challariya,
Usman Mohammad, Arjinder Singh, Jagtar Singh, Anurag Trivedi
Illustrator Subhash Vohra
Managing Editor Glenda Fernandes
Managing Art Editor Navidita Thapa

First American Edition, 2012
Published in the United States by
DK Publishing
375 Hudson Street
New York, New York 10014

12 13 14 15 16   10 9 8 7 6 5 4 3 2 1

001—180689—January 2012

A catalog record for this book is available from the Library of Congress.

ISBN 978-0-7566-8964-3
DK books are available at special discounts when purchased in bulk
for sales promotions, premiums, fund-raising, or educational use.
For details, contact: DK Publishing Special Markets, 375 Hudson Street,
New York, New York 10014 or SpecialSales@dk.com.
Printed and bound in Singapore by Tien Wah Press

Discover more at
www.dk.com

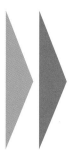

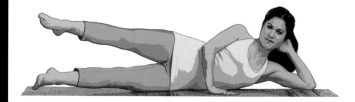

Contents

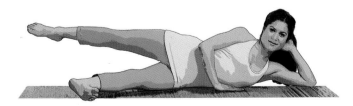

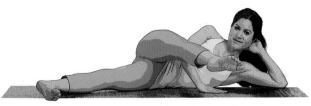

Foreword

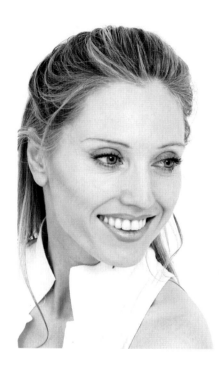

During the course of my 15 years' experience as a personal trainer, I have taken on board all the key issues that women face when it comes to health, fitness, weight loss, and getting in better shape. Women often say they don't have time to fit in exercise, don't know where to start when it comes to getting fitter, can't find an activity they enjoy doing, or they're not getting the results they want from the exercise they're doing. As a personal trainer, it's my role to help them out. However, not everyone is in a position to have one-on-one sessions with an expert, which is why I, along with leading Pilates and yoga experts Elisa Withers and Graham Stones, and fitness writer Kelly Thompson, have designed this book to act as your very own personal trainer.

What makes this book different from other fitness books is the wide range of choice it gives. We have divided exercises into two main categories, both of which everyone needs for complete fitness: cardio to give your heart a good workout and sculpting to tone your body. Within these categories we provide a vast choice of different types of activity. Cardio includes walking, running and jogging, cycling, swimming, and aerobics and dance, while sculpting encompasses resistance training, stretching, Pilates, and yoga.

The aim of providing such variety is to maximize your chances of finding at least one activity that you really enjoy, which will not only make you more motivated, but also give you more scope for varying your activities in order to keep things fresh. For each activity, we outline the main reasons it's good for you before going on to explain exactly how to do it, just as would happen in a personal training session.

To make things as easy as possible for you, we also provide a wide range of tailor-made workouts for you to choose from. These range from 10 minutes to 1 hour in length so that you can fit them in no matter how pushed you are for time. We've provided a choice of 45 cardio workouts at three different levels of intensity—gentle, moderate, and intense—so that all fitness levels are catered for. And we've created 30 sculpting and quick-fix workouts to target the key body areas and address the main concerns that affect women, whether clothes-based such as Little black dress or Skinny jeans, body-based such as Fabulous abs or Dream legs, goal-orientated such as Ten-years-younger, or time-based such as Lunch break workout. By doing three to five of these cardio workouts and three of the sculpting workouts a week, coupled with healthy eating and plenty of rest, you should start to see—and feel—the fitness results after just three to four weeks!

My hope is that this fitness book will provide you with all the information, motivation, practical guidance, and inspiration that you need to lead a healthier life, achieve the body you've always wanted, and both feel and look fitter and younger. Enjoy!

Lucy Wyndham-Read

Introduction

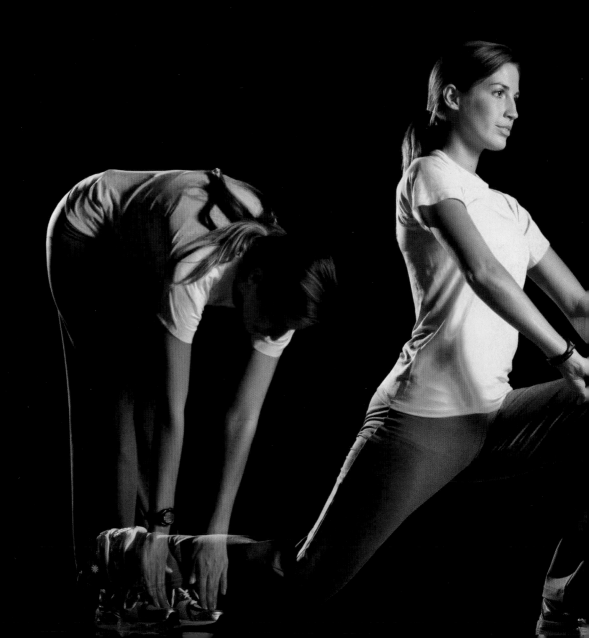

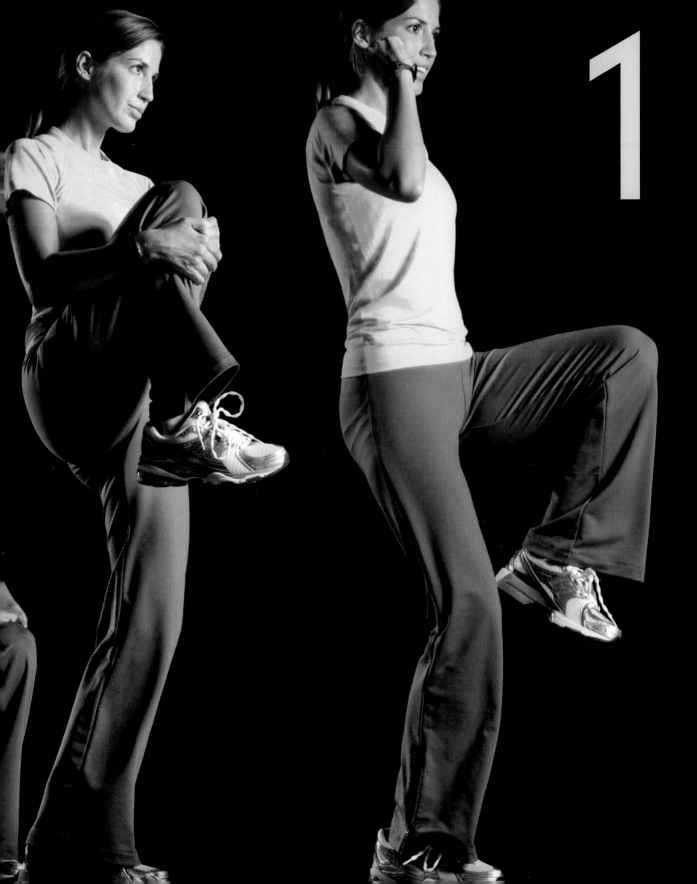

1

How to use this book

This book has been specially designed to enable you to take charge of your own fitness and get the body you've always dreamed of, all in the comfort of your own home. It sheds light on the fundamentals of a wide range of exercise types and empowers you to identify the activities that you are likely to enjoy the most—and that will therefore get you the results you want!

Discover the exercise essentials

First, read the entire Introduction (pp.10–51) since it will deepen your understanding of what exercise is and how it works. It will also provide you with the knowledge to make smart decisions about the best exercise for you, not only according to your personal tastes and lifestyle requirements, but also your body type, fitness level, and of course, crucially, your goals and desires.

Explore your exercise options

The substantial Cardio (pp.52–97) and Sculpting (pp.98–247) chapters that follow the Introduction form the bulk of the book—the building blocks for the

Workouts (pp.248–327)—which are made up of exercises from these two chapters. The Cardio and Sculpting chapters will equip you with the know-how to tackle a wide range of exercise types safely and effectively, finding out along the way exactly what each one is most useful for. This portion of the book could be viewed as your fitness DIY manual if you like—in preparation for the toolkit (workouts) still to come.

The Cardio chapter comprises sections on five key activities for you to choose from in order to burn off calories and increase your aerobic fitness: walking, running, cycling, swimming, and aerobics and dance.

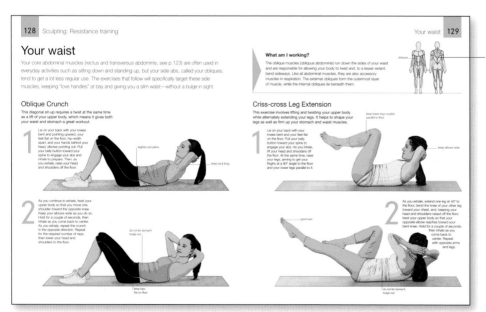

The anatomical diagrams highlight the muscles being used both on the front and back of the body, where relevant.

The Sculpting spreads feature an extensive range of resistance, stretching, Pilates, and yoga exercises. The chapter is broken down into various body areas so that you can focus on the exercises that are specific to your needs.

Each section offers information on that discipline's benefits, equipment, technique, and form, as well as step-by-step guidance on particular exercises that will enhance performance in your chosen area. So get going and enjoy!

The Sculpting chapter includes sections on four exercise types for you to choose from in order to tone and firm up your body: resistance training, stretching, Pilates, and yoga. Each section will shed light on the key benefits and principles of that particular activity so that you can decide which one is best for you. Page after page of invaluable, step-by-step exercises are then presented, which work from upper to lower body as you progress through each section.

Use your exercise toolkit

The Workouts section then draws together many of the exercises from the Cardio and Sculpting chapters to provide you with the ultimate fitness toolkit—in the form of 75 specially designed workouts for you to mix and match according to your needs. Whether you're looking

to lose some weight, flatten your tummy, firm up your arms, increase your confidence, boost your energy level, or all of the above, you will find a way to achieve it here. Four types of workout are included in this section:

- Universal—a warm-up and cool-down, and optional relaxation
- Cardio—a choice of walking, running, cycling, swimming, and aerobics and dance workouts at three intensity levels
- Sculpting—a choice of 20 workouts, combining elements of resistance, stretching, Pilates, and yoga
- Quick fixes—a choice of seven workouts to be done when you have a little unexpected spare time or need an instant boost.

See pp.250–51 for guidance on how long each workout will take, how to most effectively combine the various workouts, and how long your new, personalized exercise program will take to give you the fitness results—and the trim, toned, enviable body—you've always wanted!

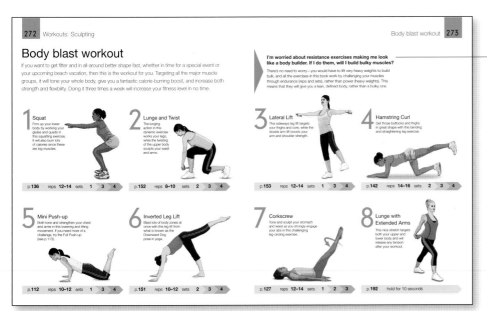

The question and answer features offer practical advice on tackling problem areas, allowing you to get the most out of your workout.

The workouts include cardio programs that really get your heart going, sculpting routines to tone and strengthen your body, and quick-fix exercises to fit in whenever you've got a spare moment, as well as warm-up and cool-down stretches.

What is exercise?

Exercise is, quite simply, any activity that involves physical exertion, however gentle or intense. Different types of exercise challenge your body in different ways to keep you feeling and looking your absolute best throughout life—and who doesn't want that? So read on to discover how you can become the fittest and healthiest you have ever been, and have a beautiful, sculpted body, too.

A route to optimal health

In days gone by, when people farmed their own lands and did their daily tasks by hand, the physical nature of their lives meant there was no need for extra exercise in order to keep their weight down and their bodies healthy. Day-to-day life in our current age of convenience and technology, on the other hand, is often comparatively sedentary, with us spending more and more time sitting—whether in cars, on trains, at desks and computers, or on the sofa watching television—which can leave us feeling unfit and out of shape. Sound familiar? If so, read on. This book will gently lead you out of this rut and into the realms of optimal health and fitness.

What do I need to do?

It's important to combine three different types of exercise in order to achieve a healthy, balanced body:

- **cardiovascular**—for the health of your heart
- **strength and endurance**—for muscle efficiency
- **flexibility**—for the mobility of your joints and muscles.

However, this doesn't mean that you need to spend hours on end working out in a gym or sweating it out on a treadmill. Instead, this book provides you with a wide range of varied exercises and workouts covering all three bases above, which you can do within short time frames—anything from about ten minutes upward. And you don't even have to leave the comfort of your own home if you don't want to! There's also no need to worry if you're not the athletic type—the suggestions cater for all fitness levels and tastes, from gentle walks, rejuvenating swims, nourishing stretches, and relaxing yoga postures to invigorating cycles, challenging runs, energizing dance steps, strengthening resistance exercises, and strong Pilates moves. After all, the main function of doing regular exercise is to be as fit as possible for the demands of everyday life. If you want to enhance your performance in a particular sport, fantastic. But wanting simply to have more energy for your children, tone up before your summer vacation, or feel more confident in your skinny jeans are also great reasons to exercise.

Exercise helps you to stay flexible. Yoga movements, such as Downward Dog shown here, are especially good for stretching your muscles and keeping your joints mobile.

What are my options?

In the pages that follow, you will find guidance on a range of the most popular and effective forms of exercise: walking, running, cycling, swimming, and aerobics on the cardio side; and resistance exercises, stretching, Pilates, and yoga on the strength and flexibility side. However, there are countless other exercise options that would complement the workouts in this book, such as racquet sports, ball games, martial arts, water sports, or anything else that appeals to you.

The key is to find the activities that not only you enjoy the most, but that also seem most likely to get you the fitness results you want—whether that's a flatter tummy, slimmer arms, or more energy and stamina. It's also important to incorporate physical activity into your everyday routine as much as you can by following some simple steps, such as:

- walking or cycling, rather than driving
- taking the stairs instead of the elevator
- being aware of posture and alignment (see p.32) when doing daily tasks such as cleaning, gardening, DIY, and even when just sitting on your office chair.

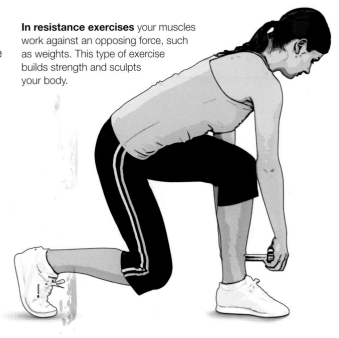

In resistance exercises your muscles work against an opposing force, such as weights. This type of exercise builds strength and sculpts your body.

The more aware you remain of your desire for health and fitness, the more healthy choices you will automatically make—in terms of both exercise and nutrition (see pp.48–51). Soon, taking the healthy option will become automatic. As you start to see positive results, you'll also be motivated to continue with your new way of life.

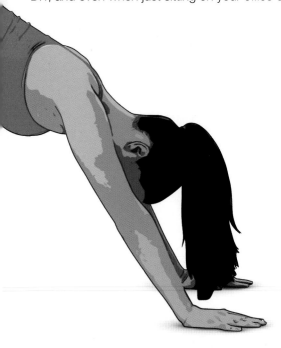

A sample healthy day

- Gentle stretches in bed (see Morning wake-up workout, p.314–15)
- Cereal and fruit for breakfast
- Cycle to work and take the stairs once you're there
- Homemade soup or salad for lunch, then a brief walk
- Stretching sessions as breaks from work (see Computer workout, pp.316–17)
- Nuts, seeds, and fruit for snacks
- Water and herbal tea for refreshment
- Cycle home from work
- Rice, fresh vegetables, and fish for dinner
- Sculpting workout, such as "Little Black Dress" (see pp.278–79) or active household chores in the evening
- Pre-bed relaxation time, whether a hot bath or reading an inspirational book

Why exercise?

We all know that exercise is good for us, but it's helpful to remind ourselves from time to time of the many specific ways in which it can enhance your life. When you really consider the wide range of benefits, it becomes hard to understand why anyone wouldn't incorporate exercise into their daily routine!

The feel-good factor

Regular exercise gets your heart pumping, your lungs working harder, and your joints and muscles working through a wide range of movements, not only boosting the efficiency of all your body's systems (see pp.20–23), but also making you feel more vibrant and dynamic. It therefore improves not only your physical fitness, but also your mental and emotional fitness, leading to an overall enhanced quality of life.

Restoring balance

With today's ultra-busy lifestyles, when we constantly have to multitask to cope, we often place ourselves under excessive stress to get everything done. Such stress can lead to our bodies being on high alert all the time, with soaring levels of adrenaline and other hormones, as the sympathetic nervous system (see p.22) instigates what is known as the "fight or flight" response in readiness for the perceived need for urgent action. This involves, among other things, an accelerated heart rate, faster breathing, and slower digestion, which, when sustained over a long period of time, can lead to exhaustion and burnout.

Regular exercise can help to rebalance your system under such circumstances. An intense workout such as a challenging run or Body blast (see p.272) will provide an outlet for what would have been the natural conclusion of a real "fight or flight" situation: physical activity. A less strenuous exercise session, on the other hand, such as a gentle walk or a relaxing yoga session, will help to turn off the "fight or flight" switch, thus restoring your body to a calm and healthy state.

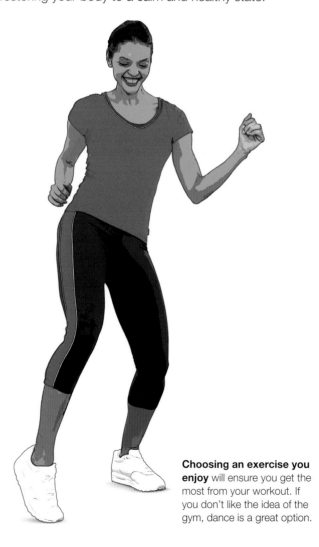

Choosing an exercise you enjoy will ensure you get the most from your workout. If you don't like the idea of the gym, dance is a great option.

Training your brain

Regular exercise can boost your brain as well as your body. After all, getting your heart pumping harder boosts your circulation, which increases blood flow to your brain as well as to your muscles and other tissues around the body. The awareness needed to do many of the exercises in this book will also help to keep your mind sharp and fresh. In technical terms, doing such exercises increases the action of your proprioceptors—specialized receptors in tendons and muscles that link your body and brain—making you aware of your body position and movements.

Getting into a "happy groove"

Research shows that exercise releases endorphins and other "happy hormones" in the body, which promote a feeling of well-being and vibrancy. This, in turn, is likely to make you want to exercise even more—bringing you into a cycle of positive action.

Lifestyle benefits

Regular exercise gives you the chance to:
- spend time with friends or on your own
- get in better shape
- manage your weight
- boost your energy levels
- get stronger
- build your stamina
- become more flexible
- improve your coordination
- increase your mobility
- develop your balance
- enhance your posture
- alleviate stiffness
- reduce stress levels
- increase your focus
- become more confident
- lift your spirits
- enhance your body image and self-esteem
- fight the aging process
- live healthier for longer

Physiological and health benefits

Regular exercise can help to:
- make your heart work more efficiently
- re-balance your nervous system
- strengthen muscles
- enhance circulation
- define muscles
- stabilize joints
- strengthen bones
- boost metabolism
- increase lung capacity
- reduce body fat

Regular exercise can also help to reduce the risk of chronic problems such as:
- high blood pressure
- osteoporosis
- back and joint pain
- coronary heart disease
- stroke
- some cancers
- type 2 diabetes

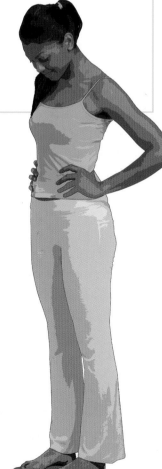

Weight loss is a key motivating factor for many people when it comes to exercise. Exercising regularly does help control weight but what you eat is important, too.

Principles of training

A successful fitness routine should combine elements of aerobic exercise to increase cardiovascular capacity and/or weight loss; resistance training to promote strength, endurance, and muscle definition; and stretching to maximize mobility and flexibility. It's important to know some underlying principles of safe and effective training before you start.

How often?

The amount and level of exercise that you need to do will depend on your age, general health, current level of fitness (see pp.34–39), your activity preferences, and what you want to achieve. Don't worry if you haven't exercised in a while—begin gently and you'll soon get back into the swing of it. Every workout in this book—whether Cardio (see pp.258–69), Sculpting (see pp.270–311), or Quick-fix (see pp.312–27)—offers three levels of intensity (gentle, moderate, and intense), from which you can choose. If your aim is to get fitter as well as slimmer and more toned, it's generally best to do:

- Cardio at least 3–5 times a week
- Sculpting (strength and flexibility) 3 times a week—on alternate days
- Quick-fix (strength and flexibility) in any spare time slots.

Be consistent with your exercise: doing five 20-minute sessions a week is more beneficial than doing nothing all week and then a one- or two-hour blast.

Before doing any exercise involving jumping, such as skipping (which can be done with or without a rope), it's best to do a low-impact warm-up first.

When?

There are no hard and fast rules about when to exercise: do it any time that works for you—both to suit the natural rhythm of your energy and your schedule commitments. For many people, however, first thing in the morning can be a good time to fit in an exercise session—not only because they haven't yet used up much energy, but also because they haven't gotten started with the many tasks of the day, which can end up causing that "I'm too busy for a workout" feeling. A morning workout also provides a sense of achievement for the rest of the day. The down side is that you might be quite dehydrated in the morning, so drink plenty of water or some fresh juice before you start anything.

Whatever time you find most beneficial to exercise, never do it on a full stomach. Leave at least two hours between eating a meal and starting a workout. It's fine, however, to have a small, healthy snack, such as a banana, 20–30 minutes before exercise if desired.

How much?

The intensity of each workout you do is entirely up to you, based on your individual needs: your current fitness level, what your goals are, and how seriously you want to commit to getting in better shape. When it comes to resistance exercises, intensity depends on how many repetitions (reps) you do in a row before resting as well as on the number of sets of repetitions you do. For

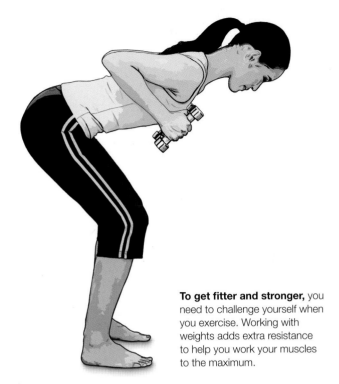

To get fitter and stronger, you need to challenge yourself when you exercise. Working with weights adds extra resistance to help you work your muscles to the maximum.

nerve impulses travel to your muscles (thus enhancing control and coordination), a warm-up also gradually increases your heart rate and body temperature. It also reduces the chance of injuries occurring and increases the overall effectiveness of the workout. It's also important to do a cool-down (see pp.254–55) after any workout to bring your body back to its pre-exercise state. This not only normalizes your heart rate and body temperature, and helps to remove lactic acid (a by-product of vigorous exercise) from your body, but also provides a chance to increase your flexibility since your muscles are warm and pliable at this stage—this is why cool-down stretches are often more intense than warm-up ones.

Apply the overload principle

It's essential to challenge your body in order for it to adapt, develop, and become fitter and stronger. If you don't, you won't see results. So when we say in this book to move "as far as is comfortable" or to hold "for as long as is comfortable," we mean to the point of maximal challenge without any discomfort or pain. This "point of challenge"—where you feel like you can't physically do any more—is the stage at which the most effective strength work can be done, so urge yourself to do "just a little bit more" at this point if you possibly can—do just a few more reps or hold the pose for a few more seconds in order to really get the most from your body, as is also suggested for the strength tests on pp.36–37. This "overload" principle works on the idea that for any physiological system, whether the muscles, skeleton, heart, or lungs, to improve its function, it has to be exposed to a load larger than it normally has to deal with.

example, you might squat 10 times (10 reps), take a break, then do 10 more reps. This is two sets. When it comes to yoga, stretching, and Pilates, generally it's about how long you hold a position, which can be measured by counts or number of breaths, one breath being an inhalation and an exhalation. If you are "unfit" or "below average" in the fitness ratings (see p.39), you'll probably want to start with low-intensity workouts and work up to more vigorous ones once you feel stronger and have more time.

Warm-up and cool-down

It's crucial to do a warm-up (see pp.252–53) before any workout so that your body is prepared for the more demanding movements to come. As well as limbering up your joints and muscles, and raising the speed at which

*It's essential to **challenge your body** in order for it to become fitter and stronger, so always work to your point of maximal challenge—where you feel you can't do any more—but never continue if you feel discomfort or pain.*

Listen to your body

Whatever form of exercise you are doing, be sure to find and work at your own level, no matter what anyone else is doing around you. Some rules of thumb are:

- never force a movement or position
- slow down a little if you are breathing heavily or feel overheated
- stop if you experience any real discomfort.

If a sculpting exercise seems too challenging, consider how to bring the intensity down a notch. For example, do fewer reps or sets, or hold the position for a shorter time than advised; try the exercise without weights if you're currently using weights; or alter your position, where appropriate, to make the movement less extreme, such as by bending your knees slightly in a forward bend.

Conversely, if an exercise doesn't feel challenging enough, try doing more reps or sets, or holding the position for longer; adding weights or increasing the size of the weights you're using (see also p.106); or altering your position, where appropriate, to make the movement more difficult, such as by doing a deeper squat. It's best to consult a fitness professional if you're unsure about how to adapt the level of an exercise to suit your needs.

Vary your activities

People often stick to the same fitness routine week-in, week-out because it's what they know and within their comfort zone. Yet this is rarely the most effective approach. It's important to add variety to your exercise program—not only to keep you from getting bored and giving up on it, but also to ensure that you challenge yourself in different ways. Otherwise, your body will soon adapt to the physiological demands of a repetitive workout and you'll no longer see results—a phenomenon known as reaching a "plateau." Varying your workouts also reduces the chance of over-use injury.

Recognize the value of rest

It's essential to get enough sleep each night to give your body time to recover from day-to-day demands, so experiment to find how much is optimal for you. Getting less than this amount can lead to reduced concentration, slower reaction time, a feeling of sluggishness, and an inability to handle stress. Adequate sleep, on the other hand, will leave you feeling rejuvenated and ready for anything. You must also leave rest days between sculpting workouts to give your body time to repair and ready itself for further progress (see p.104).

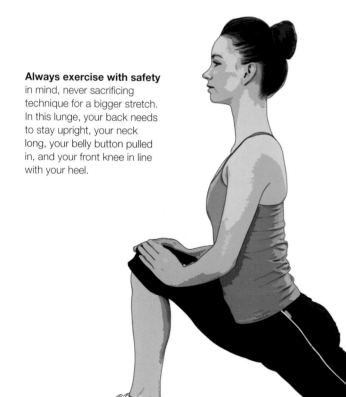

Always exercise with safety in mind, never sacrificing technique for a bigger stretch. In this lunge, your back needs to stay upright, your neck long, your belly button pulled in, and your front knee in line with your heel.

Exercise safely

Always

√ do a warm-up routine before you start any workout (see pp.252–53).

√ maintain the natural alignment of your spine (see p.23) throughout all movements—the back of your neck should be long, your back curving naturally, and your pelvis slightly tucked.

√ pull your belly button toward your spine to engage your abdominal muscles—this will give your lower back adequate support, build core strength (see p.37), stop your stomach from bulging, and encourage good posture.

√ move slowly and with control during every movement, both going into and coming out of positions. This not only maximizes safety, but also increases the effectiveness of each exercise.

√ remember to breathe—it may seem obvious, but people sometimes get so carried away thinking about good technique that they accidentally hold their breath.

√ exhale on the movement involving most exertion and inhale on the return movement—guidance is given within the steps for each sculpting exercise.

√ work at your own pace—only do as much as is comfortable for you and feel free to adapt movements according to your needs, whether you need something less or more challenging (see left).

√ drink plenty of water to stay hydrated (see p.51).

√ finish exercises symmetrically—do the same number of repetitions on each side.

√ stop exercising if you experience any discomfort or pain at any time, or if you become faint, dizzy, or have difficulty breathing.

√ do a cool-down routine (see pp.254–55) once you have completed any workout.

Never

X exercise on a full stomach.

X ignore your medical conditions or fitness level*.

X exercise to a point of discomfort or pain (see p.17).

X hunch up your shoulders as you exercise, since this will collapse your chest and cause bad overall posture, as well as a wrinkled chest!

X over-arch your back, since this can create unhealthy compression and tension.

X allow your stomach to bulge out as you exercise.

X bend your knees farther forward than your toes or "lock" your legs when they are straight; either action will put undue pressure on your knees.

X sacrifice good technique for more reps, sets, or length of time held—doing an exercise incorrectly not only reduces its effectiveness, but also increases your chance of injury.

X overdo it so much in one session that you feel too weak for the next one; instead, try to adopt a measured and moderate approach.

X compare yourself to others—every individual's needs and capacity are unique so trying to move at someone else's pace could be detrimental to you.

X underestimate the importance of adequate rest: your body needs time between sculpting workouts to restore and repair itself, so rest is just as important as exercise.

Note: If you have health issues or any doubt regarding the suitability of any of the exercises in this book, be sure to consult a doctor before trying them.

How your body works

Before starting any kind of exercise program, it is useful to understand how your body works and how it will therefore benefit from the physical activity you are about to start. Of the body's many incredible systems, the ones most directly affected by regular exercise are the skeletal, muscular, cardiovascular, respiratory, nervous, and endocrine systems.

The skeletal system

Your skeleton is made up of an amazing 206 bones that keep you upright, protect your organs, allow you to move (bones are the levers of all movements), and store essential minerals. All your bones, except one (the hyoid bone in the neck), meet with other bones to form joints.

Some joints, like those in the skull, are immovable and are joined by fibrous tissue. Others, such as the vertebrae in the spine, are only partially movable; these are connected by pads of cartilage. Most of the joints in our bodies, however, are complex, freely movable joints, called synovial joints.

Synovial joints are lubricated by synovial fluid, which helps to absorb the shock of any high-impact movements. In addition, the ends of the bones in a synovial joint are coated with smooth cartilage that provides cushioning and allows your joints to move without discomfort. The whole joint is stabilized by ligaments that connect the bones. All these structures allow movement to occur, but it is your skeletal muscles (see right) that provide the power. When a muscle contracts, it pulls on tendons, which connect the muscle to bones, moving the bones in the desired direction.

The muscular system

We know that muscles enable movement, but how exactly do they do this? The answer is that they alternately contract (shorten) and relax (lengthen).

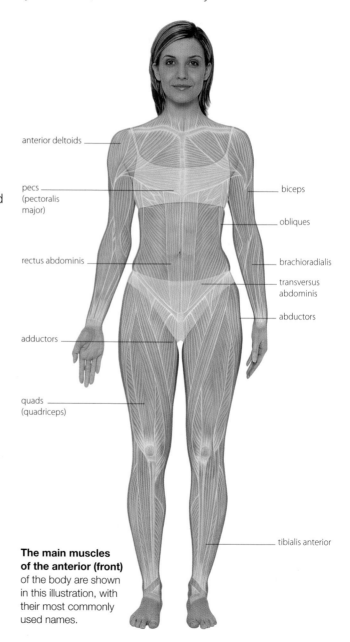

anterior deltoids

pecs (pectoralis major)

rectus abdominis

adductors

quads (quadriceps)

biceps

obliques

brachioradialis

transversus abdominis

abductors

tibialis anterior

The main muscles of the anterior (front) of the body are shown in this illustration, with their most commonly used names.

__The way our bodies move is amazing__—we can run, jump, throw, and perform many other complex actions—all made possible by the coordinated interaction of our bones, muscles, tendons, ligaments, and nerves.

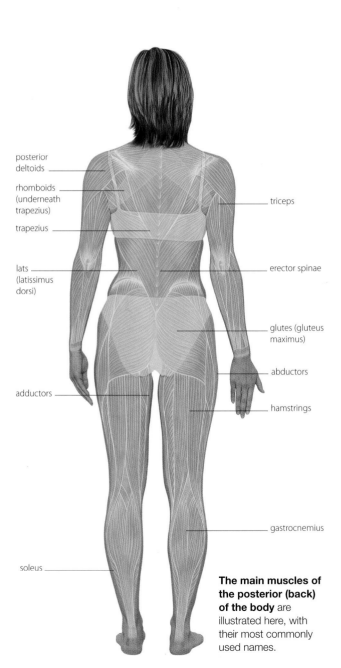

posterior deltoids

rhomboids (underneath trapezius)

trapezius

lats (latissimus dorsi)

adductors

soleus

triceps

erector spinae

glutes (gluteus maximus)

abductors

hamstrings

gastrocnemius

The main muscles of the posterior (back) of the body are illustrated here, with their most commonly used names.

Connected to your muscle fibers are nerves that carry messages to and from your brain, and blood vessels that carry energy in the form of oxygen to your muscles and waste in the form of carbon dioxide away from them. The human body contains three types of muscle:

- cardiac muscle—in the heart
- smooth muscle—in the walls of internal structures, such as the intestines
- skeletal muscle—attached to bones.

Cardiac muscle works to pump blood around your body, determining your cardiovascular fitness (see p.35). Smooth muscle works, among other things, to keep essential substances moving through your body. However, it's skeletal muscle that is responsible for giving your body its shape, holding it upright, stabilizing your joints, and enabling your bones and therefore your body to move. Every external movement that you make, no matter how small, is therefore a result of skeletal muscle.

While cardio and smooth muscle are involuntary, which means that they aren't under your conscious control, skeletal muscle is a voluntary muscle, meaning you can control when and how you use it. Given that we each have more than 600 skeletal muscles in our body, it would be somewhat tricky to try to actively think about how to use them all each time we work out! However, there are certain key muscle groups that are particularly useful to be aware of when exercising (see left). With regular use of a wide range of your skeletal muscles via the workouts in this book, you should gradually see an increase not only in how long each muscle can contract for and how much weight it can support (endurance and strength), but also in how much each muscle can stretch before returning to its normal state (flexibility).

The cardiovascular system

The term "cardiovascular" simply refers to your heart and all your blood vessels. Your heart beats on average an incredible 100,000 times a day. Every single minute, it pumps all your body's blood—about 9 pints (5 liters)—through a system of arteries, veins, and capillaries in order to provide your organs, muscles, and nerves with the oxygen they need to function and to take away carbon dioxide and other waste products.

It's no wonder then that it's so crucial to keep your heart fit and strong. But how can this be achieved? Well, the walls of your heart are made of a special cardiac muscle (see p.21), found nowhere else in the body. This muscle is immensely powerful and enables your heart to act as a vital double pump, contracting and relaxing alternately in order to squeeze oxygen-rich blood into your arteries and around your body, while at the same time pumping used blood to the lungs for more oxygen (see The respiratory system, below). The heart has its own pacemaker, which produces electrical impulses that spread through the heart, stimulating contraction.

Like any muscle, your heart needs to be regularly challenged in order to function at its best. And it's only through physical exercise—or, specifically, cardio (or aerobic) exercise—that this is possible (see pp.52–97).

The respiratory system

The main functions of your respiratory system are to:
- supply your blood with the body's essential fuel, oxygen
- remove the waste product carbon dioxide from your blood.

So how exactly does this work? It all starts when you breathe in. The oxygen that you inhale through your nose travels down to your lungs, where it diffuses into your bloodstream. From here, it's transported to your heart, where it is pumped around your body for use as fuel. Meanwhile, carbon dioxide, which is created as a by-product of your body's activity, is carried by your blood to your heart, where it is pumped into your lungs and exhaled through your mouth.

Full, deep breathing is therefore a must if you are to remain healthy and active throughout life. Good breathing (see p.33) also enhances performance in most forms of exercise since it provides your muscles with increased oxygen, which they need to work harder.

The nervous system

Your nervous system is made up of your brain and spinal cord (central nervous system) and the many nerves branching out from your spinal cord to the rest of the body (peripheral nervous system). Electrical impulses within your nerve cells (or neurons) trigger the production of chemicals called neurotransmitters, such as serotonin, which send all the vital messages between your central nervous system and everything else in your body, including your muscles, telling them what they need to do when. The nervous system has two parts:

- **Sympathetic:** "fight or flight"
This prepares your body for emergencies by increasing your blood pressure, heart rate, and breathing rate, and sending blood to your muscles in readiness for action. It is dominant when you are very active and/or stressed.

*Good breathing **enhances your performance** during most forms of exercise since it provides your muscles with increased oxygen, which they need in order to work harder.*

- **Parasympathetic:** "rest and digest"
This restores your energy by keeping your blood pressure, heart rate, and breathing rate at a low level, and focusing on your body's many vital underlying functions, such as digestion. It is dominant when you are at rest or engaged in relaxing activities.

Over-stimulation of one system or the other can, with time, lead to imbalance in the body. However, regular exercise of the right kind can help to restore this balance—vigorous exercise such as intense cycling or running workouts can help to rev up your sympathetic nervous system, if required, while gentle activities such as slow walks and swims, and nourishing yoga sequences, can help to activate the relaxation response of the parasympathetic system.

The endocrine system

The primary responsibility of your endocrine system is to keep your body in balance (homeostasis). It does this by the release of hormones from various organs and tissues around the body that help to regulate, among other things, mood, energy, fertility, metabolism (which affects weight control), and growth.

However, hormone levels can become out of balance for all sorts of reasons—such as during times of heightened stress or anxiety, when it's the "time of the month," or if you are going through menopause. Luckily, research suggests that regular exercise can help to balance hormones. Physical activity can, for example, encourage the release of more endorphins, which reduce tension and anxiety, and help to promote a positive frame of mind.

Exercise can also help to balance levels of the sex hormones estrogen and testosterone, as well as those of growth hormone, which is particularly useful for anyone over 40, since your natural levels of these hormones tend to decrease as you age.

The all-important spine:

Your spine is made up of a series of bones, called vertebrae, which are connected by disks and ligaments that provide both cushioning and mobility. Your spine has many vital functions—it:
- supports your body, keeping it upright
- enables upper body movement
- acts as a shock absorber
- protects the spinal cord.

The spine's four main sections give it a slight "S" curve when viewed from the side. The cervical area curves slightly inward, the thoracic spine slightly outward, the lumbar slightly in, and the sacrum and coccyx slightly out. It's crucial to keep these natural curves in place not just when exercising but all the time, since they enable the spine to absorb and deal with the many stresses placed on it as we move. Retaining these curves is what we mean by good posture (see p.32).

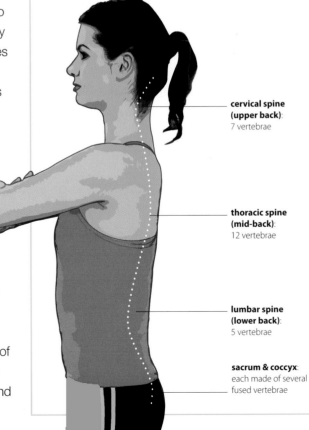

cervical spine (upper back):
7 vertebrae

thoracic spine (mid-back):
12 vertebrae

lumbar spine (lower back):
5 vertebrae

sacrum & coccyx:
each made of several fused vertebrae

How your body moves

All body movement involves the interaction of your bones and muscles: your bones, which meet at joints, are moved by the action of your muscles. In order to get the best results from the exercises in this book, it's useful to have an understanding of the different types of movement that can take place so that you know which activities work which body zones—and how.

Planes of movement

There are three overall planes of movement in which your body can move:

- **sagittal**—forward and backward
- **lateral** (also called frontal)—sideways
- **transverse**—rotation.

Most of our day-to-day activities, including walking, going up and down the stairs, and sitting down and getting up, tend to involve movement in a sagittal plane only (forward and backward). This means that, for many of us, the muscles on the front (anterior) and back (posterior) of our bodies are worked frequently, while the muscles on our sides—responsible for sideways and rotational movements—are somewhat neglected.

Likewise, many traditional exercises, such as squats, lunges, and push-ups, move in a sagittal plane. Although these are great exercises in themselves, it's essential to move in all three planes for a full-body tone. Think of your body as a Russian doll: you start off a certain size and, by doing sculpting exercises that target your muscles and joints from every angle, you can gradually trim down the outer layer to become the next-size-down doll. If, however, you always just do sagittal movements, you won't be drawing in the muscles from your sides. Another good analogy is that a body worked only in a sagittal plane is like a gift that you have wrapped neatly on two sides but left messy on the other two.

Varying your movement

It's a good idea to ensure a balanced range of movement when choosing which workouts to do from within this book. When it comes to cardio, walking, running, and cycling all work you in a sagittal plane, while swimming and aerobics/dancing can work you in all three planes, depending on which stroke you choose to swim and which dance moves you choose to do. You may therefore want to vary your Cardio workouts (see pp.258–69) from time to time to ensure that you target your body from all angles. For example, you could do a walking, running, or cycling workout for 3–4 weeks and then switch to a swimming or aerobics/dance workout for the next 3–4 weeks. You may also want to vary your swimming strokes as much as possible.

When it comes to the Sculpting and Quick-fix workouts (see pp.270–327), you will see that these have been specially designed to incorporate the widest range

*Think of your body as a Russian doll: you start off a certain size and, by doing sculpting exercises that **target your muscles and joints** from every angle, you can gradually trim down the outer layer to become the next-size-down doll.*

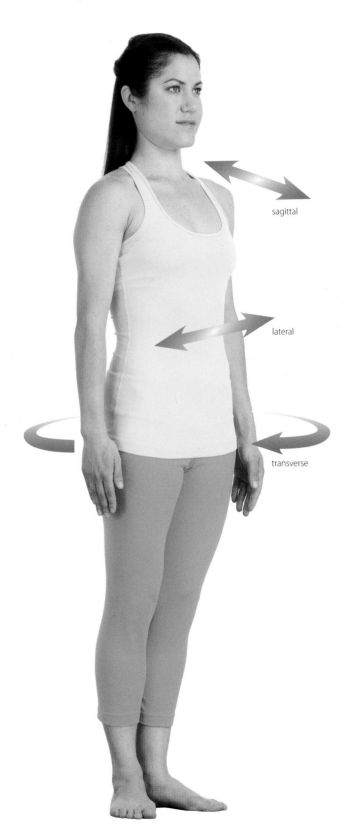

sagittal

lateral

transverse

of movement possible, whether of the whole body or around isolated body parts, so all you need to do is choose the ones that appeal to you most. The Skinny Jeans workout (see pp.282–83), for example, works the lower body in all three planes of movement:

- sagittal: e.g. Lunge Kick—kicking forward and lunging backward
- lateral: e.g. Side-squat Kick—lifting your legs to the side
- transverse: e.g. Side-lying Leg Circle—moving each leg in a sweeping circle.

Types of movement

The three planes of movement described above can be further broken down into several main types of movement, named according to the direction in which they cause your muscles and joints to move in relation to the central line of your body—whether you're standing, sitting, or lying.

   The exercises in this book will have you doing a combination of all these types of movement and will therefore give your body a healthy, balanced workout. The main types of movement are:

Sagittal

- Flexion—forward movement
- Extension—backward movement

Lateral (or frontal)

- Adduction—sideways movement toward center (inward)
- Abduction—sideways movement away from center (outward)
- Lateral flexion—sideways movement of the upper body and neck (side-bending)

Transverse

- Medial rotation—twisting movement toward center (inward)
- Lateral rotation—twisting movement away from center (outward)

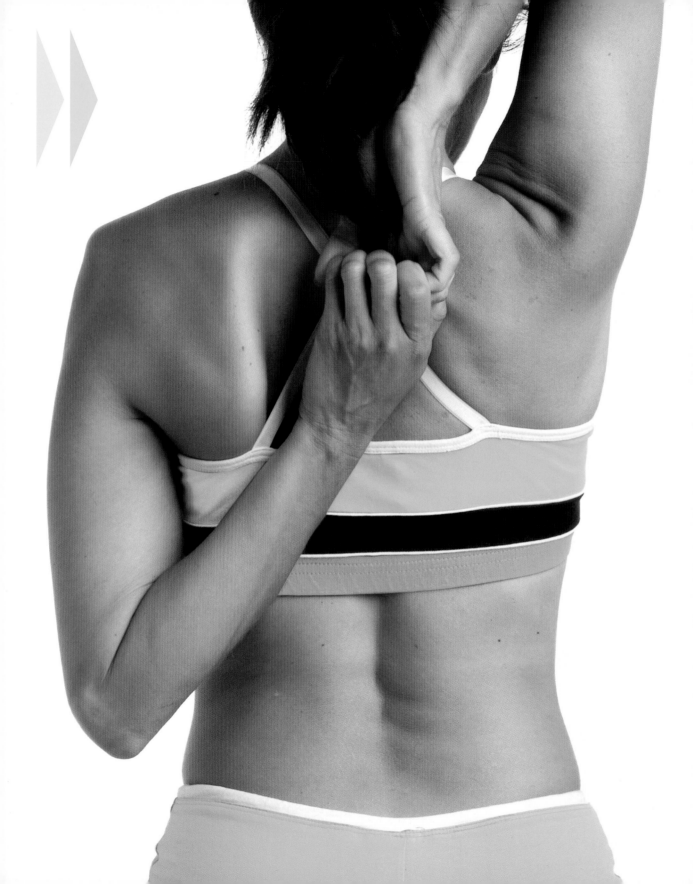

Know your body

It's important that any exercise you do matches your ever-changing fitness and lifestyle needs. Otherwise it won't be a safe, effective, and enjoyable way of producing the results you want—whether that's increased cardio capacity, a slimmer waist, or more toned arms and abs. The pages that follow will give you the tools you need to be able to choose the most appropriate exercise for your own unique body by encouraging you to:

- get to know your body shape

- realistically evaluate your weight

- identify your fitness needs according to your age

- become more aware of your posture

- recognize the importance of full, deep breathing

- establish your current level of cardio fitness

- assess your levels of strength and flexibility

- consider which types of exercise best suit your personality

Assessing your body

Before you can create an effective exercise program, it's crucial to gain a good understanding of your body and its needs. Keeping regular track of your weight, BMI (body mass index), and waist and hip circumference, as well as establishing which frame and type of body you have, will help you to decide what your fitness priorities should be.

Weigh yourself

Your changing body weight can be a useful point of reference if one of your aims is to lose weight. However, it's important to remember that decreased weight doesn't necessarily equate to a smaller waist or hips; you'll need to do area-specific exercises to target particular body zones. Also, keep in mind that muscle is heavier than fat so positive changes may be occurring within your body even if your weight is not decreasing. It's best to weigh yourself first thing in the morning, before you've had your first meal of the day. Many people prefer to do it naked or in their underwear to get the lowest reading possible.

Work out your BMI

Your BMI (body mass index) is an approximate measure of whether you're a healthy weight for your height. Use the following formula to determine your BMI score: BMI = weight in kg / height in meters squared, e.g. 61kg ÷ (1.62m x 1.62m) = 23.28 Then use your score to check which category you fall into:
• below 18.5: you may be underweight, so could be over-training or eating an unbalanced diet (see pp. 48–51); consult a medical expert.
• 18.5–24.9: you are a healthy weight for your height, so maintain this in order to look and feel your best.

Apple

Women with this body type store most of their fat around their mid-section. It is therefore important to supplement lots of fat-burning cardio work at the appropriate level with stomach, waist, and chest exercises to define these areas.

Suggested workouts:
• Bikini body (pp.284–85)
• Beautiful back (pp.286–87)
• Fabulous abs (pp.292–93)
• "Apple" (pp.298–99)

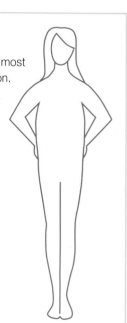

Pear

Women with this body type store most of their fat around their hips, thighs, and buttocks. It is therefore important to supplement lots of fat-burning cardio work with specific lower body exercises.

Suggested workouts:
• Skinny jeans (pp.282–83)
• Ultimate butt (pp.294–95)
• Dream legs (pp.296–97)
• "Pear" (pp.300–01)

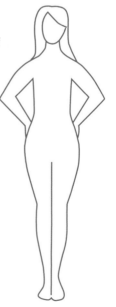

• 25.0 and above: you may be overweight and therefore at increased risk for certain health problems, so work toward losing weight. This score can, however, class you as "overweight" if you have very dense bones or a large body frame, or if you are particularly muscular (since muscle is heavier than fat). So only ever use it as a rough guide in conjunction with how you feel and how you look in the mirror—preferably naked. And if you do ever fall slightly into the "overweight" category, there's no need to panic or feel bad. Instead, simply use it as motivation to work toward feeling lighter, fitter, and healthier.

Measure your waist and hips

Your health could be at greater risk depending on where you carry the most weight. For instance, fat around your mid-section (where most of your vital organs are) creates a greater risk of cardiovascular issues and diabetes than fat around your thighs. It is therefore important to assess your body fat distribution. You can do this by establishing your waist-to-hip measurement. When measuring, don't suck in your tummy or pull too tightly on the tape.

Calculate your waist-to-hip ratio:
• Measure the narrowest part of your waist—usually just above the belly button, e.g. 28in (71cm)
• Measure the widest part of your hips, e.g. 38in (96.5cm)
• Divide your waist measurement by your hip measurement, e.g. $28 \div 38$ $(71 \div 96.5) = 0.74$

Analyze the results:
• A ratio of less than 0.85 = your waist and hips are in healthy proportion, so work toward maintaining this.
• A ratio of 0.85 or more = you are carrying too much weight around your mid-section. Aim to eat more healthily, increase the amount of cardio exercise you do, and focus your sculpting work on your mid-section.

Establish your body type

Knowing your approximate body type, based on your body's proportions, helps you to decide which workouts will be most beneficial for you. Below are four of the most common body types. Which one, or combination, do you most identify with?

Ruler

Women with this body type are slim, lean, and straight-up-and-down. To create feminine curves, focus on stomach and waist-slimming exercises; to build strength do total body workouts.

Suggested workouts:
• Body blast (pp.272–73)
• Ultimate bust (pp.288–89)
• Fabulous abs (pp.292–93)
• "Ruler" (pp.302–03)

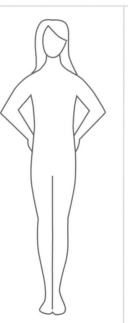

Hourglass

Women with this body type are in good overall proportion, with a nipped-in waist, which creates a lovely curvy figure. To maintain this shape, it's important to do regular, well-balanced workouts.

Suggested workouts:
• Little black dress (pp.278–79)
• Core Pilates (pp.274–75)
• Total body yoga (pp.276–77)
• "Hourglass" (pp.304–05)

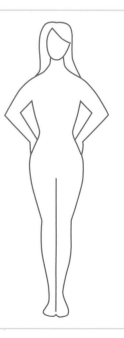

Exercising throughout life

Getting older—it happens to us all. And with it comes a lot of physical changes. Knowing what to expect of your body as you age—what is likely to happen and why—means that you can take action to help lessen or delay the changes, keeping you both looking and feeling younger and fitter for longer. After all, the right level of exercise can boost health and fitness, whatever your age.

Attitudes to aging

There are two main ways to think about your age:
• chronological—based on your date of birth
• biological—based on your physical fitness level and your ability to cope with life's daily demands.

While there's nothing you can do to change the former, research has shown that regular exercise can delay the latter by up to 12 years! Regular, moderate exercise is also associated with a decreased risk of many health disorders (see p.15). The key is to choose activities that suit both your current level of fitness (see p.39) and your age (see box far right) to counteract the main changes that take place over the years.

Starting to exercise when you're young will make it easier for you to maintain optimal health and fitness throughout life.

Cardio capacity

Women begin to lose cardio fitness around the age of 35, with aerobic power falling by up to half by the age of 60, so it becomes all the more important to incorporate adequate cardio exercise (see pp.52–97) into your everyday life as you get older.

Muscle mass and strength

Women lose 6–9 percent of their muscle mass every ten years after the age of 30, so resistance training (see pp.102–53) becomes all the more important at this stage in order to stay fit and healthy for daily activities, such as climbing the stairs or lifting and carrying heavy objects.

Bone mass and strength

Bone mineral density (BMD) starts to decline at about the age of 30—more bone starts to be lost than is made and levels of minerals, such as calcium, decrease. Again, this makes resistance training particularly important as you get older in order to avoid the onset of osteoporosis (brittle bones due to loss of bone mass).

Tissue elasticity

The gradual loss of elastin means that high-impact activities that take joints beyond their normal range of movement, such as squash, should be avoided in later years. However, regular stretching (see pp.154–93), Pilates (see pp.194–219), and/or yoga (see pp.220–47) all help to minimize loss of flexibility.

*To counteract the main changes that take place over the years so that you stay looking and **feeling younger and fitter for longer**, the key is to choose activities that suit both your current level of fitness and your age.*

Confidence and balance

The many physical changes linked to aging can cause a loss in confidence when it comes to moving around, which can lead to hesitant balance. To counteract this, it's important to ensure good posture (see p.32) because healthy alignment encourages balance. It's also important to maintain your strength via resistance training to create a solid foundation from which to move.

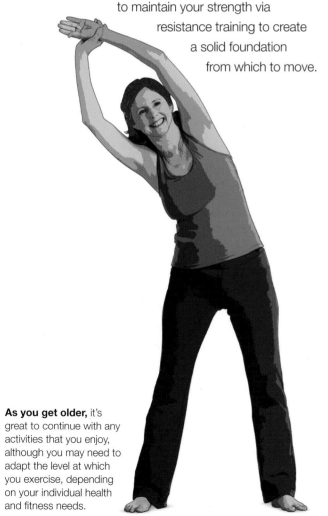

As you get older, it's great to continue with any activities that you enjoy, although you may need to adapt the level at which you exercise, depending on your individual health and fitness needs.

Respecting the stages of life

Exercise at any age can revitalize you both inside and out. But, regardless of your age, it's important to take into account your key needs at that stage.

In your 20s: Now is the time to lay the groundwork for a lifetime of fitness, so establish what you like and what balance of different types of exercise works for you.

In your 30s: Ensure you are doing enough cardio training during this time since it can start to get harder to shift weight, especially around the tummy area, as you get older, which means you could become at increased risk for heart disorders.

In your 40s and 50s: Keep up both your cardio and resistance training to keep your metabolism high. Consider upping your resistance training during these years since weight-bearing exercises can help to slow down loss of bone mass. Regular moderate exercise can also help with some of the symptoms of menopause, such as sleep disturbances.

In your 60s and beyond: For some people, it's best to avoid high-impact exercise such as running, which can be detrimental for stiff or brittle bones. Gentle forms of exercise, such as swimming, which helps to maintain mobility, and yoga, which helps to maintain flexibility, can be more beneficial. Studies show that women of this age who exercise moderately for one hour a week are less likely to develop arthritis (inflammation of the joints).

Note: If and when you become pregnant, consult your doctor for information on how to adapt your fitness routine throughout not only your pregnancy, but also your postpartum period.

Assessing your posture

Good posture is an essential part of safe and effective exercise. However, it is also a fundamental aspect of everyday life since it promotes balance and healthy alignment throughout your body. It gives you an increased sense of openness and freedom, making you look and feel taller, younger, and more confident.

Importance of natural spine alignment

Maintaining a nice, neutral posture, with the natural curves of the spine forming a slight "S" shape (see p.23), reduces stress on your spine, hips, and knees. It prevents any lower back pain, ensures a stable position from which your joints can work at their optimal level, and also counteracts the force of gravity, which can otherwise cause you to start stooping with age. It's a good idea to make time every morning to check your posture in a mirror and, if necessary, amend it in order to encourage self-awareness. When done regularly, this self-assessment will encourage you to adopt good postural habits (see below) without even thinking about it. In the beginning, however, it's important to make a conscious effort every day until you get used to it.

It's not only important to maintain a good spine alignment while standing, but also while sitting and lying down—the same rules apply to all.

Standing tall

It can be useful to visualize a piece of thread constantly attached to the top of your head, pulling you upward. This will help you to maintain a sense of length throughout your body.

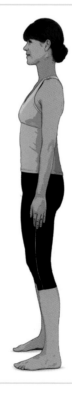

Good posture
- lengthened neck
- chin neither tucked in nor jutting out
- shoulder blades pulled back and down
- open chest
- naturally and subtly curved spine (see p.23)
- abs engaged
- pelvis tilted neither forward nor backward

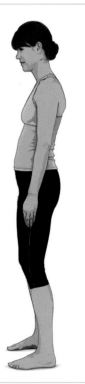

Poor posture
- neck bent forward
- head dropping forward
- rounded shoulders
- collapsed chest
- overly curved spine—most visible in the lower back
- bulging stomach
- pelvis tilted backward

Tip: A good way to instantly improve slouched posture is to imagine that someone has dropped an ice cube down your back. If that happened for real, it would soon make you stand up nice and straight!

Assessing your breathing

Breathing is our constant companion—we wouldn't survive without it for more than a few minutes. Inhalation gives our body the essential fuel (oxygen) that it needs to function, and exhalation eliminates the toxins (particularly carbon dioxide) produced as we go about our daily business (see p.22). Why then do we often pay little or no attention to how we breathe?

Importance of deep breathing

For thousands of years, spiritual seekers and yogis have realized not only the physical, but also the mental and spiritual benefits of breathing. Yet in modern-day society, many people do not breathe "well." Instead, they "shallow breathe"—short, sharp breaths into the top of the chest rather than slow, deep ones into the belly. Subtly look around you the next time you're on a train or bus—the inhalations of most people will probably be so shallow that you will hardly see their stomach or chest moving. They are only "half-breathing."

This is a real shame since slow, deep breathing not only maximizes your intake of oxygen and your elimination of waste products, which enhances all your body's functions, but it also helps to:
- increase energy levels and stamina
- relieve physical tension
- boost mental focus
- reduce stress and anxiety
- promote a sense of calm and equilibrium
- improve overall mood
- enhance overall fitness.

How well do you breathe?

It's useful to assess from time to time how you yourself breathe—to see if you, too, take this vital function for granted. So follow the steps on the right to get a sense of how true deep breathing feels. Compare it to how you normally breathe to establish what adjustments you need

to make, if any, to maximize the use of your breath. After all, breathing is one of the few automatic functions that we can consciously control, so we should make the most of it! It's important to use full breathing both during everyday actions and during exercise, since physical activity further increases your body's need for oxygen.

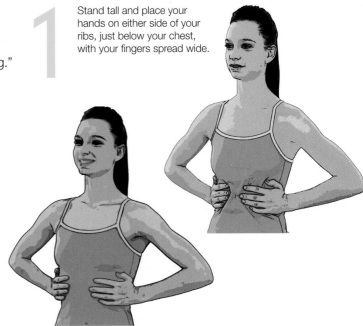

1 Stand tall and place your hands on either side of your ribs, just below your chest, with your fingers spread wide.

2 Take a slow, deep breath through your nose and, as you do so, feel your stomach gradually expand and your hands on your rib cage lift slightly. When you feel like you can't take in any more air, slowly breathe out through your mouth, feeling both your rib cage lower and your stomach deflate, until you feel like you have expelled all air. Do this several times.

How fit are you?

Before you start an exercise program, you need to establish your current level of fitness. This will enable you to be realistic about what you would like to achieve and by when, and will also indicate which types and level of exercise are most appropriate for you. Assessing your fitness personality can also help you to determine what type of exercise may suit you best.

Assessing your fitness

The tests on the following pages cover the three main aspects of fitness: cardiovascular, strength, and flexibility. Simply note how you do in each test and we will then assess the results together on p.39. It's important to remember that while the relationship between high levels of fitness and good health is strong, the two are not synonymous. The self-assessments that follow are indicators of your fitness only, not of your health. The only person qualified to assess the latter is a medical expert, so be sure to consult your doctor if you have any concerns about your health.

What "fitness personality" are you?

Different personality "types" tend to be suited to different types of activity. It's therefore worth assessing which of the fitness types below you most associate with, since it can help you to decide which forms of exercise you might enjoy the most. Intensity is measured on a scale of 1–10, with 10 being the most challenging (see also p.57).

Personality type	Preferred types of exercise	Preferred location	Main aims	Preferred level of intensity	Sample suitable activities
"Take-it-easy"	low impact, calming, and rejuvenating, possibly with a mind-body-spirit focus	mainly indoors	overall well-being	4–5	gentle to moderate walks or swims, relaxing yoga
"Get-up-and-go"	combination of low- and high-impact, with the possibility of social interaction	indoors and outdoors	more energy, improved cardio fitness, a firmer body	5–7	moderate cycling or aerobics, Pilates
"Let's-do-it!"	high-speed, high-energy, and high-impact, possibly with a competitive element	mainly outdoors, in all weathers, and on all terrains	physical challenge, stress release, extreme fitness	7–8	running, hill-climbing (whether walking or cycling), working with heavier weights

Test your cardio fitness

Cardiovascular fitness, also known as cardio or aerobic fitness, is about how fit your heart is. You can check this by measuring your Resting Heart Rate (RHR) or by measuring how quickly your heart rate slows down after exercise, called your heart rate recovery time.

Heart Rate Recovery Time test

Step 1: Establish your Resting Heart Rate (see right).
Step 2: Step up and down on a high step for 3 minutes.
Step 3: Sit down for 30 seconds, then check your pulse again to establish your new heart rate.

What do the results mean?
The lower your heart rate in Step 3 above, the shorter your Heart Rate Recovery Time and the higher your level of cardio fitness (see p.39 for more details).

How often should I take this test?
Redo the test after 3–4 weeks of regular cardio workouts (see pp.258–69) to see if you are getting more cardio fit.

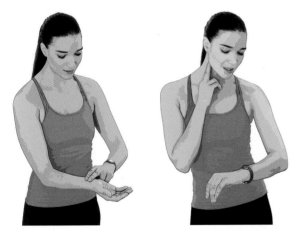

You can take your pulse by placing your index and middle fingers either on your inner wrist or the side of your neck, whichever works best for you. Use your watch to time yourself.

Establishing your Resting Heart Rate

Your Resting Heart Rate (RHR) is a measure of how many times your heart beats per minute when you are at rest, and is therefore a useful way of checking your approximate level of cardio fitness at any time. RHR is also used as a baseline marker when you are carrying out the Heart Rate Recovery Time test (see left).

How do I measure my heart rate?
Hold one hand with your palm facing upward and place the index and middle fingertips of your other hand at the base of your thumb on your inner wrist, on what is called the radial artery. If you can't feel anything, press harder or move your fingers around until you find your pulse. Count it for 15 seconds, using a watch or phone to keep time, then multiply the result by 4 to establish your heart rate. Alternatively, you may find it easier to take your pulse on the side of your neck, just below your jawbone, on what is called the carotid artery.

When should I check my RHR?
If using RHR on its own, the best time to check it is when you wake up in the morning, since this is often when your body is at its most relaxed. However, any time when you've been resting for at least 10 minutes and you're not stressed is fine. It's best not to have recently consumed any caffeine-based drinks or other stimulants since they can artificially raise your heart rate.

What do the results mean?
In general, the lower your RHR, the more cardio fit you are (see p.39 for more details). However, RHR varies with age, overall health, and weight, so a cardio fit heart rate is not the same for everyone. Nevertheless, by establishing your RHR before starting a new fitness routine, you can use it as a benchmark to see how you're progressing. If your heart rate lowers with regular workouts, this can mean you're getting fitter. If it's not changing, you need to increase your workout level.

How often should I take it?
Monitor your RHR as often as you like. However, despite the fact that every workout counts, don't expect any real difference until about four weeks into a regular routine.

Test your strength

It's important to keep your body strong enough to handle the daily demands placed on it. The exercises below test the strength of your three main body areas: your upper, core, and lower body. For each, see how many repetitions (reps) are possible before you feel like you can't do any more: about 8–9 on the Rate of Perceived Exertion scale (see p.57). Then, push yourself to do a few more—this is the "point of challenge" (see also p.17).

What do the results mean?
The more reps you can do, the stronger you are in that body area (see p.39 for more detailed results).

How often should I take this test?
Carry out the three test exercises again after 3–4 weeks of regular sculpting workouts (see pp.270–311) to see if you are becoming stronger and fitter.

The Upper Body Strength test

1 Get onto all fours on the floor. Place your palms on the mat directly under your head, with your hands slightly wider than shoulder-width apart. Move your knees slightly backward, looking downward so that your neck, back, and upper legs form a straight line. Inhale to prepare.

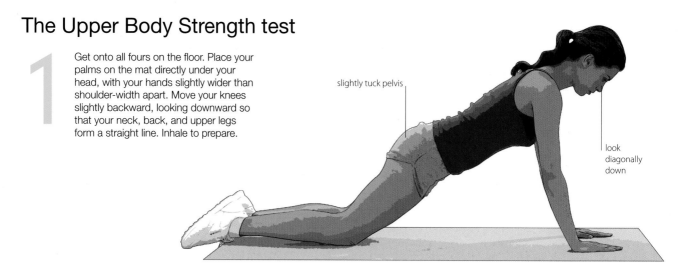

slightly tuck pelvis

look diagonally down

2 As you exhale, bend your arms to lower your body toward the floor, allowing your elbows to move out toward the sides. Hold for a couple of seconds, or as long as is comfortable. As you inhale, push yourself up until your arms are once again straight, but not locked. Do as many reps as you can until you reach the "point of challenge" (see above).

Once you can relatively easily do 25–30 reps of this push-up, try the test with Full Push-ups (see p.113).

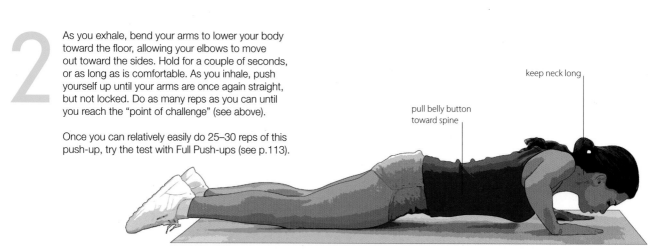

keep neck long

pull belly button toward spine

The Core Body Strength test

1 Lie on your back with your knees bent and pointing upward. Keep your feet flat on the floor, hip-width apart. Place your hands behind the base of your head and pull your belly button toward your spine to engage your abs. Inhale to prepare.

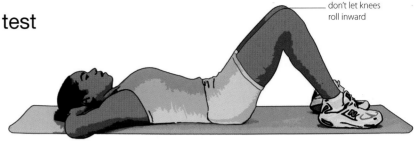

don't let knees roll inward

2 As you exhale, raise your head and shoulders off the floor as far as is comfortable, making sure that your abs are fully engaged. Hold for a couple of seconds. As you inhale, slowly lower yourself. Do as many reps as you can until you reach the "point of challenge."

Once you can relatively easily do 60–70 reps of this sit-up, try the test with your arms extended straight above your head instead of behind it.

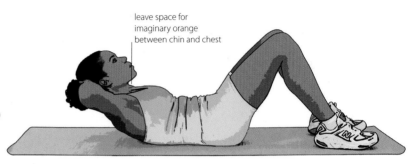

leave space for imaginary orange between chin and chest

The Lower Body Strength test

1 Stand against a wall with your feet hip-width apart and parallel, and your arms relaxed by your sides. Walk your feet slightly away from the wall so that you can bend your knees to a right angle without moving your feet. Inhale to prepare.

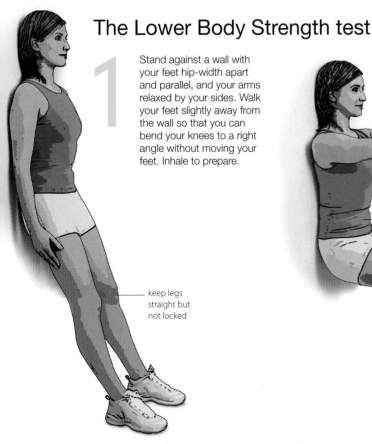

keep legs straight but not locked

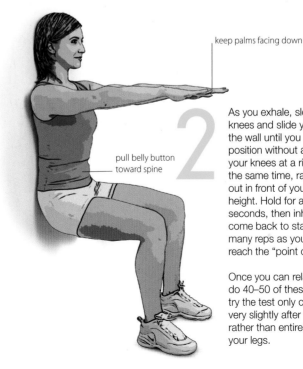

keep palms facing down

pull belly button toward spine

2 As you exhale, slowly bend your knees and slide your back down the wall until you are in a sitting position without a chair, with your knees at a right angle. At the same time, raise your arms out in front of you at shoulder height. Hold for a couple of seconds, then inhale as you come back to standing. Do as many reps as you can until you reach the "point of challenge."

Once you can relatively easily do 40–50 of these wall squats, try the test only coming up very slightly after each squat, rather than entirely straightening your legs.

Test your flexibility

Stiff, inflexible muscles can affect the way you look and feel. But they can also, ultimately, restrict your range of movement, thus decreasing your quality of life. The Seated Flexibility test below will let you assess your current flexibility (mainly in the hamstrings and back) so that you know whether it is something that you particularly need to focus on.

The Seated Flexibility test

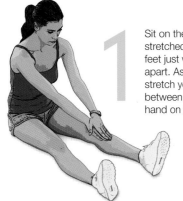

1 Sit on the floor with your legs stretched out in front of you and feet just wider than hip-width apart. As you inhale, start to stretch your arms forward between your legs, with one hand on top of the other.

What do the results mean?
The farther forward you can reach, the more flexibile you are (see right for specifics).

How often should I take the test?
Redo after 3–4 weeks of regular sculpting workouts to assess your progress, since all workouts include elements of stretching. For rapid progress, redo after 3–4 weeks of regularly doing the Flexibility workout (see pp.324–25).

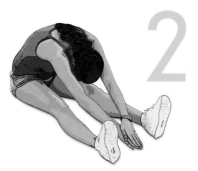

2 As you exhale, reach your hands as far forward as you can on the floor, tucking your chin toward your chest as you do so. Hold for a few seconds. Note how far your fingertips can reach—your knees, shins, ankles, toes, or farther? Repeat 3 times. Use the farthest you can reach to assess your flexibility (see below right).

What does it all mean?

Now it's time to assess the results of your various fitness tests: cardio, strength, and flexibility. Referring to the Fitness test results (right), first find where your result for each test falls in the relevant chart. Then scan along to see which fitness category this puts you in—fit, above average, average, below average, or unfit— and how many "points" you score for this.

Once you know your fitness level and how many points you have in each category, add them all up. Then have a look at the last chart, which gives "your overall score," and see which category of overall fitness you fall into. This provides you with a guide to which intensity of workouts is most suitable for you at the moment.

"Fit" or "Above average" shows that you have good overall fitness, so aim to maintain or increase this with "moderate" to "intense" workouts from pp.248–327.
"Average" means you are doing well but would benefit from improved overall fitness, so work at a "moderate" level for 4–6 weeks to move up a fitness category. If one particular type of fitness is dragging down your overall score, work on that area specifically.
"Below average" or "Unfit" should not make you feel disheartened. Use this information as a motivator and you'll be amazed at how quickly you can increase your overall fitness. Start with "gentle" workouts for 4–6 weeks, focusing particularly on areas in which you scored poorly.

Fitness test results

The charts on this page give the results for the cardio, strength, and flexibility fitness tests outlined on pp.35–38. For how to use and interpret these results, see What does it all mean? (below left).

Your cardio fitness (from p.35)

Fitness level based on Resting Heart Rate	Beats per minute during rest
Fit = 5 points	Below 65
Above average = 4 points	65–74
Average = 3 points	75–79
Below average = 2 points	80–84
Unfit = 1 point	85 or higher

Fitness level based on Heart Rate Recovery Time	Beats per minute after 3 minutes stepping and 30 seconds rest
Fit = 5 points	Below 80
Above average = 4 points	80–109
Average = 3 points	110–119
Below average = 2 points	120–139
Unfit = 1 point	140 or above

Your flexibility (from above left)

Fitness level based on Seated Flexibility	Distance reached in seated forward bend
Fit = 5 points	Past your toes
Above average = 4 points	Your toes
Average = 3 points	Your ankles
Below average = 2 points	Halfway down your shins
Unfit = 1 point	Your knees

Your strength (from pp.36–37)

Fitness level based on Upper Body Strength	Push-up reps until "point of challenge"
Fit = 5 points	More than 20
Above average = 4 points	16–20
Average = 3 points	11–15
Below average = 2 points	6–10
Unfit = 1 point	0–5

Fitness level based on Core Body Strength	Sit-up reps until "point of challenge"
Fit = 5 points	More than 50
Above average = 4 points	41–50
Average = 3 points	31–40
Below average = 2 points	16–30
Unfit = 1 point	0–15

Fitness level based on Lower Body Strength	Wall squat reps until "point of challenge"
Fit = 5 points	More than 45
Above average = 4 points	31–45
Average = 3 points	21–30
Below average = 2 points	11–20
Unfit = 1 point	0–10

Your overall fitness score

Fit	25–30
Above average	19–24
Average	13–18
Below average	7–12
Unfit	6

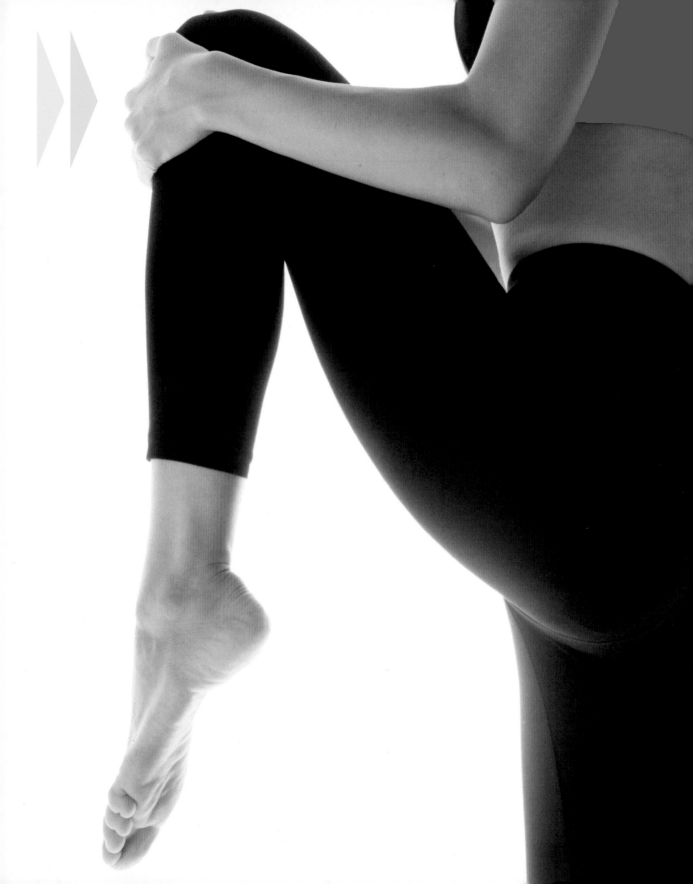

Getting started

As with many things in life, the hardest part of getting in shape can often simply be knowing where to start. After all, there's so much choice and it can easily feel like we have so little time, what with all the other pressures on our everyday schedules. The pages that follow will give you the tools you need to make regular exercise an instant and achievable reality by encouraging you to:

- develop a positive relationship with the notion of exercise

- establish exactly what you want—and by when

- choose the activities that will enable you to attain this

- commit to specific times and activities

- start exercising with belief and determination

- remain positive and motivated

- assess your progress on a regular basis and amend your regimen as required

- combine all this with healthy eating

Making exercise work for you

Most of us can't deny that we feel much better—simultaneously more relaxed and energized—after exercise. Yet it can often be so hard to get started. The key is to make exercise as simple and enjoyable for yourself as possible so that when the time comes, you don't have to give it a second thought—you can just get up and go. Below are some ways to help you to do this.

Make friends with exercise

It's all too easy to think of exercise as yet another thing on a long to-do list, which can make it feel tedious and tiring before we even start. If you feel this way, it's important to turn this attitude around and instead see exercise for what it really is—something positive and energizing that, if you choose to do it regularly, will help you to get the most out of your life. After all, it's up to you whether or not you want to feel and look better, and the very fact that you're reading this book suggests you do!

Choose activities that you enjoy

The good news is that there's an enormous amount of choice when it comes to ways of getting in better shape. However, this in itself can initially feel a bit overwhelming when trying to put a fitness plan together: Where do I start? Which activities will help me to lose weight? Which exercises will blast which body parts? This is where this book comes in, so dive in to get the lowdown on a wide range of options. Then, crucially, take time to choose a combination of workouts (see pp.248–327) that will not only give you the results you want, but will also appeal to you the most. Doing the activities that you enjoy most will maximize your chances of sticking to them!

Plan where you'll exercise

Many of the workouts in this book can be done pretty much anywhere, but in order to establish an easy, regular routine for yourself it's a good idea to decide in advance where you would like to and are able to carry out each component of your fitness program:

• For walking, running, and cycling workouts (see pp.260–65), it's best to plan the routes you'll take so that you know the distances and terrains will meet your intensity needs and that you can complete them in the time you have available.

• For swimming workouts (see pp.266–67), think about where you'll do these. Is a pool near home or work better? If you're lucky enough to have access to a lake or the ocean, how long will it take you to get there and how safe is it, bearing in mind that conditions can vary?

• For dance/aerobics and sculpting workouts (see pp.268–311), prepare an area in your home that will provide you with both enough space and privacy to move freely and with confidence—preferably somewhere that is neither too cold nor too warm.

• For quick-fix workouts (see pp.312–27), make use of whatever space you have available to you when you have time to fit them in.

Shut out the external world

It's important that you treat your exercise time as valuable space for yourself. Aim to allocate specific amounts of time for your workouts so that you never feel rushed or distracted while doing them. Turn off your phone and computer so that you can fully focus on your own well-being and fitness. Only if you give 100 percent will you get 100 percent, both physically and psychologically.

Gather the equipment you need

This book has been designed so that you need minimal equipment. However, there are a number of things that you need for almost any exercise regimen, so it's good to invest your time and money getting these together from the start so that you're all set to go.

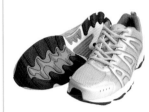

Good-fitting, well-cushioned sneakers
These should reduce stress on your joints during high-impact activities such as running, as well as fully support your ankles. Break them in around the house before you wear them to exercise.

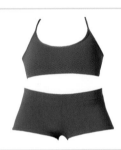

Loose or stretchy exercise clothes
There's a fantastic range of stylish sportswear these days, so enjoy experimenting to find the items in which you feel most confident.

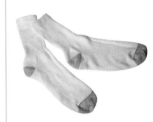

Good-quality socks
These will maximize your comfort. Ensure that they are snug-fitting so that they do not wrinkle beneath your feet when you move, causing blisters.

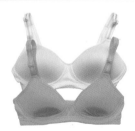

A sports bra that offers adequate support for your size and shape
A good sports bra prevents discomfort during exercise and also helps to minimize future sagging. Specialty stores may offer a personalized fitting service.

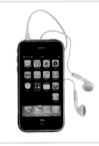

Music system
Listening to music that you love can be a great motivator as you exercise. You could play background music on your stereo or use headphones with a portable device such as an iPod or cell phone.

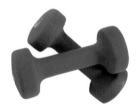

Set of hand weights
Hand weights provide increased resistance in certain exercises to give you a stronger workout. If you don't have any, two small bottles of water would be fine instead.

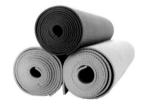

Exercise mat
This will protect your spine when you do floor exercises. Such mats are available online and at most sporting goods stores. If you don't have one, you can use a thick towel.

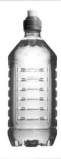

Water
Always having water on hand to sip throughout your workout as required will help to prevent dehydration (see p.51 for recommendations on how much to drink).

Occasional extras
- Cushion and/or or rolled-up towel for extra support
- Exercise ball (also called a Swiss ball)—available online and at most sporting goods stores (see p.107)
- Resistance band—available online and at most sporting goods stores (see p.107)
- Tennis ball, soccer ball, or other small- to medium-sized ball
- Firm chair to sit on, and step for certain leg and foot exercises
- Notebook and pen to keep track of your goals and progress

Planning your way to a better body

A little advance planning can mean the difference between simply having intentions about getting in better shape and turning those intentions into a reality. And goal-setting is often the best way to go about this. Experts in self-improvement often recommend setting what they call SMART goals. This means that your goals need to be specific, measurable, action-oriented, realistic, and timed.

Specific
Know what you want—and by when

It's always easier to get yourself to do something when you know exactly why you're doing it, so be clear with yourself. Write down what your main fitness goal is and by when you would like to, realistically, achieve it. *Example:* I want to look my best for our beach vacation, which is six weeks from now.

Measurable
Break your end goal into quantifiable mini-goals

Once you've established your main goal, consider what smaller steps are needed to achieve it and how you can measure these.
Example: To look my best for my vacation, I will need to:
• lose weight
• slim down my waist
• firm up my thighs, bottom, arms, and abs.
To do this, I will need to:
• assess and improve my eating habits (see pp.48–51)
• commit to doing 3–5 cardio workouts
(see pp.258–69) a week
• do appropriate sculpting workouts (see pp.270–311).
To track my progress, I will therefore set up weekly "check-ins," where I:
• make a note of my weight
• take my waist measurement
• make observations about my body in a particular outfit—preferably in my bikini.

Action-oriented
Create a fitness timetable

Don't fall into the trap of telling yourself that you'll just fit your workouts in whenever you can, because as your week unfolds they then may never happen! Instead, plan in advance specifically when you will, realistically, be able to do each component of your fitness program. Write them down in your diary—just as you would do for important meetings with other people. Choose times that not only fit in with your normal routine but that will also allow you to get the most from the exercises.
Example:

Monday 5:30pm	Body blast workout
Tuesday 7:30am	Moderate run
Wednesday 7:30am	Moderate walk
Wednesday 5:30pm	Bikini body workout
Thursday 7:30am	Moderate run
Friday 5:30pm	Dream legs workout
Saturday 3pm	Intense cycle

Realistic
Make sure your plan is feasible

If you want to succeed in achieving the goals you've set, it's essential that you maintain a strong sense of what is genuinely possible within the framework of your personality, lifestyle, energy, and fitness levels at any given time. Otherwise, you'll just be setting yourself up for disappointment.

*It's crucial to **decide on a fixed time frame** for achieving your goals so that you can really work toward those dates and assess your progress at each stage.*

Examples:

• If you're a size 16, it's unrealistic to expect to whittle yourself down to a size 10 within six weeks.

• If you struggle to get up early in the morning, there's no point in trying to force yourself to do early-bird workouts.

• If you have a demanding job, with 15-minute lunch breaks, don't try to convince yourself that you'll fit in a whole Lunch-break workout (see pp.318–19) every day.

Timed

Establish by when you need to do what

It's crucial to decide on a fixed time frame for achieving goals you have set—both the main one and the mini ones along the way—so that you can really work toward those dates and assess your progress at each stage.

Example: If I want to feel and look my best when I go on vacation in just over six weeks' time, I need to start a six-week fitness regimen next week, and I therefore have a few days to get a plan up and running.

Today:

• I will add all my fitness appointments to my diary.

• I'll highlight my end date in pink—to spur me on.

• I'll prepare my workout space and/or routes as well as gather any equipment that I need.

Tomorrow:

• I'll write down the results of my first "check-in" (see Measurable, left)—making a point of comparison for my other results.

• I'll add "check-in" times to my diary for the same time each Sunday for the next six weeks.

Day after tomorrow:

• I'll start my fitness program!

If you realize at any point that you're not sticking to your plan, assess why this is—have you been lazy or slack? Or were your goals unrealistic in the first place? If the former, make a fresh commitment to yourself with the knowledge that you don't want to let yourself down. If the latter, set yourself a new set of more achievable goals that will free your mind to enjoy the exercising.

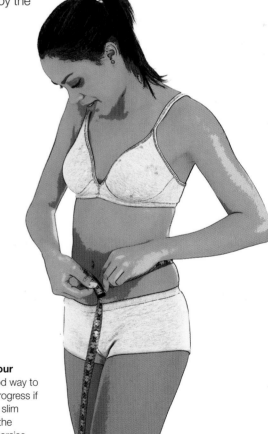

Measuring your waist is a good way to assess your progress if your goal is to slim down around the middle with exercise. Don't pull too tightly on the tape when you are measuring.

Keeping motivated

There are going to be times during any exercise program when your energy and enthusiasm start to flag, and you'll feel like missing sessions or even giving up altogether. It's essential to have some tricks up your sleeve that you can draw on during such times in order to keep you firmly on the fitness track.

Focus on the positive

Remind yourself of the things that you like most about exercising. Make a list of these even if there are only one or two. For example: "It gives me time to myself," "It gets me out in the fresh air," "It makes me feel less stressed," or "I feel more confident about myself afterward." Use these thoughts to spur you on.

Use visualizations

Keep in mind your overall goal (see pp.44–45) and visualize yourself achieving this. Imagine where you are, what you are wearing, how you feel when you achieve it—satisfied, confident, beautiful, strong. Allow yourself to bask in this feeling and use it to drive yourself forward and out of your rut.

Keep an exercise diary

Write down on a daily basis not only what you did during that day's exercise but also how you felt— both while doing each activity and afterward. Take a moment to identify what you were doing when you felt your best and why you think this was the case, so that you can tap into this again if ever your enthusiasm is waning. Keeping a record of your fitness progress also works as a reminder of how much you are doing, which it can otherwise be easy to underestimate.

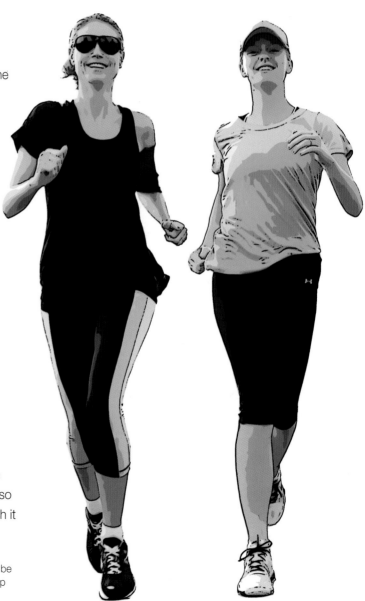

Exercising with someone you're friends with can be motivating since you'll encourage each other to keep going. Potentially, you'll also have a chance to talk!

*Imagine how you feel when **you've achieved your fitness goals**— satisfied, confident, beautiful, strong—and allow yourself to bask in this feeling to drive yourself forward.*

Recruit an exercise buddy

Arranging to do at least some of your exercises with a friend, neighbor, or like-minded colleague can be just the boost you need at times to stop your fitness plan from faltering. As well as giving you a chance to spend some valuable time with someone you like, it encourages you not to miss sessions, since you won't want to let that person down.

Get some fresh air

Sometimes bringing your exercise into the great outdoors—whether your backyard or a local park— can give you a much-needed pick-me-up. Being outside and breathing in the fresh air can give you an increased sense of freedom, movement, and energy.

Sign up for a charity event

Committing to a cause greater than yourself can give you the extra focus you sometimes need to challenge yourself to the max with your training. And collecting sponsorship from your friends and family can really boost your determination, since you'll feel you owe it to both your sponsors and your chosen charity to do the best you possibly can. If there's an element of competition to the event, it might spur you on even more—especially if you're a "Let's-do-it!" personality type (see p.34).

Create a new playlist

If you enjoy music, the simple act of choosing new songs to exercise to can sometimes give you the extra encouragement you need to keep training. While it's important that you remain focused to ensure you work out safely, uplifting music can give your mind a welcome distraction. Music also causes your brain to release the chemical dopamine, which boosts your mood.

Rejuvenate your workout wardrobe

Sometimes, if you're lacking in enthusiasm, it can help to treat yourself to a new item of exercise gear, whether a colorful top or a nice water bottle— anything that you will look forward to wearing or using, in order to help you to get off the couch!

Reward yourself

When you find during your regular exercise "check-ins" (see p.44) that you're making progress, be sure to give yourself due recognition. For instance, decide that if you continue to progress in the same way within the next two weeks, you'll treat yourself to something nice, such as a relaxing massage, a self-pampering night, or a new dress for your vacation. It's always nice to have something to look forward to!

Keep it fresh

Once you have met your initial fitness goal—whether to fit into your new jeans or feel confident about your body on the beach this summer—it's important to stay motivated so that you'll maintain your new-found body shape and increased energy. Otherwise, you'll be back to square one. You'll need to reassess your fitness needs, create a new, sustainable program about which you feel excited, and potentially also consider new options, such as attending local classes and joining local clubs in order to keep you moving forward.

The basics of good eating

The food you eat is the fuel that drives you. It is therefore essential to provide your hard-working body with a healthy diet to keep it in optimal working order and top physical condition. Forget about all the fad diets and "miracle" weight-loss plans out there, and instead simply put your time and effort into ensuring a balance of the right types of food, in the right amounts, and at the right times.

What does my body need?

You need to provide your body with energy, in the form of calories, as well as a combination of specific nutrients in order to stay fit and healthy, mainly:
- carbohydrates—for instant energy
- fats (both saturated and unsaturated) —as a longer-term source of energy
- protein—to build and repair body tissues
- fiber—to enable bowel efficiency
- vitamins, such as A, B1, B2, B6, C, D, and E —to help with all kinds of bodily functions
- minerals, such as calcium, iron, magnesium, potassium, and zinc—to assist all kinds of cellular activity and to help regulate metabolism.

Because each of these components is found in different foods, it's essential to eat a wide and varied diet.

Which foods should I avoid?

Although it's often easiest to just grab the first fast food available in the midst of today's hectic lifestyle, it's vital to think about longer-term health, preventing illness rather than having to cure it later. Avoiding the following foods will help you to stay healthy:
- Processed foods
- Fast foods
- Foods high in salt, sugar, or saturated fats
This is not to say that you can't have the occasional treat, whether it's pizza or doughnuts. Just don't get into the habit of eating these foods too often.

Counting calories

No matter how healthy the food you eat, you won't get fitter or lose any weight if you eat too much. One way of assessing how much you need to consume is by means of calories (kcal). An average man needs around 2,500 calories a day, and an average woman needs around 2,000 calories a day.

Most store-bought items have the calorie content listed on them, which means it can be easy to keep track of approximate intake. However, the recommended amounts above are mere guidelines since each person needs to adapt the amount they eat to match their own lifestyle requirements. The key to maintaining weight is to burn off (through cardio exercise) the same amount of calories as you consume, and the key to losing weight is to burn off more calories than you consume.

Serving size

If you don't want to count calories, you can monitor how much you eat by being aware of serving size. Below are guidelines to the ideal amounts of specific food types for a moderately active, average-sized person to eat in any given meal (although you don't need to include both fish and meat in one meal):
- vegetables—as many as you want
- fish—a piece the size of a checkbook
- lean meat—a piece the size of a deck of playing cards

• pasta, rice, cereal, grains, or potatoes—a serving the size of a clenched fist

• cheese or other dairy products—a serving the size of a small matchbox.

If you feel you need to cut down on your serving size but are finding it tough, try the following:

• Keep serving size in mind when preparing your meal, so you don't make too much in the first place.

• Use a smaller plate than usual so that it doesn't look too empty when placed in front of you.

• Eat slowly to give your brain a chance to register when you're full.

Planning ahead

In order to ensure a varied, balanced diet and to minimize the chance of last-minute unhealthy meals, it's a good idea to plan your meals in advance. Choose a regular day each week or two to set your menu, then make your shopping list based on this. Your weekly menus should include the following foods:

• at least five servings of fruit and vegetables a day, including a maximum of two or three pieces of fruit due to their high sugar content.

Note: a "serving" is any of the following:

   1 medium-sized fruit or vegetable;
   3 heaping tablespoons of cooked vegetables;
   5 fl oz (150 ml) fruit or vegetable juice.

• a moderate to generous amount of potatoes, wholegrain cereals, bread, rice, and pasta.

• a moderate to generous amount of legumes, such as black beans, chickpeas, cannellini beans, kidney beans, lentils, peas, and soy beans.

• a moderate amount of dairy products, such as low-fat milk, low-fat cheese, low-fat (or soy) yogurts, and free-range eggs.

• a moderate amount of poultry, fish, and shellfish, such as skinless turkey and chicken (the skin contains a lot of fat), including at least one or two servings of oily fish, such as mackerel, sardines, salmon, herring, or fresh tuna and trout.

• a moderate amount of seeds and nuts to eat as snacks or use in cooking, such as pumpkin, sesame, sunflower, flaxseed, poppy seeds, almonds, brazil nuts, cashews, hazelnuts, peanuts, pecans, pine nuts, pistachios, and walnuts.

• a moderate amount of oils, for both cooking and to make dressings, such as olive, vegetable, and canola.

• a small amount of red meat—lean cuts such as pork fillet or rump, or fillet steak are healthiest (with the excess fat trimmed off before cooking).

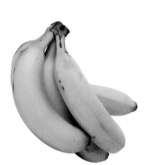

Bananas are a good all-around food, providing energy, fiber, potassium, and vitamins B6, C, and A.

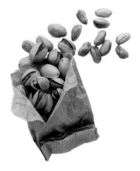

Nuts are a convenient, high-protein snack, but they are high in fat so you need to limit the amount you eat.

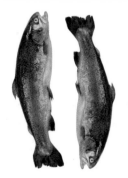

Fish is a good source of protein and many vitamins; oily fish are high in healthy omega-3 fats.

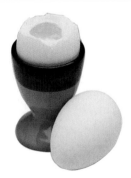

Eggs make a quick and nutritious meal, supplying vitamins D and A, as well as several B vitamins.

When should I eat?

Everyone's natural rhythm is different when it comes to the best times to eat, but on the whole it's best to aim for either three evenly spaced-out meals a day, or five to six smaller ones. This will provide you with a steady supply of energy throughout the day.

Always try to have breakfast since this is the meal that prepares you, energetically speaking, for the rest of the day; without it, you are more likely to want to snack later in the day. A healthy breakfast could be:
• a bowl of wholegrain cereal with low-fat milk, strawberries, blueberries, and a sprinkling of seeds
• a slice of wholegrain toast and a poached egg
• a homemade juice or smoothie.
Or if you're in a rush, a piece of fruit, such as a grapefruit, an apple, or an orange, is a good, easy solution.

If possible, have a substantial lunch and a light dinner, especially if you usually don't get to have dinner until late in the evening. Although it's tempting to eat on the run at

A healthy, wholesome breakfast is important to prepare you for the day, so always leave enough time for this. Wholegrain cereal with low-fat milk is quick and easy.

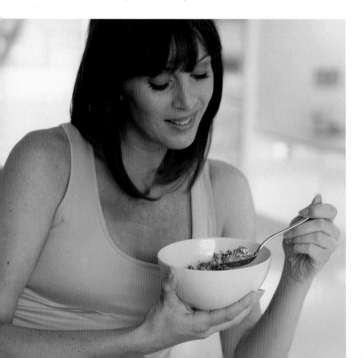

lunchtime, grabbing a sandwich as you dash between appointments, it really does make a difference if you can make the time to sit down for even just 15 minutes and focus solely on the act of eating, without rushing. This gives your body time to start digesting the food before it has to divert its attention again to other activities.

Avoid eating meals very late at night because there won't be enough time before bed for your body to work off any of the calories consumed, which means that fat may be stored more easily. Eating late can also have a negative impact on your sleep.

Is it okay to snack?

Constant "grazing" can wreak havoc with fitness and weight-loss plans, so try to keep snacking to a minimum. If and when you get an urge for a snack between meals (and let's face it, this will probably happen!), ask yourself if you're genuinely hungry or if your desire for food might stem more from feelings such as boredom or stress. If the latter, try to figure out how you could make yourself feel better without eating. Maybe, some herbal tea or a quick stroll as a break from whatever you're doing would help instead. But if you really are hungry, opt for a "smart snack," such as a piece of fruit or a handful of nuts, seeds, dried apricots, or berries, rather than a sweet treat, like chocolate, cookies, or cake. A banana, for example, will give you a quick energy boost and is high in fiber, a nice juicy orange is packed with vitamins and minerals to give you a lift, and a handful of nuts or seeds is rich in both minerals and "healthy" fats.

A few more substantial snack options would be:
• celery and carrot sticks with low-fat hummus
• rye bread with low-fat cottage cheese
• rice cakes with finely chopped tomatoes and olive oil.
But be sure to keep portions minimal: a snack should be just that! And avoid false friends, such as commercial cereal bars, which are often classed as "healthy snacks" but can have more calories than a chocolate bar!

Staying hydrated

Water makes up about two-thirds of the weight of a healthy body, and we need it to help our body to perform all its most fundamental functions. Yet we lose water all the time—mainly through sweat and urine. To stay hydrated and healthy, it is therefore important to keep replacing the water that we lose.

In moderate climates, aim to drink six to eight glasses of water or other healthy liquids (see below) every day, but you will probably need more than this when the weather is hotter and when you're more physically active, so be sure to tune into what your body tells you. Try to avoid, however, waiting until you feel parched before taking a drink because your body will already be suffering by this stage. It is a good idea to carry a bottle of water with you at all times to sip at throughout the day.

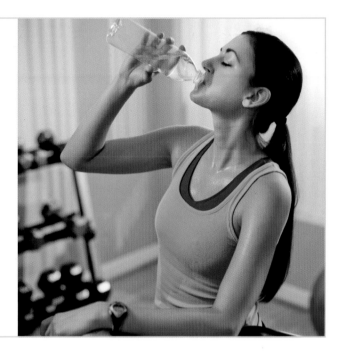

During periods when you're exercising a lot, you might feel a need to snack more often. Because you're burning extra calories, it's important to ensure that you're eating enough carbohydrates in your main meals to provide you with the energy you need. However, if you still need more, you could have a substantial carb-rich snack, such as a wholegrain bagel with low-fat peanut butter and a banana, an hour or two before your workout to give yourself an energy boost.

What can I drink?

Water is the best fluid to drink, but we often don't drink enough. Research done by the *European Journal of Sport Science* has shown that although the majority of sportspeople tend to drink enough water during their workouts to stay hydrated, they often still wake up the next morning dehydrated. This emphasizes the importance of drinking enough both before and after workouts—as well as throughout each day (see above).

When it comes to liquids other than water, avoid:
• carbonated drinks due to their high sugar content, which can throw blood sugar levels off kilter and contribute to weight issues
• caffeine-based drinks, such as tea, coffee, and cola, which can over-stimulate the body
• alcohol, which is high in calories as well as potentially hazardous to your health when taken in excess.

Instead, opt for fresh fruit juices and herbal teas. When buying fruit juice, check that it doesn't have added sugar since fruit is already naturally high in sugar.

Although it's tempting to eat on the run at lunchtime, it really does make a difference if you can **make the time to sit down** *for even just 15 minutes and focus solely on the act of eating, without rushing.*

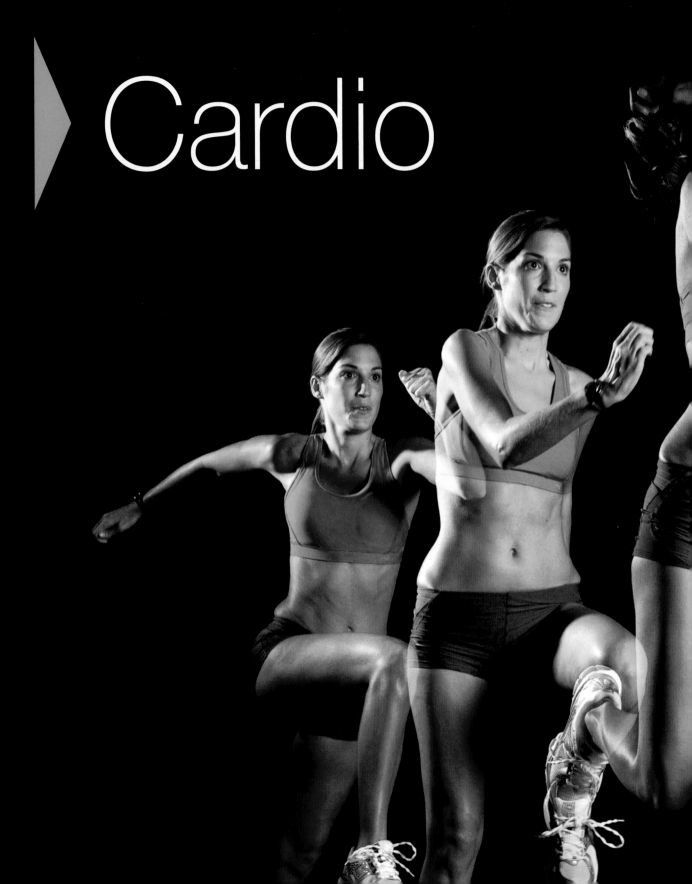

Cardio

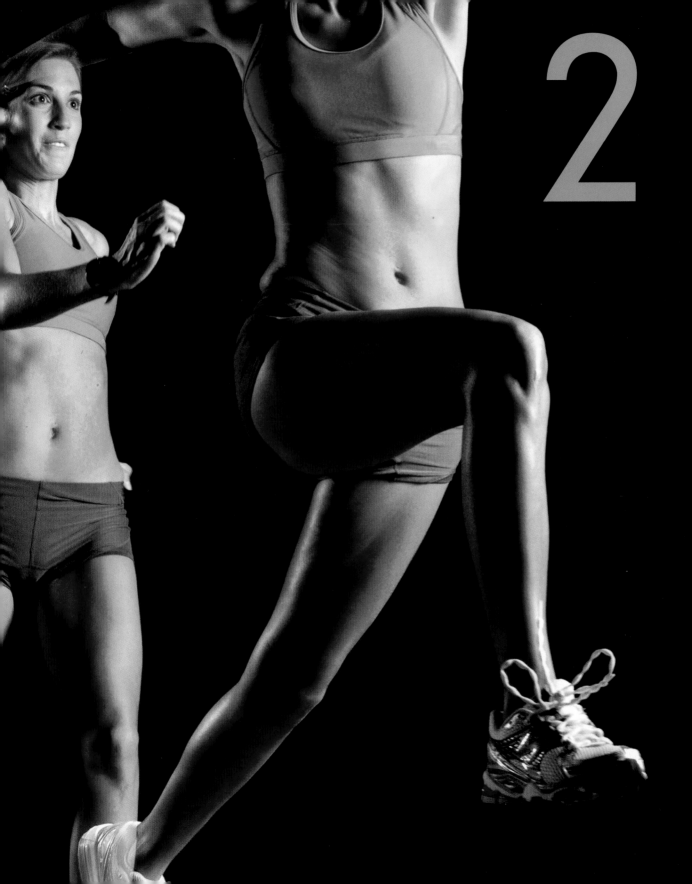

What is cardio exercise?

Cardio is a term you may be familiar with, but what does it really mean? Put simply, cardio is short for cardiovascular, which refers to the body system that has the heart at its core (see also p.22). Cardio exercise is therefore any type of exercise that gets your heart beating faster than usual for a sustained period of time. It's also known as aerobic exercise.

The benefits of cardio

Cardio, or aerobic, activity involves the continuous, rhythmic contraction of large muscle groups. It includes an enormous array of activities from skipping, cycling, and hula-hooping, to playing tennis and football, and doing athletics. The main forms of cardio exercise covered within this book are, however, walking, jogging and running, cycling, swimming, and aerobics and dancing—popular solo activities that can be done almost anywhere at whatever level of intensity suits you, with optimal fitness results. The key is simply to choose, and commit to, the activities that appeal to you most.

Any of these activities will not only boost the health of your heart, increasing your all-around cardio fitness, but will also burn off calories and therefore fat, enabling you to manage your weight. Plus, they will help to keep stress at bay, combat anxiety and depression, increase energy levels, enhance your mood, boost circulation and complexion, keep you feeling younger in both body and mind, and reduce the risk of health issues such as high blood pressure, high cholesterol, and heart disease.

How much? How often?

The 2011 American College of Sports Medicine guidelines recommend either doing a 30-minute, moderate-to-intense cardio workout at a pace that works up a light sweat, five days a week, or a 20-minute vigorously intense cardio workout three days a week. These sessions can even be broken down into 10-minute

blocks throughout the day if necessary in order to fit them in, as long as they are done in addition to standard daily physical activities. However, for the average adult, this amount of exercise is more about maintaining good health and preventing disease than building fitness.

To lose weight and improve fitness, 30–60 minutes of moderate-to-intense physical activity five times a week is more likely to be necessary.

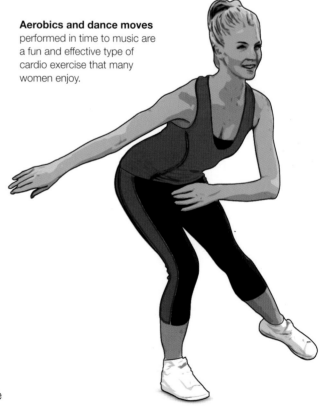

Aerobics and dance moves performed in time to music are a fun and effective type of cardio exercise that many women enjoy.

*Cardio activity will not only boost the **health of your heart**, increasing your all-around cardio fitness, but it will also burn off calories and therefore fat, enabling you to manage your weight.*

High-impact exercise

High-impact exercise is any action that involves you raising or coming off the floor in a jumping motion, whether with one or both feet. Such movements, called plyometric exercises, rely on the tendons in the lower limbs to propel you upward, and include jogging, running, and any skipping, jumping, or bounding moves in an aerobics or dance session. High-impact exercise is great for building lower-limb strength as well as for pushing you into an intense cardio zone. And contrary to popular thought, a certain amount of high-impact work can be good for the bones and help to prevent or delay the onset of diseases such as osteoporosis. High-impact workouts tend to be particularly suitable if you have, or identify with, a "Let's-do-it" fitness personality (see p.34).

Low-impact exercise

Low-impact activities include walking, swimming, cycling, non-jumping dance and aerobics moves, and resistance, stretching, Pilates, and yoga exercises. These forms of exercise, which involve little or no impact and therefore raise the heart rate less than high-impact work, tend to be more suited to "Take-it-easy" and "Get-up-and-go" fitness personality types (see p.34). However, despite not working the heart as hard, they still provide an effective fitness workout, with the added bonus of less risk of injury. They are particularly useful for older people, prenatal and postpartum women, and anyone who is overweight or new to exercise, as well as for anyone recovering from injury.

Before and after a cardio workout

On page 17, you'll have discovered the importance of warming up before a workout in order to prepare your cold, stiff body for the activity ahead. So before doing any of the forms of cardio exercise recommended in the pages that follow, leave time to do the Universal warm-up (see pp.252–53).

It's also essential to do a cool-down at the end of a cardio workout in order to gradually bring your heart rate and temperature down to normal and to flush out the adrenaline and lactic acid that have built up in your body. This will prevent both dizziness and post-exercise muscle ache, so be sure to leave time for the Universal cool-down (see pp.254–55) at the end of every cardio session.

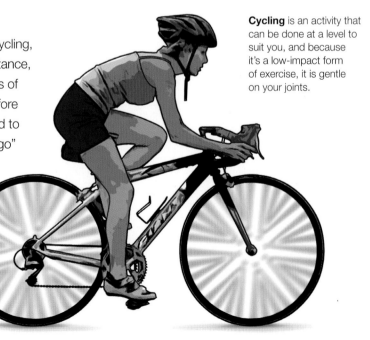

Cycling is an activity that can be done at a level to suit you, and because it's a low-impact form of exercise, it is gentle on your joints.

How hard should I work?

Cardio exercise is all about working the heart, so it's important to have some way of knowing just how hard this vital organ is working. You don't need specialist equipment to do this—just listen to, and monitor, the best "machine" you've got: your body. Paying attention to the way you're talking, how you're feeling, and how fast your heart is beating will give you all the feedback you need.

Deciding at what level to work

It's important to bear in mind when deciding which level to work at that different intensity levels will be suitable for you at different times—depending not only on your fitness personality (see p.34) and fitness level (see p.39), but also on your mood, energy levels, time available, and current objectives.

Talk test

One way of assessing how hard you're working during a cardio session is to do what is called the "talk test,"

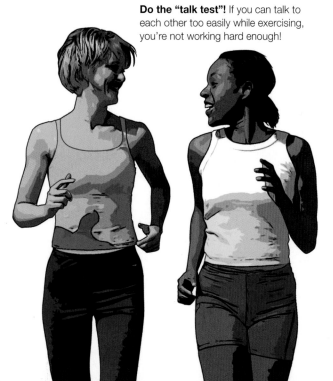

Do the "talk test"! If you can talk to each other too easily while exercising, you're not working hard enough!

where you try to talk out loud as you continue to do your movements:

• If you can talk too easily, you need to work harder.

• If you can talk with a bit of effort, you're working at a "gentle" level, using oxygen and in your aerobic zone. You should be able to train in this zone for quite a long period of time. However, if you're very overweight or have done no exercise for months or years, even five minutes can feel like a long time. This pace is a good starting point for any training.

• If you're able to talk but unable to have a full-blown conversation, you're working moderately to intensely with oxygen (aerobically), but getting close to your threshold with anaerobic exercise (without oxygen). For most people, it's good to train in this zone for between 10 and 40 minutes at least once a week.

• If you can't talk at all, you're in the anaerobic zone— a high-intensity zone that you'll only be able to maintain for a short period of time. This is the zone that sprinters run in. If you're relatively fit, you're likely only to reach this "intense" zone during bursts of extreme speed or effort. However, if you're very unfit, you may reach this zone quite quickly, in which case you will benefit from building up your aerobic fitness by working at a "gentle" pace first.

Rate of Perceived Exertion

Another method of assessing how hard you are working is by establishing your Rate of Perceived Exertion (RPE) at any given point. Also known as the Borg scale, this uses a number scale to rate the intensity of any exercise you do, based on how you feel while doing it. Borg originally used a scale of 0–14, but this is simplified to 0–10 here—where 0 is completely inactive and 10 is working to your max. The great thing about this scale is that it's individual: your gentle pace might be another person's max.

Dancing and aerobics can involve moves in which we jump off the floor. These high-impact moves really increase the intensity of the workout we get.

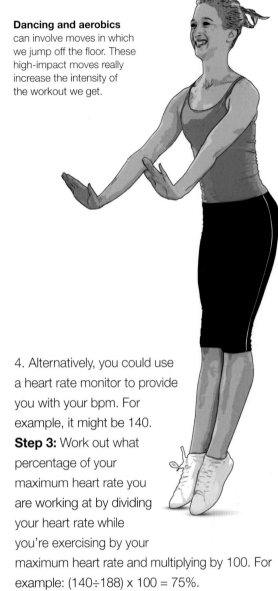

Scale for Rate of Perceived Exertion (RPE)

• **0–4** Exercise feels easy. This "gentle" zone is appropriate for people who are new to exercise, very unfit, overweight, or recovering from injury.

• **4–8** Exercise requires moderate to intense effort and makes you hot, sweaty, and breathe more heavily. For most people, this is the appropriate zone to work in when doing the cardio workouts (see pp.258–69):

    4–5 effectively works your entire body

    5–7 gives both really good toning and fat-burning

    7–8 challenges your body's systems more strongly.

• **8–9** Exercise requires intense focus and effort. This is the zone in which professional sportspeople and athletes tend to work out, but which is good for us to dip into now and then.

• **9–10** Exercise requires your absolute maximal effort—you're doing the activity as fast and hard as you can. This is the zone that professional sportspeople work in when competing.

Heart rate training zones

Another way of assessing whether or not you're working at a suitable intensity for you is based on your heart rate while you exercise:

Step 1: Establish your Maximum Heart Rate (MHR) by subtracting your age from 220. For example, if you're 32, your MHR would be 220–32 = 188.

Step 2: Take your pulse while you're exercising, either at your wrist or neck (see p.35), by counting the number of heart beats during a 15-second period and multiplying by

4. Alternatively, you could use a heart rate monitor to provide you with your bpm. For example, it might be 140.

Step 3: Work out what percentage of your maximum heart rate you are working at by dividing your heart rate while you're exercising by your maximum heart rate and multiplying by 100. For example: (140÷188) x 100 = 75%.

Step 4: Familiarize yourself with the recommended heart rate training zones and see which of the four RPE categories you fall into. Most workouts in this book should be done at between 60–85% of your maximum heart rate if you want to lose weight and improve fitness:

• 60–65% of max heart rate = 4–5 on the RPE scale

• 65–80% of max heart rate = 5–7 on the RPE scale

• 80–85% of max heart rate = 7–8 on the RPE scale

• above 90% of max heart rate = 8–10 on the RPE scale.

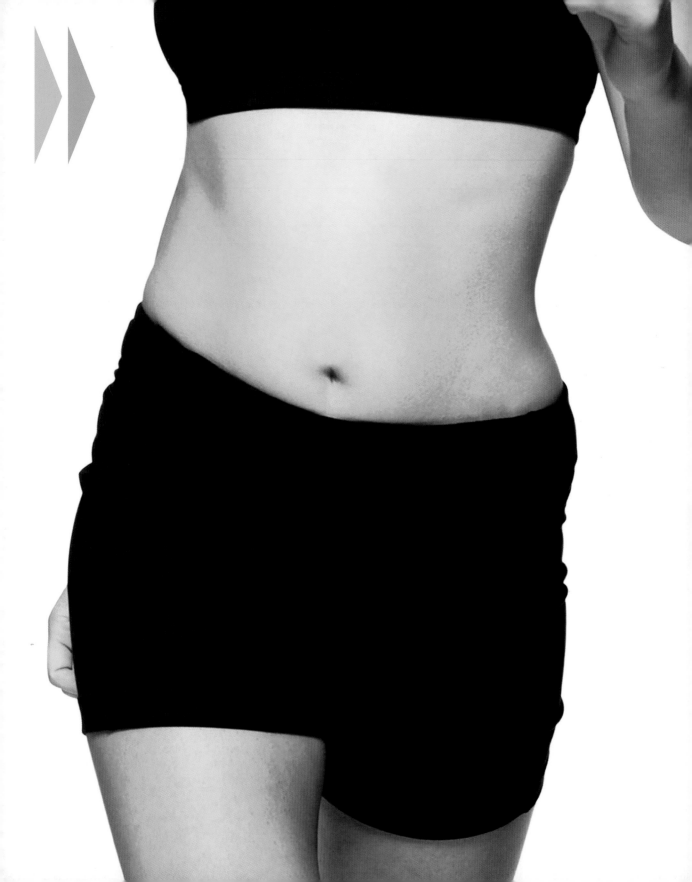

Walking

Walking is one of the simplest forms of exercise to fit into a busy lifestyle—it can be used as a way of getting you from A to B, and as a way of maintaining or enhancing cardio fitness levels. The pages that follow will give you the lowdown on the various types and levels of walking. Whichever approach you take, walking will:

■ boost your cardiovascular system by working your heart

■ help you to burn off calories and therefore to control your weight

■ tone your legs, since walking involves mainly lower body muscle action

■ keep your joints mobile, without straining them during high-impact activities

■ give you time to yourself to restore balance in your mind as well as in your body

■ create a healthy sense of forward movement in your life

■ get you out in the fresh air if you choose to walk outside

■ help the environment if you walk to your destination instead of drive

The fundamentals of walking

Whether you take gentle walks in the local park, power walk to and from work every day, or go for long hikes in the country, walking is a great, natural way to enhance both your health and your fitness. Although it's, generally speaking, a low-impact form of exercise, you can still alter the level of intensity as desired via speed and incline to get your heart really pumping and therefore burn off fat.

Moving ahead

On top of the physical benefits of walking, it could be thought of as a form of "meditation on the move," since time spent walking can help clear the mind. Placing one foot in front of the other is also a good metaphor for moving forward in life, which can increase motivation.

What to wear

One of the beauties of walking is that you don't need to spend a fortune on gear. However, it's important that you dress appropriately since you may need to be ready for all kinds of weather. Below are some guidelines:
• Choose items made from specialist, lightweight material that will wick away perspiration and provide adequate ventilation.
• Opt for stretchy material and elasticated waists on your shorts or pants—for comfort and ease of movement.
• Opt for flat-lock seams to avoid chafing.
• Wear layers so that you can add or remove items for temperature control.

Assessing your gait

Before investing in a new pair of walking shoes, it helps to have an understanding of your manner of walking—or your gait. It's best to have this assessed by an expert in a specialist sports shoe store, but a more general way to make an approximate assessment is the "tread test." This involves looking at the areas that are most worn down on the soles of your current walking shoes:

• If just the inside of the sole is worn down, you have a low arch and your foot "pronates" (rolls inward excessively).
• If your sole shows balanced wear between its two sides, you have a balanced gait, as each foot lands on the outside of the heel and rolls slightly inward to absorb shock.
• If just the outside of the sole is worn down, your foot "supinates" (rolls outward excessively).

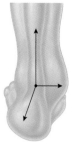 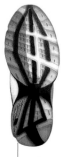 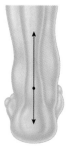 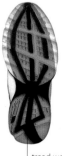 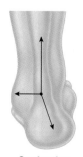 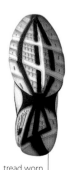

| **Pronation** (left foot) | tread worn on inside | **Neutral** (left foot) | tread worn evenly | **Supination** (left foot) | tread worn on outside |

Flexibility is key

As well as providing adequate support and protection, your walking shoes must be flexible enough to allow a deep bend through your foot during the "push-off" movement between one step and the next.

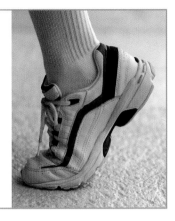

To get the perfect fit it's a good idea to go to a specialist store, where they will both accurately measure your feet and get you to walk on a computerized treadmill to analyze your gait. Shoes for people whose feet roll inward (pronators) are likely to have high arches, extra heel lift, and firm mid-soles; while those for people whose feet roll outward (supinators) will have extra cushioning under the ball of the foot.

• Wear wind- and waterproof jackets on cooler and wetter days.
• Wear high-visibility items on darker days and in the evenings.
• Wear good-fitting socks and walking shoes.
• Wear a peaked cap and sunglasses to keep the sun off your face on hot days; also apply UV protection.
• Consider wearing a fanny pack to carry keys, your phone, emergency money, and other essentials.
• Carry a bottle of water for rehydration purposes; you can now get ones with built-in handles for ease.

Choosing your shoes

Walking shoes need to provide both comfort and support, allow freedom of movement throughout the whole foot, and, to a lesser extent, act as shock absorbers. The main features to look for are:
• Lightness and flexibility—to allow a full range of motion through the feet (see above).
• Heel cushioning—to support the heels as they land.
• Low heels—to avoid overworking the shins.
• Adequate arch support—to ensure a balanced gait (see left).
• Cushioning for the ball of the feet—to enhance comfort during the "push-off" movement (see p.62).
• Spacious, rounded toe areas—to give the toes room to spread out.

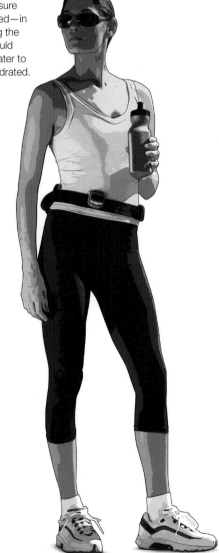

Before you go for your walk, make sure you're well equipped—in addition to wearing the right gear, you should carry a bottle of water to avoid getting dehydrated.

How to power walk

Power walking allows you to work at a higher intensity than normal walking and will therefore burn more calories. It's the same as normal walking but with more pronounced and purposeful leg and arm movements, which can increase your speed from an average 3mph (5km/h) to 5mph (8km/h). It takes a little technique to get it right, but power walking will help you reap fantastic fitness rewards.

Technique tips

Below are some tips for how to position and use your body in order to get the most from your power walking sessions:

Head, shoulders, and chest: Draw your head up tall, your shoulders back and down, and ensure that your chest is lifted to achieve a sense of length and poise throughout your body.

Abs: Pull your belly button toward your spine so that the movement really comes from the core, and is therefore safe and strong.

Hips: Keep your pelvis and hip area as relaxed as possible so that you can stride freely with your legs.

Arms and hands: Bend your arms to 90° at waist level and "pump" them from the shoulders to propel each stride forward, keeping them bent at 90° as you do so. If your left leg is forward, your right arm should be forward, as if punching diagonally upward (palm facing inward), and your left arm back, as if elbowing someone behind you!

Hands: Cup your hands in a relaxed way, so that they make loose fists. As your arms swing, they should move in an arc shape from your waist up to about shoulder height in front of you.

Feet: Land each foot heel-first and roll through onto your toes, from where you can "push off" dynamically for the next step, to create a sense of momentum.

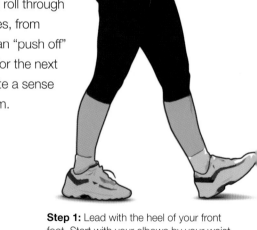

Step 1: Lead with the heel of your front foot. Start with your elbows by your waist and your forearms parallel to the floor. Keep your body upright.

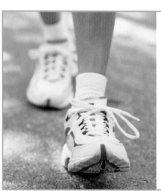

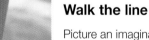

Walk the line

Picture an imaginary line stretching out in front of you and aim to walk along this, a bit like a tightrope. This means placing each foot directly in front of the other as you walk.

Things to avoid

- Don't slouch your shoulders, let your chest collapse, let your belly stick out, or look down as you walk.
- Don't over-stride: keep your steps within a comfortable range of motion.
- Don't twist your hips: keep them level and facing forward. It can help to visualize the front of your hip bones as the headlights on a car.

- Don't allow your arms to swing across the central line of your chest, or out to the sides.
- Don't let your front hand go higher than shoulder height when pumping your arms.
- Don't let your back hand dip below your waist as you propel yourself forward with your arms.

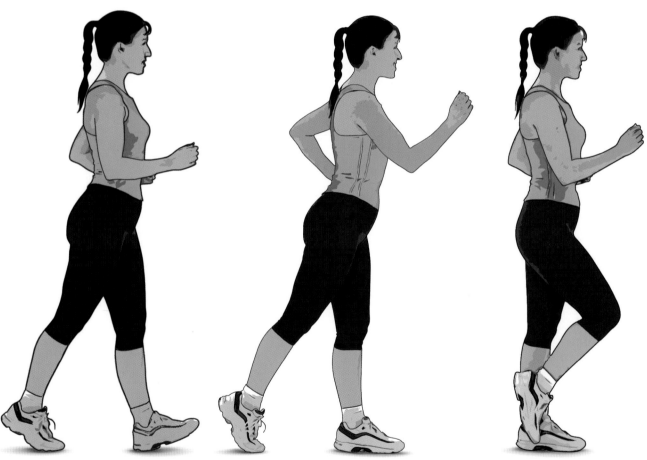

Step 2: Allow your back heel to come off the floor as the toes of your front foot gradually lower. Start to move one bent arm forward and the other backward. If your left leg is forward, your right arm should be forward, and vice versa.

Step 3: Transfer your weight fully onto your front foot as you raise the heel of your back foot off the floor, ready to push forward again off the ball of the back foot. At this "push-off" point, your pumping arms should be at their highest. Keep your abs engaged to maintain balanced posture.

Step 4: Lift your back foot and keep your toes close to the ground as you bring it beside your other foot, before striding it forward, heel first, as in Step 1. Note that your moving leg is bent while your supporting leg is straight. At the same time, start to switch the position of your arms, moving your front arm backward and your back arm forward.

Getting the most from your walking

To get the most from any walking you do, it's a good idea to plan your route in advance and have particular goals in mind, whether speed-related, distance-related, or both. Another way to enhance your walking experience is to regularly do a few walking-specific exercises between workouts to increase your fitness, so see guidance on p.65.

Choosing your route

Once you've decided when you're going walking and how much time you have available, it's a good idea to plan where to go so that you can ensure it meets both your timing and fitness needs. This will also allow you to walk with a sense of ease and purpose once you're on your way, without worrying about getting lost or not getting back in time for other commitments.

If you live in a city, you'll probably want to consider local parks, canal and river trails, and routes that take in local historical or architectural sites. Whereas if you live in the country or on the coast, check out local beaches, woods, and other dedicated public walking trails, especially in areas of particular natural beauty. A walk always seems to go by much faster when you have interesting things to look at along the way!

Wherever you choose to walk, ensure that you include some hills, if appropriate, to increase the intensity of your workout. Also think about the terrain on which you would like to walk: a hard, even surface, such as concrete, will provide stability but be slightly more harsh on your joints; an uneven grassy or gravelly surface means you'll have to pay more attention to balance; and a soft surface, such as sand, will make you work considerably harder.

Finally, always take safety into consideration: if you'll be walking on your own, choose well-populated routes. Alternatively, you might prefer to arrange to go walking with a friend or as part of a local group.

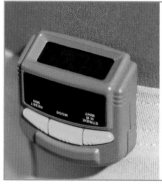

Counting your steps

Wear your pedometer (see below) attached to the waistband of your pants or clipped onto a belt around your waist, since movement will be sensed here.

Using a pedometer

A pedometer is a handy gadget that will count the number of steps you take, work out the distance you have covered, the speed you are walking at, and even how many calories you have burned off. As such, it can be a great tool to keep you motivated during any walking workouts you choose to do! However, it is also useful to wear one as you go about your daily activities. Here are some recommended goals to work toward:

- **3,000 steps a day** = good starting point for getting fit
- **6,000 steps a day** = will keep diseases related to obesity and inactivity at bay
- **10,000 steps a day** = the "magic number" set by leading health and fitness professionals to help you to lose weight and maintain a healthy heart.

It's not as hard as it at first might seem to get up to the desired 10,000 steps: take the stairs instead of the elevator, walk to the store rather than drive, or simply take a walk around the block!

Quad and Ankle Stretch

The bent leg lift in this exercise will stretch out the front of your thighs (known as your quads), while the lifted heel will strengthen your ankles and calves, as well as stretch down the front of your shins.

1 Stand tall with your feet hip-width apart and parallel. Inhale to prepare. As you exhale, lift your right foot off the floor, take hold of your ankle with your right hand, and raise it toward your buttocks until you feel a good stretch down the front of your right thigh. Keep a slight bend in your supporting leg and a slight tilt in your pelvis throughout. Hold for 10 seconds.

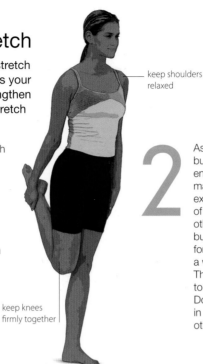

keep shoulders relaxed

keep knees firmly together

2 As you inhale, pull your belly button toward your spine to engage your abs and gain maximal stability. As you exhale, rise up onto the ball of your foot, keeping your other foot as close to your buttocks as possible. Hold for 5 seconds, holding onto a wall for balance, if needed. Then slowly return your heel to the floor as you inhale. Do Steps 1 and 2 10 times in total. Then repeat on the other side.

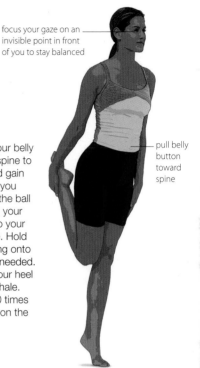

focus your gaze on an invisible point in front of you to stay balanced

pull belly button toward spine

Walker's Lunge

The quads are the large muscles on the front of your thighs responsible for extending your legs at the knee when you walk. This exercise will stretch and strengthen these muscles, adding more power to your stride.

1 Stand tall with your feet hip-width apart and parallel, and your hands on your hips. Take a stride forward with one leg, keeping your hips and feet facing directly forward and both heels on the floor. Look forward as you do so.

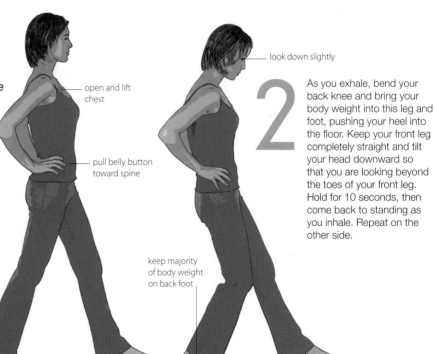

open and lift chest

pull belly button toward spine

look down slightly

keep majority of body weight on back foot

2 As you exhale, bend your back knee and bring your body weight into this leg and foot, pushing your heel into the floor. Keep your front leg completely straight and tilt your head downward so that you are looking beyond the toes of your front leg. Hold for 10 seconds, then come back to standing as you inhale. Repeat on the other side.

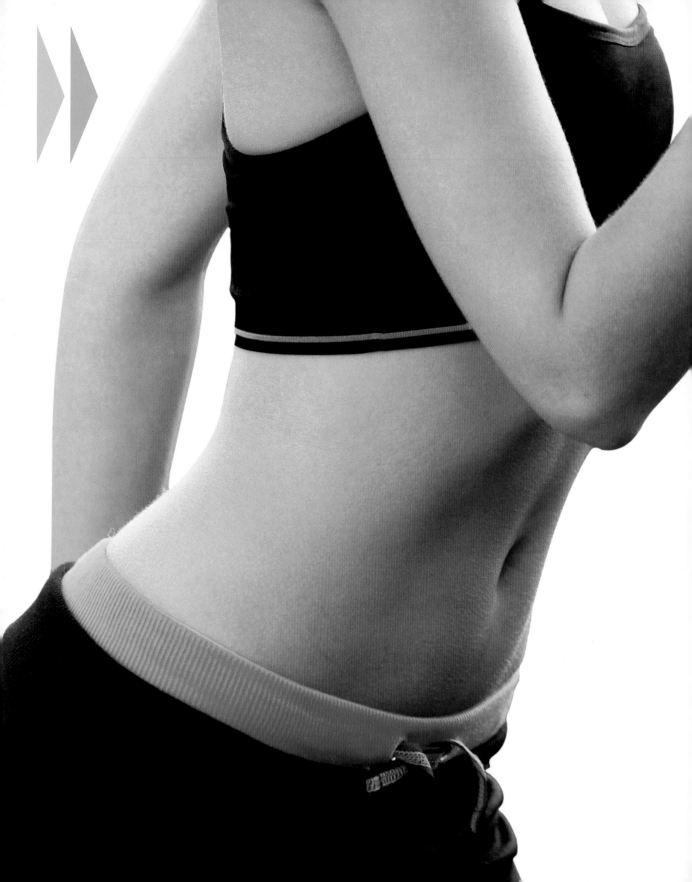

Running

Regular jogging or running is one of the best ways to stay fit. More than 40,000 people run the New York City Marathon every year, and more and more people are taking to pounding the streets (or treadmill) with their feet—whether for a charitable cause, physical fitness, or pure enjoyment. The pages that follow will give you insight into how to benefit the most from running but, whatever your approach, it will:

- boost the health of your heart by temporarily making it work harder

- burn off serious calories, helping with weight loss, if desired

- help to slow down the loss of muscle and bone density that occurs with age

- provide a form of "meditation on the move," helping you to declutter your mind

- alleviate stress—you can literally "run off" your worries

- enhance your mood, since it boosts the number of endorphins in your system

- give you a chance to get time on your own or meet new, like-minded people

- get you out in the fresh air, which will help to reinvigorate your system

The fundamentals of running

As the king of cardio, running is quite simply the most effective way to lose weight: you can burn more calories per hour running than doing any other form of cardio workout. However, like any form of exercise, it can be performed at different levels of intensity, depending on your wants and needs—from slow jogs to intense sprints, and short runs to long-distance ones.

Getting started

The beauty of running is its simplicity: a good pair of running shoes and some basic gear to protect you from the elements is all you really need to get started. Here is some advice on acquiring these.

What to wear

All the same principles apply to choosing clothes for running as for walking (see pp.60–61). In summer, you'll need shorts and a tank top or T-shirt, a peaked cap, UV protection, and sunglasses designed to stay on while you're on the move. In winter, you'll need full-length base-layers, a wind- and waterproof lightweight jacket, a hat, and lightweight gloves. You may also want to try out compression socks, tights, and tops, which are designed to boost blood flow where it's needed and therefore help with recovery after a run. Other optional gear includes:
• a water bottle or hydration system that you wear on your back like a backpack
• a fanny pack or belt to carry keys, money, and other small essentials
• an armband for an MP3 player or phone (some of which double up as GPS systems).

Choosing shoes

It's essential to invest in a good pair of sneakers before doing any running, so make a trip to a specialist running or sports store to discuss your needs and try on a range of models. Trained staff are likely to analyze your gait (see p.60)—the way in which you move your feet when running. This will determine whether your feet have a tendency to pronate (roll inward), supinate (roll outward), or neither—each of which creates a certain set of sneaker requirements. The sales staff should also discuss with you the type of running you'll be doing (on- or off-road) and the type of runner you are— a heel striker or toe striker (see p.70), since this will affect what is best for you. Be sure to take heed of the advice that you are given, try on the range of shoes that they recommend, and take your time making your choice.

Never run in a shoe designed for any other sport—it simply won't provide the cushioning, support, and stability that the repetitive action of running requires. After all, your foot absorbs up to

Make sure you dress suitably for the weather conditions and always take a bottle of water to keep hydrated.

A good pair of sneakers is the most important investment you can make if you are eager to take up running.

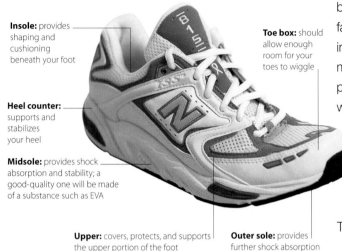

Insole: provides shaping and cushioning beneath your foot

Heel counter: supports and stabilizes your heel

Midsole: provides shock absorption and stability; a good-quality one will be made of a substance such as EVA

Toe box: should allow enough room for your toes to wiggle

Upper: covers, protects, and supports the upper portion of the foot

Outer sole: provides further shock absorption and durability

but don't worry, it gets easier and more natural the more you run and the fitter you become.

Elite runners tend to use a two-two breathing pattern: breathing in for two steps and out for two steps. Using a faster rhythm than this—one-one, for example—can be inefficient as it leads to increased work for the breathing muscles. The key is to experiment with different breathing patterns during your first running sessions to see what works best for you. As a starting point, you could try a four-four pattern—breathing in for four steps and out for four steps—to get used to moving in harmony with your breath, then adjust the rhythm according to your needs. Once you have found a pattern that suits you, practice it until it feels like second nature. This should take only a couple of weeks.

four times your own body weight with each step that you run. Sophisticated, shock-absorbing materials are continually being updated by manufacturers, and you'll pay more for sneakers whose midsoles (see above) are made with substances such as EVA (ethyl vinyl acetate), which essentially forms a layer of tiny bubbles that provides the foot with much-needed cushioning, or Brooks DNA, which responds to the amount of force placed on the foot and disperses the pressure, providing the perfect level of resilience.

Finally, it's worth mentioning the option of lightweight, "minimalist" shoes, which fit like gloves and are based on the principle that our feet need to feel the ground beneath them and be able to move as freely as possible in order to be strong and effective. Most of these are designed with sophisticated, puncture-resistant soles.

Effective breathing

Whatever intensity of running you do, one thing you'll need to master is how to breathe well (see p.33) while on the move. Most beginners struggle a little with this,

Sports bra

For women, sports bras are a must for all high-impact exercise. The support that they provide not only makes running more comfortable, but also helps to prevent potential back pain and any long-term sagging of the breasts. Normal bras reduce breast movement by around 35%, but a good sports bra achieves closer to 60%. Some sports bras are a typical bra shape, while others are more like a cut-off tank top; some have over-the-shoulder-style straps while others have a racer-back style (see below). It's best to be measured professionally to ensure that you wear the correct size.

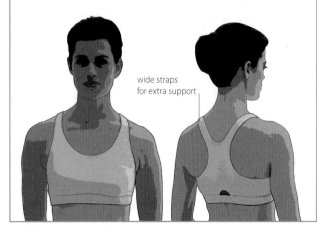

wide straps for extra support

How to run well

There's no such thing as the perfect running style. If you watch a race, you'll see that no two runners move in the same way. Fast or slow, there is no "right" way. However, taking into account the advice below will increase your awareness of how you run and will allow you to fine-tune your style and therefore boost your running efficiency and capacity.

Technique tips

Your body type and size tend to determine the length of your stride, and your stride length and frequency combined then determine how fast you run. But whatever your natural body type, stride length, and pace, the advice that follows will help you to get the most from your running and minimize your chances of injury.

Upper body: Keep your chest open, shoulders back and down, head tall and forward-facing, and belly button pulled toward your spine to engage your abs.

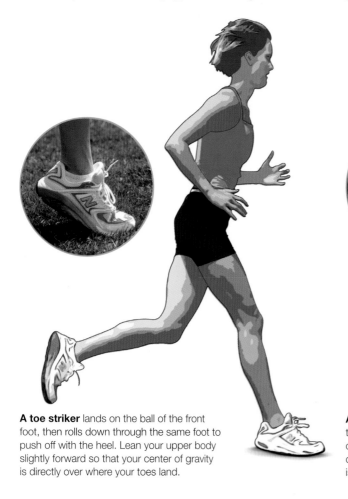

A toe striker lands on the ball of the front foot, then rolls down through the same foot to push off with the heel. Lean your upper body slightly forward so that your center of gravity is directly over where your toes land.

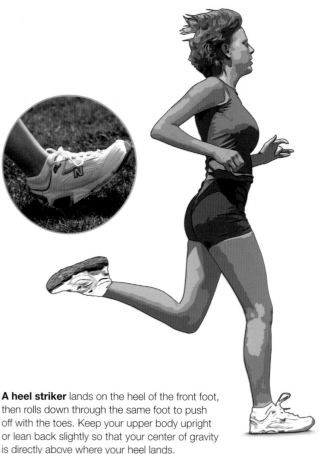

A heel striker lands on the heel of the front foot, then rolls down through the same foot to push off with the toes. Keep your upper body upright or lean back slightly so that your center of gravity is directly above where your heel lands.

Adapting stride length to vary pace

Long stride. If you have a long, lean body, lengthening your normal stride is a good way to increase your pace. However, don't overstretch yourself.

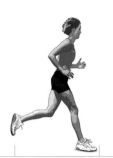

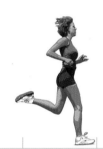

Short stride. If you are short but strong, it's better to quicken the number of normal-size strides that you take to increase your pace.

Legs: Drive your legs from your core abdominal muscles, imagining that strings are drawing your kneecaps forward as you move.

Arms: Bend your arms at approximately 90° and keep them relaxed as you move to complement your natural running form. The opposite arm to leg should always move forward.

Hands: Imagine holding a potato chip, without breaking it, between the thumb and index finger of each hand so that your hands are in a slightly cupped shape without being clenched.

Feet: Some runners, called "heel strikers," land on the heel of their front foot and roll forward to push off from their toes, as per the technique for power walking (see pp.62–63). Others, called "toe strikers," land on the toes of their front foot and push off from their heel. Simply do whichever comes most naturally to you.

Things to avoid

- Don't slouch your shoulders, let your chest collapse, your belly stick out, or look down.
- Don't over-think: over-analyzing your technique or trying too hard to get it right is likely to result in a jerky, mechanical action that will slow you down and make you more prone to injury. Simply be aware of the main technique factors, then try to relax into them.
- Don't forget to breathe: breathe deeply every few strides so that your movements start to work in harmony with your breath (see also p.69).
- Don't tense your body: relax your face, jaw, shoulders, and fists since these are the particular areas that tend to tighten up when running if you don't remain aware of them.
- Don't over-stride: keep your steps within a comfortable range of motion to avoid any unnecessary strain.

Getting the most from your running

To get the most from your running, it's best to vary your routes, terrains, and the pace at which you run. Also consider your aims—whether you want to stay healthy, lose weight, or build your fitness for an event. It's also helpful to regularly do a few running-specific exercises between sessions to prepare the key muscles involved in running for optimal action, so see the guidance on p.73.

Choosing your route

As when planning walking workouts (see p.64), it's important that your running routes match both your timing and fitness needs. There are many terrains for you to choose from: flat, hilly, concrete sidewalks, gravelly paths, grassy trails, an athletics track, or a trusty treadmill. And, as with most things, variety is the key to success.

Running off-road is generally gentler on the joints than pounding the pavements, so try to include at least some off-road running in your training regimen. If, however, you do run regularly on the same pavement route, make sure that you switch sides of the road from time to time so that if one side is at an angle, you're not always having to use your body in the same way to compensate for this, which could lead to misalignment or injury.

Be sure to include some hill running in your fitness program if you want to really work your heart and muscles harder and boost your strength. As you go up the hill, you'll target your hamstrings and glutes (the back of your thighs and butt), and as you go down, you'll fire up your quads (front thighs).

Track training can also be useful. And don't worry— it's not just for elite athletes. Most athletics tracks offer recreational sessions for a small fee. And the fact that their surfaces are specifically designed to absorb shock makes them particularly useful for faster interval training (i.e. running for short, fast bursts).

Varying your pace

Whatever your level, you'll benefit from mixing up the pace of your running sessions. If, for example, you want to run three times a week, do a different one of the workouts on pp.262–63 each time—one involving interval training, one at a steady tempo, and one longer off-road run. If you're preparing for a marathon, it makes sense to run long intervals (up to a mile) with short recovery periods; if you're preparing for a 5K or less, shorter intervals (up to 400m) with more recovery time will work well; or if you simply want to build cardio fitness while fat-burning, long, steady runs are more the order of the day. However, shorter runs are also worthwhile when you're short on time.

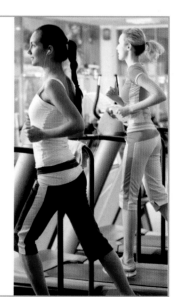

Indoor running

Treadmills are great for bad-weather days. They also absorb impact well, and their computerized feedback makes it easier to quantify your training. However, the lack of external stimulation can make running on them feel psychologically challenging, so you may prefer to mix and match treadmill and outdoor workouts.

Calf Raise

This exercise will strengthen your calf muscles, particularly the gastrocnemius in the upper part of your calf, which plays a huge part in propelling you forward when running and also in cushioning each landing.

1 Stand tall with your feet hip-width apart and parallel, resting your hands on a stable surface of about hip-height in front of you for support. As you inhale, lift one foot off the floor and wrap the toes of this foot around the back of your other ankle.

pull belly button toward spine

ensure all weight is in supporting leg

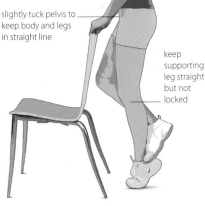

2 As you exhale, slowly lift up onto the ball of your foot, keeping the toes of your other foot wrapped behind your ankle as before. Then slowly return your heel to the floor as you inhale. Do this 10 times in total. Then repeat on the other side.

slightly tuck pelvis to keep body and legs in straight line

keep supporting leg straight but not locked

Reverse Lunge with Knee Lift

This exercise will strengthen your main upper leg muscles—your glutes, quads, and hamstrings. The balancing element of the exercise means that the hip flexors, primary movers in running, are also worked.

1 Stand tall with your feet hip-width apart and parallel. Inhale to prepare. As you exhale, take a stride backward with one foot to enter into a right-angle lunge. Keep both feet facing forward, your back heel lifted, your pelvis slightly tucked, and your upper body absolutely upright. Inhale to prepare.

do not let knee bend beyond toes

aim for lower leg to be parallel with floor

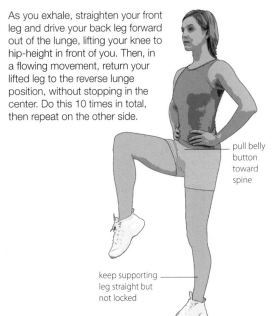

2 As you exhale, straighten your front leg and drive your back leg forward out of the lunge, lifting your knee to hip-height in front of you. Then, in a flowing movement, return your lifted leg to the reverse lunge position, without stopping in the center. Do this 10 times in total, then repeat on the other side.

pull belly button toward spine

keep supporting leg straight but not locked

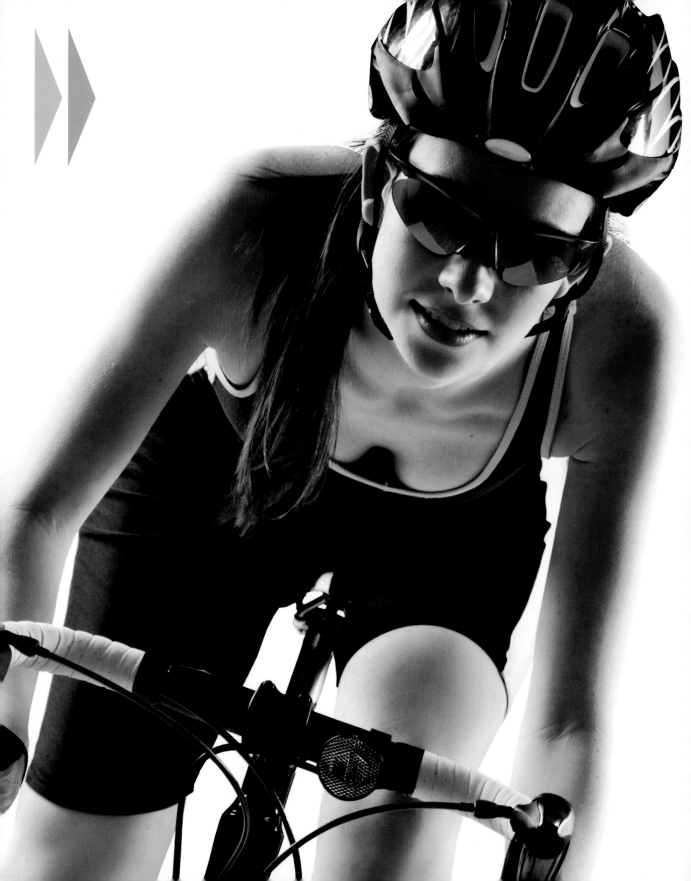

Cycling

Cycling is a low-impact, high-adrenaline sport that can take you on journeys through town and country. Not only is it sociable and good for the environment, but if you make it your means of getting from A to B, you won't have to worry about making "extra time" for the cardio aspect of your exercise regimen. The pages that follow will tell you how to get the most from cycling but, no matter what your approach, regular rides will:

- enhance the health of your heart

- burn off calories, helping you to manage your weight

- strongly activate the large muscles in your upper legs, boosting your metabolism

- provide all-over toning, since cycling works both your upper and lower body

- put minimal pressure on your bones, since your bike supports your body weight

- improve your reflexes, because you need to be ultra-alert when you cycle

- get you outdoors for some fresh air and that sense of "going on a journey"

- help the environment if you replace at least some of your driving with cycling

The fundamentals of cycling

In addition to being great for your heart and helping you to lose weight, cycling will help you to tone up all over, too. As a non-weight-bearing form of exercise, it is also more gentle on your joints than sports like jogging and running. As with all forms of cardio work, it can be done at whatever intensity best suits you at any given time, whether a leisurely cycle, an intense "spin," or a long, hilly ride.

Getting started

As well as giving you strong, shapely legs and buttocks from all the pedaling, cycling will strengthen and tone the muscles in your back, abs, arms, shoulders, and chest as you work to hold yourself upright. Of course, you'll need the right bike for the terrain you choose to travel on, plus a few other key pieces of gear, including a helmet, so review the guidance below.

What type of bike?

The type of bike you choose (see below for options) will depend on which terrain you decide to cycle on. But whatever you decide on, make sure that the frame is the right size for you and the saddle is comfortable (male and female saddles are designed differently). Staff in any good bike shop will be able to help you with this.

Indoor exercise bike?

Alternatively, or additionally, you may opt for an indoor exercise bike. This provides an alternative to outdoor cycling during inclement weather, or when you just want some variety in your workout. A turbo trainer is the best way to replicate what you do outdoors. It consists of a stand (which you attach your bike to) and a resistance unit for you to pedal against, plus speed and distance readings and additional magnetic resistance to simulate hills. But whichever type you choose, it should display the basics: distance, speed, time, calories burned, and the resistance level at which you are working. Other features may include heart-rate monitoring and pre-programmed workouts. In the same way as when you buy an outdoor bike, check for comfort, size, and stability.

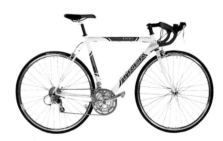

Road or racing bikes are slender and lightweight, with thin tires and dropped handlebars. They are designed for smooth surfaces and speed. When you cycle, your position on the bike means you will have to reach your arms long to hold the handlebars, and so you'll need to be reasonably supple.

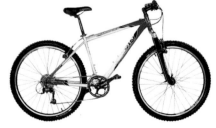

Off-road or mountain bikes have a sturdy frame and thick tires with plenty of tread and good suspension for uneven terrain. Higher handlebars means that less of a hunched-over riding position is required. There should be 3–4in (8–10cm) between your crotch and the top bar when straddling the bike.

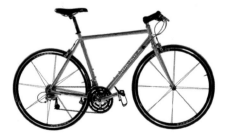

Hybrid bikes are a cross between racing and mountain bikes. They range from road bikes with flat handlebars to near-mountain bikes. However, they have thinner tires than mountain bikes, and your position on them will be more upright. These are ideal for commuting and negotiating busy roads.

What to wear

It's up to you whether you wear tight or baggy gear to cycle in, but if it's tight, make sure it's stretchy and breathable, and if it's baggy, make sure it won't catch in the spokes of your wheels. For winter cycling, whether on- or off-road, it's best to wear several thin layers for insulation, starting with a long-sleeved wicking base layer. Hands and feet should be protected from the cold by thermal gloves and socks. Whatever the season, you'll need padding in your tights or shorts to prevent a sore butt. In summer, maximal ventilation will be desired. Sunglasses should be worn on bright days not only to keep the sun out of your eyes, but also to protect them from insects and dust.

A cycling helmet is a must because it can save your life in an accident—be sure to wear it for even the shortest of journeys. When your are selecting and buying a helmet, make sure you get in-store assistance

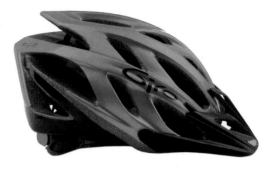

Modern cycling helmets are aerodynamic in design with ventilation holes to keep you cool, and adjustable straps and padding inside for comfort. Many have removable peaks to protect your eyes from sun and rain.

regarding the best size for you.

Specialist cycling shoes will make your ride more comfortable since they will fully support your foot for the actions required. The type you choose will depend on the type of pedals on your bike, and the type of cycling that you want them for. Staff in any good bike shop should be able to advise you on this.

Basic equipment

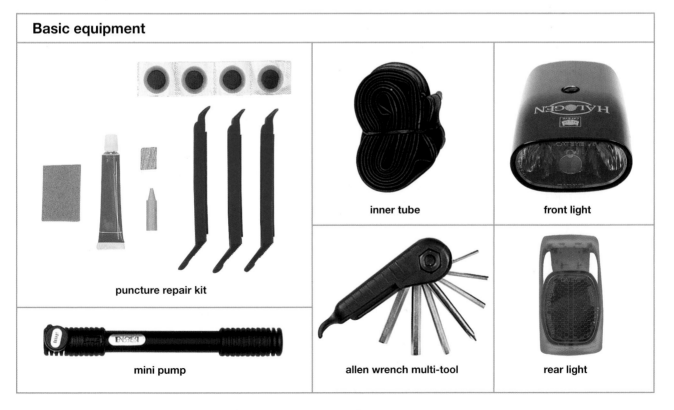

puncture repair kit

inner tube

front light

mini pump

allen wrench multi-tool

rear light

How to cycle well

All you need for cycling is a little bit of balance, a little bit of confidence, and some basic mechanical know-how regarding aspects such as riding position, efficient use of the pedals, changing gear, turning corners, and braking. So read on to learn more about these essentials if you're not already familiar with them.

Technique tips

The advice that follows will help you master the techniques of cycling. Once you have decided on the style of bike you want (see p.76) and made sure that it's the correct size for you, you can get going.

Efficient pedal use

Using the pedals of your bike well takes skill and practice. To start, angle the pedal slightly forward, since it's difficult to push downward if the pedal is pointing upward. As the pedal begins to move down, drop your heel slightly to help your leg move forward and down. As the pedal reaches six o'clock, start to pull it back up to the start position—it can help to visualize scraping something off your shoe. It's important that you make small adjustments to the angle of your feet as you move them to ensure that power is transferred to the pedals throughout the entirety of each revolution.

Riding position

It's vital to establish a safe and comfortable riding position, since this will make your bike easier to control and enhance your pedaling power.

Raise or lower the saddle of your bike so that your leg is completely straight when your heel is on the pedal at the bottom of the revolution, with your pelvis in a neutral position (i.e. in no way tilted).

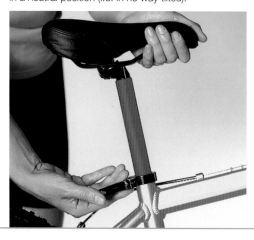

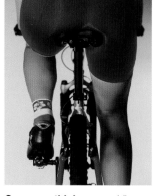

Once you think your saddle is at the correct height, make sure that you tighten the bolt underneath it for safety. Then ask a friend to stand behind you as you get on the bike and do a trial cycle in a straight line away from them. Ask them to check that your hips are not rocking as you pedal. If they are moving in this way, the saddle is too high and you will need to adjust it further.

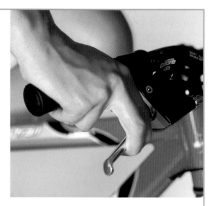

Once you're happy with your saddle height, it's important to make sure you have a comfortable arm position, too. Brake levers should be angled so that you pull on them in line with your arms. In an ideal world, you should be able to apply them easily with just two fingers. If you have to stretch uncomfortably far, you will need to adjust what is called the "reach" on your bike. You can either follow the manufacturer's instructions or ask a bike shop to do this for you.

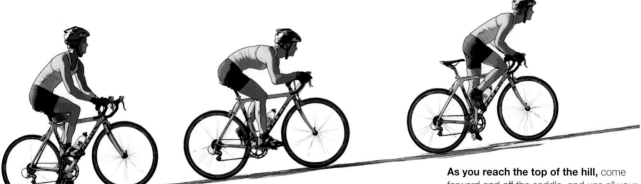

When you start climbing a hill, stay in the saddle with your weight back, selecting a low gear that will allow you to pedal quickly. Hold the handlebars on the top and close to the center. Your heart rate will already be on the rise.

As the incline increases, lean forward so that your body is almost horizontal. Push down hard on the pedals to drive you forward. Hold the top of the brake levers and open your arms slightly so that your elbows point outward. This will open your chest, allowing you to breathe more freely as the oxygen required to power your muscles increases.

As you reach the top of the hill, come forward and off the saddle, and use all your body weight to push down hard on the pedals to drive you forward for that last bit of the ascent. Your body should still be leaning forward, but not quite as much as during the previous stage.

Changing gears

Bikes have gears to allow your pedal speed (your cadence) and the effort required on your part to stay relatively steady regardless of the terrain or incline you may be on. The key thing to remember here is anticipation: always change gears just before your workload is going to change (not as it changes), whether it's a speed or gradient change that's coming up. Use low gears for uphill and high gears for downhill.

Turning corners

To successfully turn a corner on your bike, stop pedaling and lean into the corner, keeping your foot on the top revolution of the pedal—at 12 o'clock—so that you don't scrape the pedal on the ground.

Braking

Brake levers are usually on the handlebars—one front and one back brake. There are several techniques for efficient braking on a standard, two-brake bike. The most commonly taught is the 75–25 technique, which entails supplying about 75% of the stopping power to the front brake and 25% to the rear. However, some maneuvers, such as leaning into a turn and cycling on slippery or uneven surfaces, or long, steep descents, will require more rear brake force. It's always best to do a few test runs on your bike to get used to the amount of hand force—and time—required for braking before you do any serious riding, especially if you're going to be cycling in any traffic. And, no matter what, always try to brake gradually.

Things to avoid

- Don't pedal with more force on terrains such as grass or sand. Instead, shift to a lower gear if it starts to become harder to pedal.
- Don't wait for the terrain or incline to change to alter the gear—anticipate changes.
- Don't let the pedal drop to the bottom revolution when you turn a corner. That way, you can avoid it scraping on the ground as you lean into the corner.
- Don't hunch over and let your chest collapse when you're working hard. Instead, lift and open your chest to get air into your lungs.
- Don't forget to stay hydrated. However, it's best not to try to take a drink from a bottle when cycling up or down a hill in case you lose your balance.

Getting the most from your cycling

To get the most from any cycling that you do, it's important to decide what appeals to you most and what is most feasible for you in terms of terrain, length of sessions, speed, incline, and all the rest, so below are a range of options to consider. It can also be helpful to do the cycling-specific exercise (see right) between sessions to prepare the key muscles for optimal action.

Planning your routes

As with walking and running, it's important to decide in advance where you would most like to cycle and what routes will best match with your timing and fitness needs.

On-road cycling is good for speed and flow, giving the sense of a satisfying journey. Cycling on custom-built cycle tracks is a good way of unwinding, while mountain biking tends to be more about a sense of adventure.

To cycle safely in busy, built-up areas, you need to be both very competent and very confident. You'll need to get used to traveling slowly in a low gear and make safety your absolute priority. You'll also need to be extra vigilant of what other road users are doing and how this impacts your riding. Plus, balance and control will be key so that you can turn to look over your shoulder when necessary without wobbling or veering off course and raise your arm to indicate successfully when you want to turn into a side street.

If you find the idea of this too stressful, you might prefer to search out custom-built cycle paths, if you're lucky enough to have any in your area. Here, you can enjoy the same sense of freedom and movement but in a more controlled environment, whether on a canal path, around a lake, or through your local park.

Mountain biking will give you a different set of challenges—bumpy dirt tracks, gravel, tree roots, sudden steep ascents and descents. Always alter your speed before you shift onto a different terrain or gradient, and be careful not to steer too widely on corners.

Cycling on a custom-built track is another option and is a great place to practice cycling at high speed. Spinning is when you pedal as fast as you can in a low gear, while sprinting is when you pedal as fast as you can while raised up out of your saddle. Both can either be done for fun, or to help build strength and endurance.

Cycling classes

Another riding option is to join a Spinning® or other indoor studio cycling session. In these classes, the instructor will direct you to work harder by urging you to pedal faster, adjusting resistance, and getting you to work out of your saddle. Classes are highly motivating, usually with pumping music, and sometimes with "disco" lights and image projections to stimulate your senses and get the adrenaline flowing. They are excellent high-intensity workouts that will get you sweating, your heart racing, and burn lots of calories.

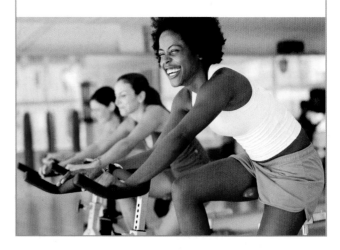

Angel Wings

This exercise will strengthen your upper body to help with a stable riding position and your lower body to help with pedal power. It will also increase spine flexibility, which is useful for the bent-over position associated with uphill cycling in particular.

1 Lie flat on your back with your arms on the floor above your head. As you inhale, feel the breath filling your lungs and abdomen. As you exhale, relax all your muscles into the floor. Stay like this for a few breaths. Then, as you inhale, really engage all your muscles and, as you exhale, stretch both your fingers and toes away from your center to create a sense of length throughout your whole body.

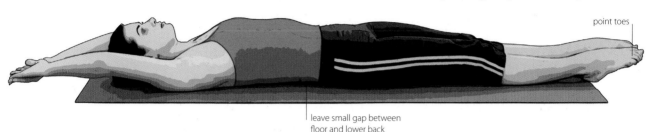

point toes

leave small gap between floor and lower back

2 As you inhale, sweep your arms from above your head to by your sides, forming the shape of "angel wings" as you do so. At the same time, lift your legs off the floor so that your knees are bent at approximate right angles. As you exhale, lift your head and shoulders off the floor, rest your gaze between your knees, and lift your arms slightly off the floor.

pull belly button toward spine

leave enough space for an imaginary orange between chin and chest

3 As you inhale, draw your feet in toward your buttocks. As you exhale, reach forward with your hands to take hold of your heels, curling your body into as much of a little ball as possible. Hold for several breaths, then unfurl your body and lengthen your legs and arms down to the floor again as you inhale. Repeat all steps 8 times. On the last repeat, hold Step 3 more intensely before relaxing into the floor.

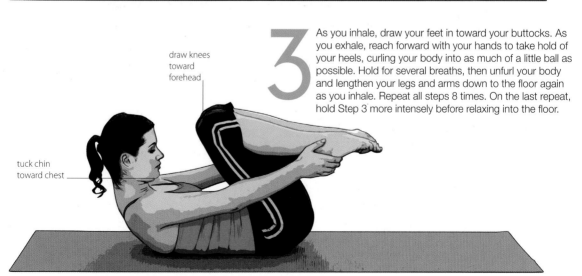

draw knees toward forehead

tuck chin toward chest

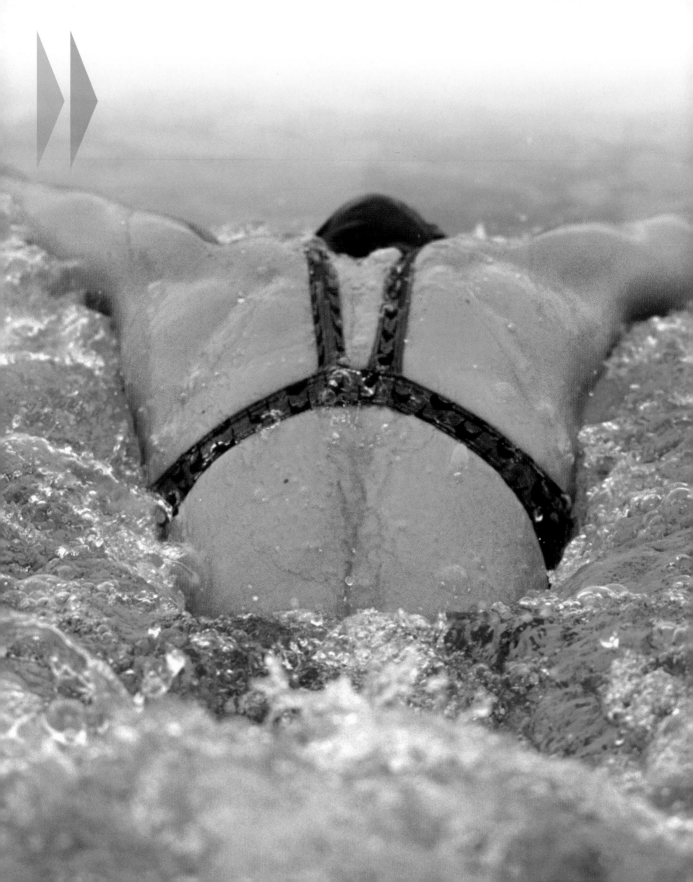

Swimming

Swimming is a wonderfully relaxing, non-weight-bearing way to burn fat, which makes it suitable for people of all ages and sizes who want to get fitter, lose weight, and improve their body shape. The pages that follow will guide you on how to get the most from swimming but, whether you do a gentle 20-minute breaststroke and backstroke session or an intense one-hour front crawl and butterfly blast, it will:

- boost your cardio fitness without risk of bone or joint injury

- help you to lose weight with its substantial calorie-burning potential

- maximize your all-around mobility and flexibility

- tone up your entire body due to the water acting as a means of gentle resistance

- improve your core strength as you work your stomach muscles to stay afloat

- encourage deep, rhythmical breathing

- create a sense of fluidity and lightness within both your body and your mind

- encourage you to relax and unwind

The fundamentals of swimming

Potentially as relaxing as it is invigorating, swimming is a fantastic way to boost your cardiovascular fitness, flexibility, and core strength, as well as rebalance your nervous system, without putting unnecessary strain on your bones and joints. Like any form of exercise, you can do it at whatever intensity best suits you, and if you vary your strokes, you'll work virtually every muscle in your body.

Getting started

Swimming requires a minimum amount of equipment, but you do need somewhere to swim of course. When starting out, swimming in a pool is the best option as conditions are controlled and the water is still. As you become more confident, you may want to explore open-water swimming, always bearing safety in mind.

What to wear

It's important to choose a bathing suit that you like the look of, that fits you well, and that gives your bust adequate support so that you feel comfortable and confident when you go swimming. There are endless options so find one that best suits you (and that won't become see-through when you get in the water!). Here's some guidance on styles:

Submerging your head in water while swimming means that you'll need to learn to breathe efficiently.

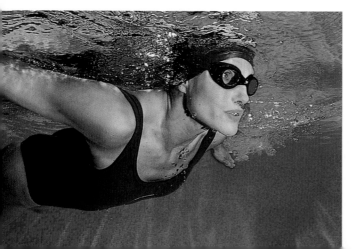

- high neck—good if you're quite flat chested
- v-neck—good if your cleavage is one of your best features and you want to draw attention from elsewhere
- halterneck—good for giving the impression of wider shoulders and a narrower waist
- racer back—good for optimal shoulder and arm movement
- wrap-over—good to accentuate a slim waist
- ruched mid-section—good to hide excess weight around the midriff
- high-leg cut—good if you have toned legs or you want to lengthen the look of your legs
- low-cut bottom (more like shorts)—good if you want increased leg coverage
- separates—particularly good if you're top- or bottom-heavy, since you can sometimes buy a different size top and bottom. For extra coverage, choose a tankini, which has a tank top (rather than bikini top) and the option of tight shorts (rather than briefs) as the bottom half.

Optional equipment

Goggles Wearing goggles prevents eye irritation from chemicals in pools. To test the fit, push the goggles on your face without doing the strap up: suction should be instant but not too tight. You can buy over-the-counter prescription goggles or have lenses made following your own prescription.

Bathing cap Wearing a cap keeps your hair out of your eyes and can make you more streamlined and

Optional equipment

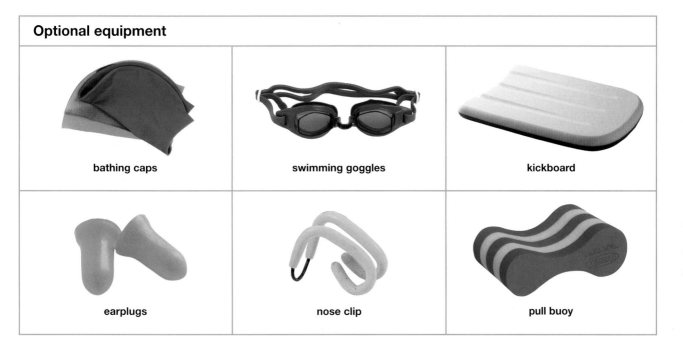

bathing caps	swimming goggles	kickboard
earplugs	nose clip	pull buoy

therefore marginally faster. Latex and silicone caps are the most commonly available. You may prefer a Lycra cap if you have long hair that gets tangled in a tight plastic cap, although your hair will get wet.

Earplugs Swimming earplugs keep water out of your ears and help to prevent ear infections, something that frequent swimmers can be prone to.

Nose clip If you find it difficult to keep water out of your nose, you might want to try using a nose clip.

Swimming aids Pull buoys and kickboards are useful for warming up. A pull buoy is held between the thighs and helps you concentrate on your upper body, while holding onto a kickboard allows you to work just your legs. Paddles, held in your hands, add resistance to build arm strength and also teach you to avoid relying on your hands to pull you through the water.

Lap timer A lap counter is a great way to keep count of the number of laps you've swum and how fast.

Music player A waterproof MP3 player, clipped to your goggle strap or shoulder strap, is a great way to combat the potential boredom of swimming laps in a pool.

Effective breathing

Breathing is something that we rarely think about in our everyday lives, but once we submerge our heads in the water to swim, we need to be ultra-conscious of how to breathe efficiently.

The big fear for most new or non-swimmers is that they will breathe in while under water, causing water to go up their nose. A good way to overcome this fear is to acclimatize yourself by dipping your face into a large bowl of water at home. At first, you might only be able to dip your face in and straight out, but gradually work up to keeping it there for longer—blowing bubbles in the water as you exhale and lifting your head to inhale.

Once you feel confident enough about submerging your head in a small amount of water, try it in the pool or ocean. When you first start swimming, let your need to inhale dictate when you bring your head out of the water and therefore the speed and rhythm of your stroke. See pp.86–87 for more on breathing technique. However, the best way to learn really good breathing technique for each stroke is to take swimming lessons.

How to swim well

Being able to swim a variety of strokes will give you more options when it comes to your workouts, which will help you maintain your interest and motivation. It will also maximize the number of muscles that you target and tone, and allow you to vary the intensity of your workout. However, each stroke requires its own particular technical knowledge. Below is a guide to the essentials.

Breaststroke

Symmetry is key to the the arm and leg movements of the breaststroke. Push your legs straight out behind you, toes pointed, then move each foot in an outward semi-circle ending at your buttocks, ready to push them backward again. At the same time, stretch your arms straight out in front of you, just under the water, then press your hands away from each other, drawing a semi-circle on each side and ending up with them in front of your shoulders, in readiness to stretch forward again.

• Breathe in as you finish each complete circle, lifting your face out of the water to do so
• Keep your shoulders and hips square

Breaststroke works your chest and triceps as you stretch forward and targets your back and biceps as you draw back; your shoulders work throughout. Your abs work hard to keep you horizontal in the water, and your legs get an effective workout, too.

Front crawl

Strong, alternate arm movement is the major force in propelling you forward during this stroke. With elbows bent, reach one arm over the top and put your hand into the water in front of your head, thumb first—the less splash the better. Stretch it forward as far as you can, slicing it through the water, and push it down toward your thigh before you lift your other arm in the same way to start again. At the same time, kick alternate legs up and down.

• Visualize trying to swim through a narrow tube without touching the sides
• Breathe on both sides, turning your head smoothly, with the side of your head resting on the water

Front crawl works lots of muscles at once. It's great for both your tummy and bottom since your abs and glutes have to work incredibly hard to keep you horizontal and moving in a straight, streamlined way. It's also useful for toning your waist as you twist to breathe.

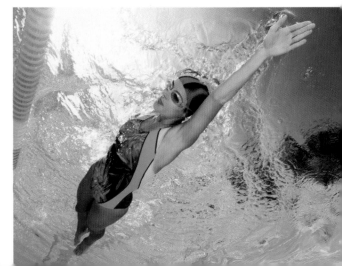

Things to avoid

- Don't be scared of putting your head under water.
- Don't let your legs relax or you'll start to sink.
- Don't let your back sag or you'll lose healthy spinal alignment and good form.
- Don't let your head come completely out of the water or your hips will drop and knock you out of alignment.

- Don't lock your legs when you straighten them out as you kick.
- Don't let your breathing interrupt your leg and arm action; instead move in rhythm with your breath.
- Avoid rough water when swimming in the ocean— it will waste your energy and could be dangerous!

Backstroke

Lying on your back as close to the surface as you can, start by putting one arm in the water straight above your shoulder, with your other arm down by your side. Slightly bend the elbow of your back arm and pull your hand below the water toward your feet until your elbow is straight, then lift it out of the water, back to its original position and repeat. Your left arm should come out of the water at about the same time as your right arm enters it. Kick your legs from the hips as you move your arms.

- Keep your chest and pelvis lifted, and your abs contracted to stay horizontal in the water
- Keep your legs together as you kick them alternately

Backstroke gives you a full-body stretch as you reach behind you. It's great for your upper body, really working your shoulders, arms, chest, and back. The kick tones your legs and bottom, elongates your hip flexors, and is fantastic for burning calories.

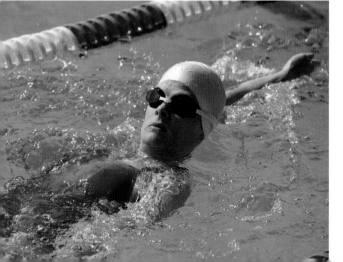

Butterfly

This involves kicking your legs together in a "mermaid tail" motion while moving your arms in large circles. Start with your arms straight, slightly behind your thighs, circle them backward, up out of the water, then forward to enter the water in front of your shoulders, and back to the start position. Keep your head in the water all the time, except when you push your chin forward so that your mouth comes out of the water to breathe in, which is best done when your arms are almost at your thighs.

- Kick your legs down as your hands go in and up as your hands come out
- Keep your head down as your arms go over the water

Butterfly is the most challenging swimming stroke for most people and is a real stamina-builder and calorie-burner. It works all the muscles in your chest, shoulders, and arms as you lift yourself out of the water each time. It's also great for spine flexibility.

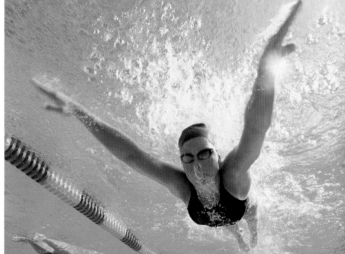

Getting the most from your swimming

To get the most from your swimming, consider all your options. Of course, you can do laps in your local pool, but you might also have a chance for open-water swimming now and then. And do you want to vary your strokes? For a holistic approach, try all of these things when possible. It can also be useful to do some swimming-specific exercises (see the guidance right).

Where to swim?

Swimming pools can be either indoors or outdoors. In a pool, the water is still, conditions are controlled, and you have the comfort factor of being able to see the bottom. It's also easy to swim in a straight line and quantify your progress by counting your laps. Most local pools will be "short course" (82ft/25m) but some are Olympic size (164ft/50m). The downside of public pools is chlorine. If you don't use chlorine-removing shampoo, swimming regularly in this type of water can make your hair very dry. These chemicals are a necessity to keep water sanitized, but wearing a waterproof bathing cap can reduce the damage.

Open-water swimming is also increasingly popular, with organized sessions held at lakes and shores across

the country. Considerations before doing this are temperature, difficulty level depending on choppiness of the water, and, of course, safety. If the water is below 57°F (14°C) you may need to wear a wetsuit to make the swim comfortable. To stay safe it's best to swim where other people are swimming, too. Or if you're on a beach, keep an eye on the lifeguard stands. Never go swimming in the ocean on your own without telling someone. Swimming in the ocean is very different than swimming in a pool so you'll need to use different techniques, most notably lifting your head a little higher so you can see where you're going, and breathing above the waves.

Mixing it up

To get the best possible workout from your swimming sessions, it's best to vary not only the strokes that you use, but also the speed at which you do them.

People often just swim up and down the pool, counting the laps. While this is great and it's rewarding to achieve more laps each week, in order to get fitter it's advisable to add sprints to your endurance work. In addition, if you just do more and more laps, you can get tired and let bad habits slip in. Doing shorter sessions at least once or twice a week with specific goals, either to work on speed or technique, can keep your approach fresh and your motivation up. Four to ten swim sprints of 10–20 seconds, with 40–60 seconds of rest between each one, will increase strength and power, and, like any interval training, will boost your fitness levels.

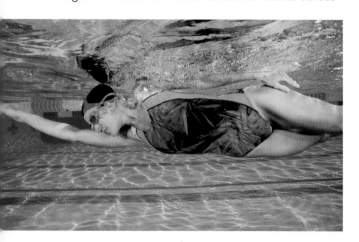

When swimming in a pool it's much easier to swim laps and use the strokes that you want if there are not too many other people around, so schedule your swims at quiet times, if possible.

Total Body Strengthener

This dynamic exercise will strengthen your back and ab muscles, which help to keep you afloat when in the water. The arm and leg work will enhance your capacity for propulsion through the water.

Lie on your tummy, with your arms slightly bent by the sides of your head and your legs stretched out behind you, wider than hip-width apart. Inhale to prepare. As you exhale, lift your head, shoulders, arms, and legs off the floor. Keeping your torso still, kick your legs in small, fast, alternate, up-down movements and move your hands alternately up and down as if splashing in a pool. Do this to a count of 30, breathing in and out rhythmically. Then relax.

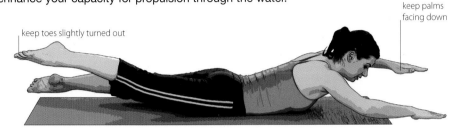

keep toes slightly turned out

keep palms facing down

Twisting Bicycle

This exercise targets your back, stomach, waist, and butt muscles, which will help your torso to rotate with control in the front crawl as your legs kick and your arms pull.

Lie on your back, knees bent and legs off the floor. As you inhale, lift your head and shoulders off the floor. As you exhale, bring one knee toward your chest, twist the opposite shoulder and elbow toward that knee, and extend your other leg out above the floor. Inhale back to center, and repeat on the other side. Do 8–16 in total—4–8 times on each side.

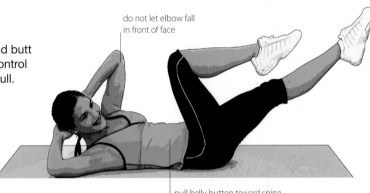

do not let elbow fall in front of face

pull belly button toward spine

Pull-over

This exercise will enhance your breaststroke and butterfly by strengthening not only your shoulders and arms, but also your back and chest—muscles that will help to boost your propulsion power.

1 Lie on your back, with your knees bent at 90°, your feet hip-width apart on the floor, facing forward, and your belly button pulled toward your spine. As you inhale, extend your arms above your head, with a weight in each hand, palms facing in.

keep arms straight but not locked

leave small gap between lower back and floor

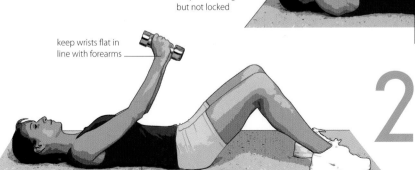

keep wrists flat in line with forearms

2 As you exhale, bring your arms up and over your chest to just above your waistline, still keeping them shoulder-width apart. Hold here for 5 seconds, then inhale as you lower the weights slowly overhead again. Keep the movements smooth and fluid. Do this forward-backward movement 10 times in total.

do not over-arch back

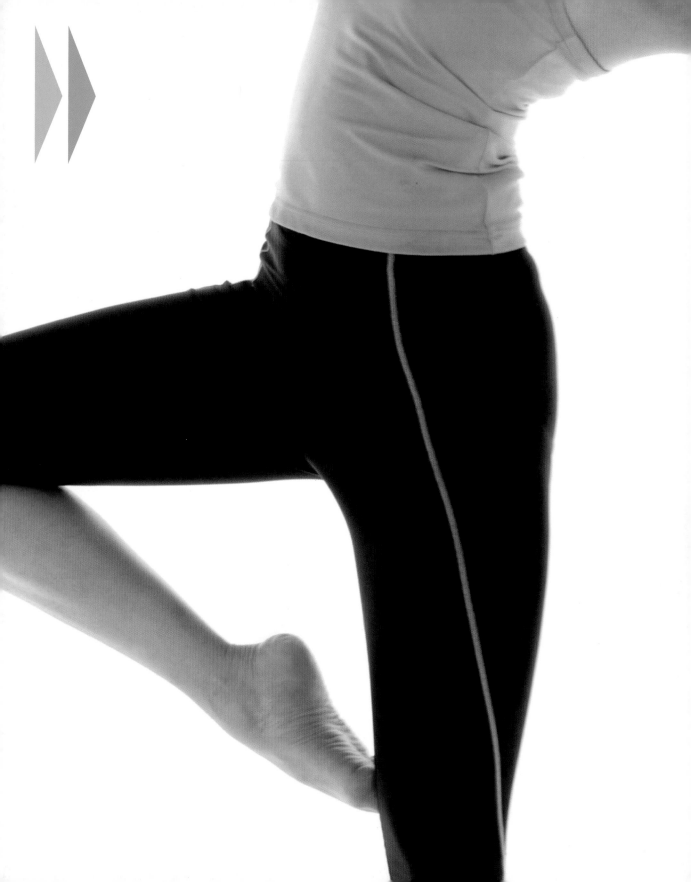

Aerobics and dance

For many people, dancing is the ultimate feel-good workout. Even better, it often doesn't feel like exercise since you're so busy focusing on the choreography. Psychologists have also shown that working out to music can help you to disassociate from the effort of cardio exercise and therefore perform more effectively. The pages that follow will help you to get the most from aerobics and dance, which will mean you can:

- boost your cardiovascular fitness

- burn off unwanted layers of fat

- sculpt your body from top to bottom

- stretch and strengthen your muscles, enhancing both flexibility and endurance

- promote the flexibility of your spine, hips, and other joints

- enhance your awareness of good posture and alignment

- improve your sense of coordination and rhythm

- increase energy levels and promote a feeling of overall well-being

The fundamentals of aerobics and dance

If listening to music makes your toes tap, aerobics or dancing could be a great way for you to lose weight and get in better shape since they both involve moving your body in time to music, which gets your heart pumping and the muscles throughout your body working. The moves don't have to be complicated, which means that you can do them either at home or as part of a class.

Getting started

Your preferred choice of aerobics or dance (see right for some examples) will depend on the type of music and movement that you most enjoy, as well as on the type of workout that you want. But whatever style you choose, the buzz you get will be similar and the fitness results can be fantastic, as long as you work yourself hard enough. One of the best things about aerobics and dance for many people is that due to the need to focus on getting the choreography right, you often don't notice just how hard you're working on your fitness.

What to wear

As with all cardio exercise, it's important to wear comfortable clothes—preferably in breathable materials—so that your body can move freely and with ease, at a comfortable temperature. Stretchy, form-fitting clothes are particularly useful for any studio-based sessions since they will allow you to see your body alignment more easily if there's a full-length mirror.

However, what you wear is likely to vary a lot depending on the type of aerobics or dance you do—each type has its own style and requirements, and many have different shoe needs in particular: for aerobics, whether normal or step, it's best to wear cross-trainers with strong ankle support, while for many other forms of dance, such as ballet, jazz, tap, Latin-American, and ballroom, specialist shoes are needed. However, if you're just starting something like ballet or jazz, you could do it

barefoot, and if you're just starting ballroom or Latin-American dance, you could opt for leather-soled shoes that will move with ease but stay on your feet as you lift and lower them. A sports bra is recommended for aerobics, but a normal bra may be adequate for many other forms of dance, depending on the intensity at which you're doing them.

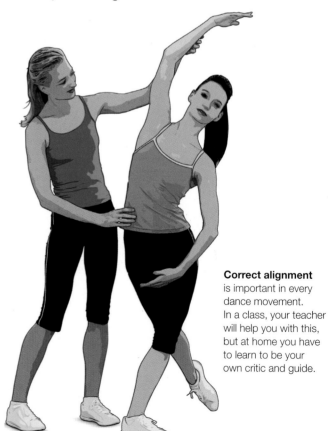

Correct alignment is important in every dance movement. In a class, your teacher will help you with this, but at home you have to learn to be your own critic and guide.

Different types

There's a wide range of options when it comes to types of aerobics and dance to choose from. Your local YMCA, gym, and independent teachers may offer a range of aerobics classes:

- standard aerobics—a choreographed aerobic workout developed with the aim of using both low- and high-impact movements to music to develop all aspects of fitness within one session: cardio, strength, and flexibility
- step aerobics—an aerobics workout as above but done while moving on and off an elevated platform, which boosts the intensity of the lower body workout and therefore increases the cardio blast
- aqua aerobics—a more gentle form of aerobics workout, done in a pool, using the water as resistance

Most classes, and any variations of them such as dance aerobics, tend to involve doing movements in sets of 4, 8, 16, or 32, in keeping with the music (see also p.95). A popular form of dance aerobics at the moment is the exhilarating Latin-inspired fitness craze Zumba®, the 2001 brainchild of Colombian fitness instructor Beto Perez. This uses four basic Latin rhythms—merengue, salsa, cumbia, and reggaeton— as its basis, is high energy and a lot of fun, and has recently taken the fitness industry by storm.

As well as these fitness-based dances there are, of course, many other forms of more "pure" dance to choose from, whether ballet, ballroom (think waltz, tango, quickstep, foxtrot, and the like), Bollywood, disco, Flamenco, jazz, Latin-American (think cha cha, jive, rumba, salsa, and the like), pole dancing, swing, or tap. A lot of these styles of dance are now offered at YMCAs and clubs throughout the country as a way of getting fitter and in better shape as well as of learning a new skill and potentially meeting new, like-minded people. Simply research and try any of them that you like the idea of and see which ones feel right for you—in terms of both music and movement style.

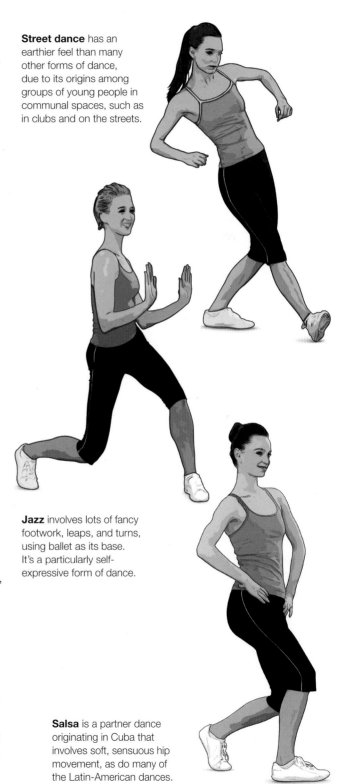

Street dance has an earthier feel than many other forms of dance, due to its origins among groups of young people in communal spaces, such as in clubs and on the streets.

Jazz involves lots of fancy footwork, leaps, and turns, using ballet as its base. It's a particularly self-expressive form of dance.

Salsa is a partner dance originating in Cuba that involves soft, sensuous hip movement, as do many of the Latin-American dances.

How to move well

Different styles of aerobics and dance require different techniques—that's what makes them all distinct from one another. However, there are certain underlying principles that apply to almost all styles—namely, learning the moves, moving in time with the music, healthy posture, balanced alignment, controlled movements, good breathing, and a sense of flow between movements.

Learning the key moves

Although the movements of professional dancers can flow so well that they seem almost unstructured, every style of dance has its own set of key moves that are used as a basis for everything else. For example, ballet has pliés (squats with turned-out feet and legs), pirouettes (spins on one leg), and rond de jambes (leg circles) among many others; aerobics has step touches, knee lifts, and heel digs; and cha cha has New Yorkers (where you step through to the side and raise one arm), Cuban breaks (where you repeatedly step diagonally back and forwards on the same foot), and hip twists (where you twist the hips and step back).

As you become more familiar with the wide range of key moves from your chosen style of dance, whether during local classes or from books, DVDs, or the Internet, it will gradually become easier for you to follow choreography in a more flowing way and also to put together your own routines at home from your favorite moves, if so desired.

It's worth bearing in mind that some teachers' choreography consists of a combination of moves that can be done to any music, as long as it's of a suitable tempo. However, other teachers create routines that are specific to individual pieces of music so that each song they play has a particular combination of moves to fit with the rhythm, feel, and sometimes lyrics of both the verses and the chorus. The former is convenient in that you can do the moves in any order you like to any music you like, but the latter is fun, too, since you can use changes in the music as memory triggers for certain moves. At first, it can be difficult to remember which moves come when but, with regular practice, it will soon become like second nature, since any good choreography should flow fairly naturally from one move to the next. It's only once you're really comfortable with all the moves in a routine that you'll be able to build up a sense of energy and momentum while doing it to get the most satisfaction and the best workout possible.

In partner dancing, it's up to the man to lead the woman, but the woman can only successfully take the lead if she is familiar with the move that he wants to maneuver her into and also if he is giving a strong enough lead-in.

Treat every dance move you do as a kind of performance, even if no one is watching. This means presenting yourself in the best way possible—smiling and with fantastic posture.

Engage the whole body with every move you make, from the tips of your toes and fingers to the top of your head, so that everything looks strong and purposeful.

Counting the beat

Most forms of dance are performed in time to music. Knowing the rhythm of the music to which you're dancing is therefore essential. Most aerobics workouts are based around music with eight-beat phrases—try listening to a few of your favorite songs to see if you can hear these musical phrases. Aerobics teachers therefore tend to design their routines to include sets of 4, 8, 16, or 32 of each move.

Other forms of dance use different types of music, so they will have different rhythms. For each one you therefore need to establish the rhythm at the outset. For example, a waltz works in phrases of three (1-2-3), while a cha cha works both on the beats and between them, known as off-beat (2-3-4-and-1—the "and" being the offbeat). Once you know the rhythm, it can be useful to practice just counting out the music before you start trying to dance to it.

Once you're more comfortable with it, it's important to anticipate the beat for each movement in order to be on time. This can seem tricky at first, but will become easier the more familiar you are with both the required rhythm and the key moves of that style of dance.

Good posture, alignment, and breathing

Good posture (see p.32) is essential during all aerobics and dance sessions because it improves the body's sense of balance and control, as well as making you look more confident and elegant. So no matter what you're doing, always try to lengthen out through your neck and the top of your head and open your chest, unless otherwise specified. Also, aim for balance between both sides of the body and be sure to breathe as deeply and evenly as you can, in harmony with your movements. Good breathing (see p.33) will maximize your sense of ease, flow, and enjoyment.

Seeing every move through to the end

To make any aerobics or dance routine look as smooth, effortless, and polished as possible, as well as to give you the optimum workout, aim to stay aware of your whole body during every movement, even if you are mainly targeting one particular body area in a given position. Your core muscles (see p.199) should be engaged at all times and nothing should be "loose" or limp, yet you should look relaxed and at ease.

Things to avoid

- Don't panic if you're having difficulty getting a move right—do your feet and legs first, then add the arm and hand movements later.
- Don't over-arch your back—pull your abs in and lengthen your tailbone down toward the floor so that your pelvis tucks under slightly, leaving just a small natural curve in your back.
- Don't lock your knees since this can cause hyperextension, and jumping on locked joints can cause injury.
- Don't let your knees bend beyond your toes because it puts unnecessary pressure on your knees.
- Don't land too heavily when you jump—try to land on your toes and roll through your feet.
- Don't forget to breathe—sometimes we can be so busy trying to get movements and alignment right that it's easy to forget the obvious; instead, keep breathing as deeply and smoothly as you can.

Getting the most from aerobics

To get the most from any dancing you do, it's important to consider what best suits your likes and needs—a local class or a home routine, partner or solo dancing, fairly simple or much more complex choreography? In the meantime, the exercises here will help to boost your capacity for hip movement and twisting throughout your body, which will be useful in many forms of dance.

Choosing where to dance

When it comes to discovering local classes, ask friends, watch out for flyers, and have a look on the Internet to see what classes you can find that both appeal to you and suit your schedule, whether at the local YMCA, gyms, dance studios, or other venues. Then try them out to see if they give you what you're looking for.

The advantage of going to a class is that you're given continuous, face-to-face guidance by an expert, which means that you can see the moves being done in front of you. You can therefore copy them more easily and get a better sense of how they flow into one other. You're also likely to be more motivated, energized, and push yourself harder when surrounded by other people doing the same activity.

However, if you'd prefer to do your aerobics or dancing in the privacy of your own home, you can follow the basic taster workouts in this book (see p.268–69) as well as any aerobics programs you like on DVDs or the Internet. Alternatively, you may find it useful to attend local classes to get you off your starting block and then supplement with your own moves at home, too.

Altering intensity

Different classes will encourage participants to aim toward different intensity levels but it's important to work at your own level within this: you should never experience extreme discomfort or pain. The main ways to increase intensity are to increase range of movement (e.g., deeper bends and longer reaches), increase the number of body parts being worked (e.g., add arm as well as leg movements), increase speed (e.g. music with a range of 120–140 beats per minute is gentle, while 160 bpm is more challenging), and change any stepping to jumping. To decrease intensity you can therefore simply do the opposite when required.

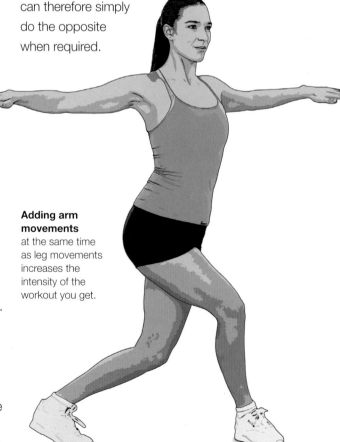

Adding arm movements at the same time as leg movements increases the intensity of the workout you get.

Salsa Swing

Practicing this salsa move will get your hips moving through a wide range of motion, so that you learn to move your lower body in isolation from your upper body. It will also tone your hips and upper legs.

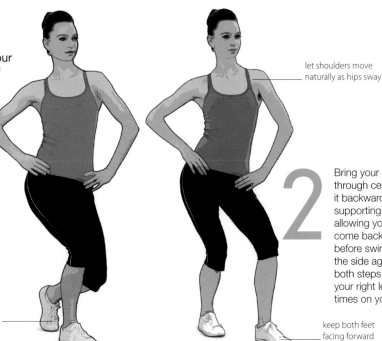

let shoulders move naturally as hips sway

1 Stand with your feet hip-width apart and your hands on your hips. Take a small step forward with your right foot, lifting the heel of your back foot off the floor. Keep both legs slightly bent and let your right hip swing out to the right side.

come up onto ball of back foot

2 Bring your right foot back through center and step it backward, keeping your supporting leg bent and allowing your right hip to come back to neutral before swinging out to the side again. Repeat both steps 8 times on your right leg, then 8 times on your left leg.

keep both feet facing forward

Twist and Shift

This twisting move will promote mobility throughout your body, which will help with a wide range of dance moves. It will also give your waist a great workout.

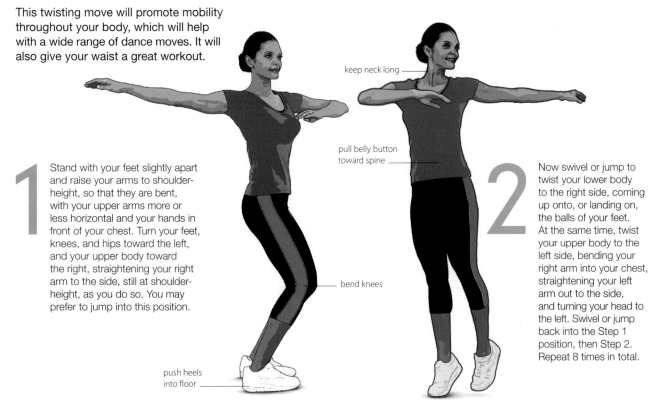

keep neck long

pull belly button toward spine

1 Stand with your feet slightly apart and raise your arms to shoulder-height, so that they are bent, with your upper arms more or less horizontal and your hands in front of your chest. Turn your feet, knees, and hips toward the left, and your upper body toward the right, straightening your right arm to the side, still at shoulder-height, as you do so. You may prefer to jump into this position.

bend knees

push heels into floor

2 Now swivel or jump to twist your lower body to the right side, coming up onto, or landing on, the balls of your feet. At the same time, twist your upper body to the left side, bending your right arm into your chest, straightening your left arm out to the side, and turning your head to the left. Swivel or jump back into the Step 1 position, then Step 2. Repeat 8 times in total.

Sculpting

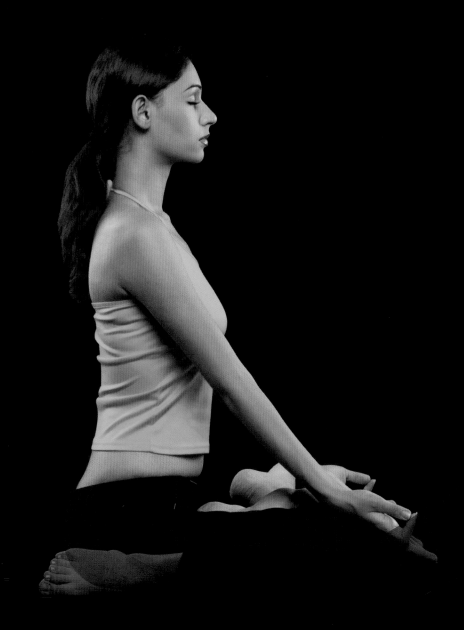

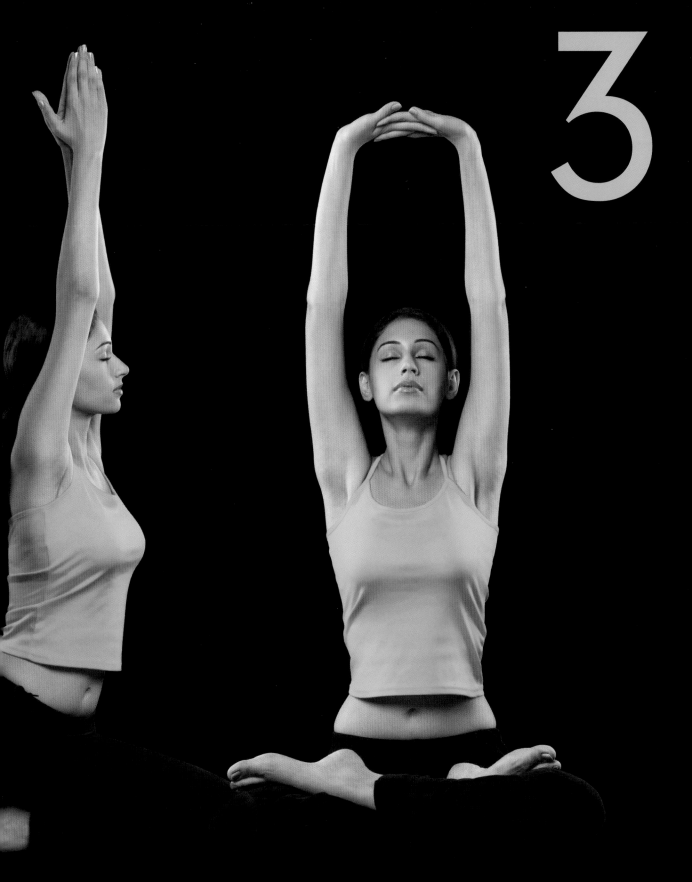

Introduction to sculpting

In simple terms, "sculpting" is exercising with a view to getting your body in better shape—in the same way that a sculptor lovingly chisels at his raw material until he transforms it into the masterpiece that he always knew it could be. So read on to discover how to become your very own fitness sculptor.

The benefits of sculpting

There's no denying that body-sculpting exercises can work wonders to firm up specific body parts, add definition where there was wobble before, and enhance your overall body shape. However, it's by no means all about physical appearance. Sculpting will also:

- strengthen your muscles, making you fitter
- enhance your stamina, giving you more staying power—both physically and mentally
- improve your mobility and flexibility
- boost your metabolism, which will help you to control your weight, as increased lean muscle mass means increased calorie-burning power
- increase your energy levels
- raise your self-confidence.

While you might start a sculpting program to improve your shape, all the above additional benefits will hopefully be motivators for you to keep at it! You should do at least three 10–30-minute sculpting workouts a week (with rest days in between) to start seeing results within four weeks. Sculpting is not, however, a substitute for a healthy diet (see pp.48–51) or regular cardio activity (see pp.52–97). A balance between all three is needed for optimal fitness benefits.

Choosing your sculpting tools

Just as any good sculptor makes sure he knows and has the right tools to create his envisioned sculpture, you too must have an understanding of the exercises that will get

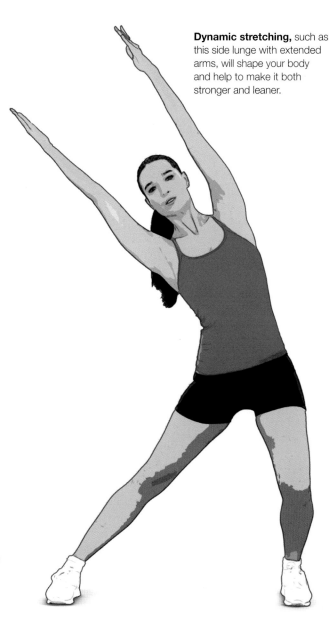

Dynamic stretching, such as this side lunge with extended arms, will shape your body and help to make it both stronger and leaner.

you the results you want. The information in the pages that follow will help with this. Detailed guidance is given on a wide range of exercises that have been selected for their sculpting capacity from four different disciplines—resistance training, stretching, Pilates, and yoga. Each of these disciplines offers particular benefits:

Resistance training (see pp.102–53) will build your strength and endurance, and make your skeletal muscle leaner, thus enhancing your body shape. For some of them, you may need equipment, such as hand weights or an exercise ball, to add resistance and therefore increase the difficulty level.

Stretching (see pp.154–93) encourages length and flexibility through your muscles, which will not only enhance your overall posture and mobility and help with toning, but will also reduce the chance of any injury during other forms of exercise.

Pilates (see pp.194–219) will work on your strength and flexibility but is particularly geared toward improving your core strength (mainly in your abs), with the aim of enhancing your overall posture and quality of movement.

Yoga (see pp.220–47) will build both strength and flexibility, not only of your body, but also your mind. It will encourage qualities such as groundedness, lightness, focus, and balance, too.

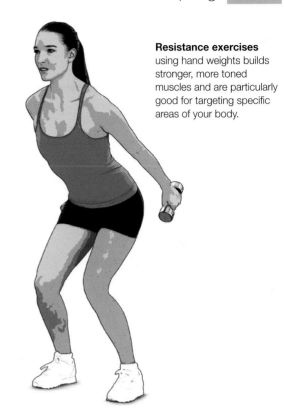

Resistance exercises using hand weights builds stronger, more toned muscles and are particularly good for targeting specific areas of your body.

Explore these sections of the book at your leisure so that when you do the suggested combinations of exercises in the sculpting and quick-fix workouts (see pp.270–327), you'll feel comfortable and understand why you're doing them. For each type of exercise, you will first learn the principles and techniques, and then be presented with clear, step-by-step exercise pages. The exercises are grouped according to the main body zones and muscle groups that they target—working from the top to the bottom of the body each time for easy reference. Happy reading…

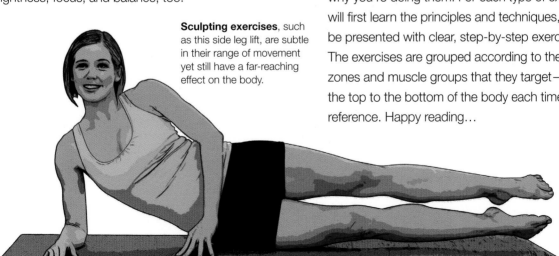

Sculpting exercises, such as this side leg lift, are subtle in their range of movement yet still have a far-reaching effect on the body.

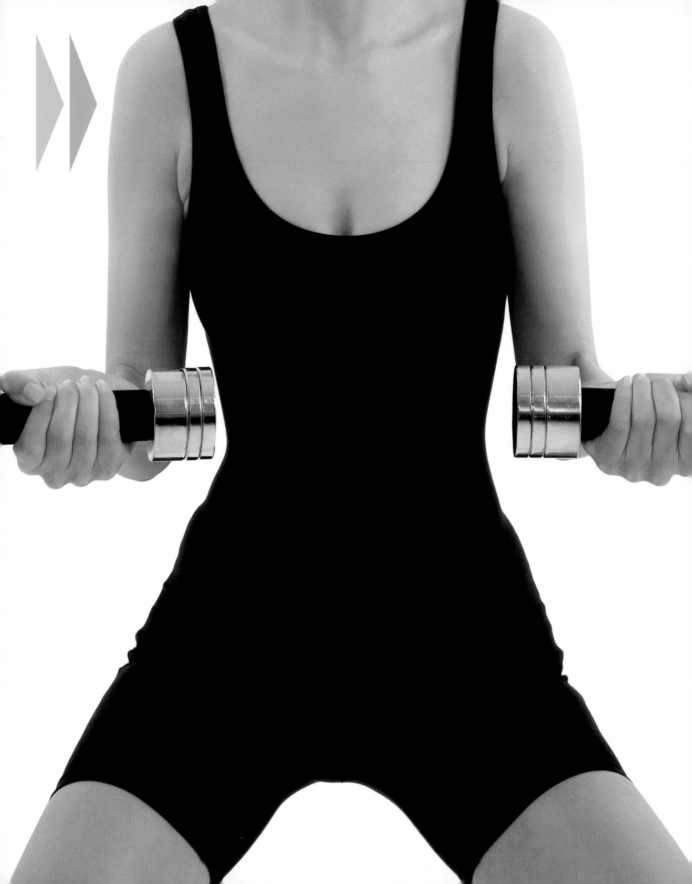

Resistance training

Resistance exercise involves working your muscles against an external resistance—whether your own body weight or fitness accessories such as hand weights or an exercise ball. Exercising in this way will define your muscles, increase your strength, and get you in all-around better shape. Don't worry—it's about firming up, not bulking up, so read on to discover a wide range of easy-to-achieve exercises that will:

- tone and shape your body so you look and feel your best

- enhance your body confidence and self-esteem

- increase your strength and stamina for everyday activities

- raise your metabolic rate, helping you to manage your weight

- improve your balance and coordination

- slow down the physical signs of aging by maintaining optimal muscular strength

- strengthen your bones to lessen the chance of osteoporosis in later life

- reduce the risk of muscular injury during physical activity

Resistance training: why and how?

Resistance, or strength, training—whether with your own body weight, hand weights, an exercise ball, a resistance band, or other fitness equipment—really is the secret weapon when it comes to sculpting your body. Regular practice of resistance exercises, such as the ones in the pages that follow, will make you stronger and fitter, as well as putting you on a path to a more toned body.

How does it work?

Exercising your muscles to their maximum capacity with some form of resistance creates harmless microscopic tears in the cells of your muscle fibers—a breakdown process called "catabolism." Amazingly, this muscle tissue then repairs itself within 48 hours—a regrowth process called "anabolism," which reforms the muscles even stronger than before. As a result, regular resistance exercise can have a wide range of benefits.

Increase your strength and stamina

Skeletal muscles consist of two different types of fiber:
• fast-twitch for bursts of power—the amount of force you can withstand in one effort
• slow-twitch for prolonged endurance—the length of time for which you can sustain a muscular contraction before you get tired.

   Because resistance exercises encourage both types of muscle fiber to break down and redevelop, an effective resistance workout will increase both your strength and your stamina, enhancing your ability to carry out all kinds of daily tasks, whether lifting heavy objects, carrying the groceries, mowing the lawn, or playing with your children.

   Resistance exercise becomes all the more important after the age of 30 when muscle mass otherwise starts to decrease (see also p.30).

Enhance your muscle tone

The good news is that getting stronger doesn't mean getting bulkier. Working your muscles via moderate resistance training builds what is known as "lean" muscle mass—giving a firmer, more chiseled musculature.

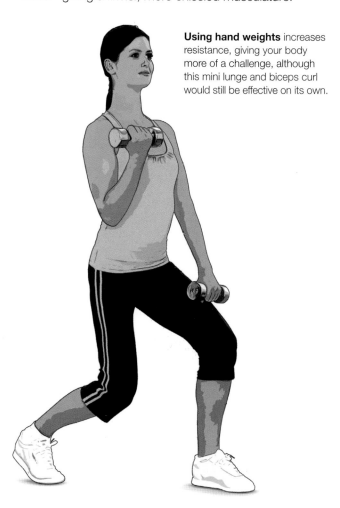

Using hand weights increases resistance, giving your body more of a challenge, although this mini lunge and biceps curl would still be effective on its own.

You'll only be able to see your newly defined abs, toned arms, or shapely legs once you shed any excess body fat via a healthy diet and adequate cardio exercise, so get going on your cardio and sculpting workouts to take your first step toward your dream body.

Raise your metabolic rate

Effective resistance training has been shown to burn calories after your workout as well as during it, and can therefore help with weight loss. It even burns calories as you sleep, since a lean body burns more calories at rest than a fatty one. This is because the muscle fibers within lean, toned muscles are more active than those in flabby, underused ones.

Build your bone strength

As well as building muscle mass, resistance training builds bone mass, which is crucial in enabling your skeletal system to support you adequately. This is particularly important the older you get, since bone mass naturally starts to decline after the age of 30, which can eventually lead to bone disorders, such as osteoporosis.

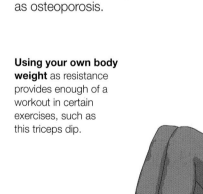

Using your own body weight as resistance provides enough of a workout in certain exercises, such as this triceps dip.

Top tips for resistance training

• Choose the most appropriate exercises for you, basing your choices on the body areas that you particularly want to tone and strengthen.
• Aim to do three sculpting workouts (see pp.270–311) a week on alternate days. Whichever of the workouts you choose, it will include a healthy dose of the resistance exercises from the pages that follow.
• Leave a rest day between resistance training sessions. This gives your body the time it needs to repair itself—it is during these vital rest periods, rather than during the workouts themselves, that your muscles get stronger.
• Move slowly and with control. Not only will this prevent injuries, but it will also give you a more effective and rewarding workout.
• Work at your own level. Never push yourself to the point of pain or discomfort and never sacrifice good technique in order to do more repetitions or sets (the number of times you do the repetitions), or to lift more weight.
• Challenge yourself to the max. You'll only see results when you apply the overload principle (see p.17). So, as soon as a certain number of reps and sets, or a certain amount of weight, starts to feel in any way easy, take your workout up a level.
• Use your breath to enhance your workout: exhale with the movement of maximal effort and inhale on the return movement.
• Respect your body's changing needs. It's natural that you'll feel less strong on some days, so don't get discouraged when this happens. Just adapt the level of your workout—whether by reducing your session time, doing fewer reps or sets, or using less resistance.

Note: No rep or set recommendations are given within the resistance training exercises that follow—only guidance on how to correctly perform each exercise. Three levels of rep and set guidance is then given for each resistance exercise within the sculpting and quick-fix workouts (see pp. 270–327): gentle, moderate, and intense.

Basic equipment

It's important to know how to use the main forms of resistance equipment in order to get the most from the exercises in the pages that follow. Hand weights, an exercise ball, a resistance band, or your own body weight can all be used as resistance and each involves its own set of considerations. Consult a medical expert before you try them if you have a history of bone or joint problems.

Your own body weight

Push-ups, sit-ups, triceps dips, and lunges are just some of the exercises in the pages that follow that involve using your own body weight as a means of resistance. The advantage of these types of exercises

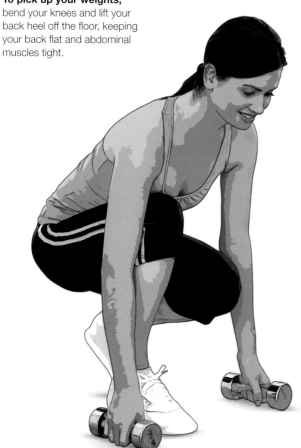

To pick up your weights, bend your knees and lift your back heel off the floor, keeping your back flat and abdominal muscles tight.

is that they can be done almost anywhere, and the amount of resistance can be altered according to your needs simply by changing your body position or lessening the range of movement, depending on the exercise. Then, when you want more of a challenge, you can progress to using one of the other forms of resistance.

Hand weights

Hand weights are an extremely effective way of adding resistance to movements that otherwise might not be particularly challenging. The fact that you can use one weight in each hand also allows you to identify, and address, any strength imbalances in your body.

Start exercising with very light weights to see how they feel. As and when they stop challenging you, progress to slightly heavier ones—even if only for certain exercises at first:

Very light = 1lb (0.5kg) each

Light = 2–3lb (1kg) each

Normal = 4–5lb (2kg) each

Heavier = more than 5lb (2kg) each.

To exercise safely with hand weights, it's important to use equal weights in each hand for balance. Keep your wrists flat. Avoid clenching your hands tightly; just hold them firmly enough to make them secure.

If using hand weights is straining your wrists in any way, you might want to try wrist weights instead—these are stretchy wrist-bands with in-built weights.

Exercise ball

Also called a Swiss or stability ball, this piece of equipment requires you to engage your muscles when exercising in order to balance safely on its slightly unstable surface. It therefore pushes you harder than if you did the same exercises on the floor or with a solid prop such as a bench. Some guidelines for using one are:

• choose a size that suits you— one on which you can sit with your feet flat on the floor and your legs at right angles

• make sure it is adequately inflated—it should be firm, with only a little give

• use it only on even surfaces

• keep away from direct heat, whether radiators or a strong sun.

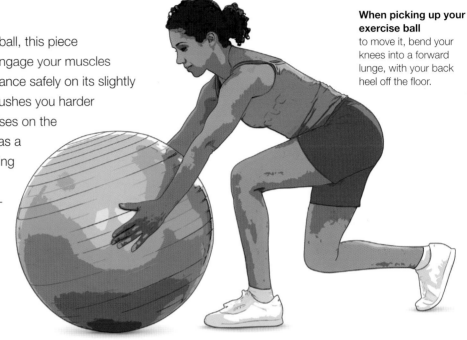

When picking up your exercise ball
to move it, bend your knees into a forward lunge, with your back heel off the floor.

Resistance band

The firm elasticity of a resistance band means that using one provides safe, progressive resistance throughout a wide range of motion. You can use one to add resistance to a body area that wouldn't otherwise be targeted in that particular exercise (such as the one below left). It also encourages you to work more slowly and increases the resistance on the return part of the exercise, as well as the movement into the main position. Alternatively, you can loop it around your feet or hands to allow you to achieve more extreme stretch positions than you would normally be able to, and therefore work your muscles harder (see p.158). Resistance bands come in a variety of thicknesses, usually graded by color: the thicker the band, the more strength is needed to stretch it. It is therefore best to start with a fairly thin band and gradually work up to using a thicker one, if appropriate.

Adjusting how close
to the ends you hold your resistance band alters its tautness, allowing you to control the intensity of the workout you give yourself.

Your shoulders and upper back

The muscles in your shoulders and upper back are often under considerable strain during everyday activities such as working at a computer, driving, or carrying heavy bags. As a result, they easily become stiff and misaligned. These exercises will not only increase your mobility and enhance your posture, but also create a lovely strong, lean shoulder line that you'll be happy to show off.

Shoulder Extension

This exercise includes forward and backward movement of your arms, flexion of your body, and rotation of your arms. As such, it offers a good all-over upper body workout.

1 Stand with your feet hip-width apart and your arms by your sides, with a weight in each hand. Pull your belly button toward your spine, bend your knees, and bend your body forward to between 45° and 90°, keeping your back completely flat. Then bring your elbows upward and backward to raise the weights to chest height, palms facing in. Inhale to prepare.

2 As you exhale, stretch one arm forward and the other backward in a slow, flowing movement—turning your arms so that, when fully extended, the front palm faces down and the back palm up. Hold for a couple of seconds, then inhale as you bring your arms in. Repeat with opposite arms. When finished, slowly roll up to standing.

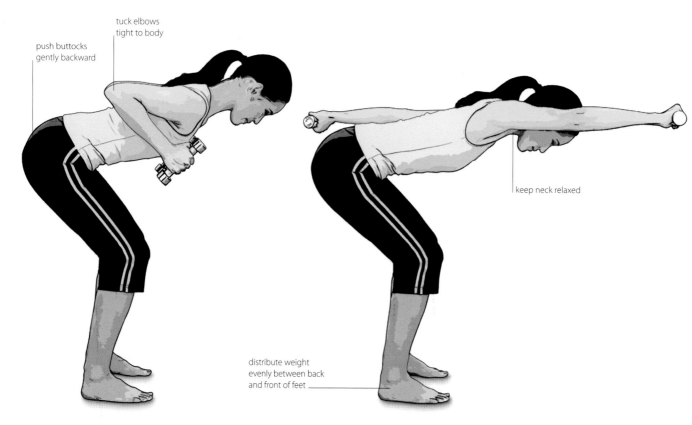

push buttocks gently backward

tuck elbows tight to body

keep neck relaxed

distribute weight evenly between back and front of feet

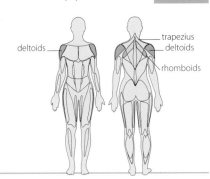

What am I working?

The trapezius, which runs from the back of your head to your mid-spine, helps to support your spine and all arm movements. The deltoids on both the front and back of your shoulders also assist all arm movements, as do the rhomboids, which lie beneath your trapezius and connect your shoulder blades to your spine.

Front Raise

This exercise is particularly good for the front of your deltoid muscles. It keeps your shoulders strong and your inner upper arms trim and toned in readiness for sleeveless summers.

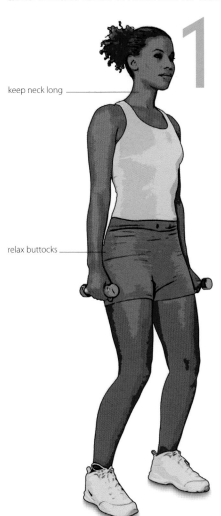

keep neck long

relax buttocks

1 Stand with your feet hip-width apart and your arms by your sides, with a weight in each hand. Imagine there is a piece of thread pulling you upward from the top of your head to enhance your posture. Pull your belly button toward your spine to engage your abs and bend your knees slightly. Inhale to prepare.

relax shoulders

2 As you exhale, slowly raise your arms diagonally away from your body until they reach shoulder height. Keep the rest of your body still as you do so, and keep your arms straight but not locked. Hold for a couple of seconds, then inhale as you slowly lower your arms back down to your sides.

keep weight through heels

External Rotation

This exercise tones the back of your shoulders via your deltoids and rhomboids. It also reinforces your rotator cuff muscles, which protect your shoulder joint from injury.

1 Lie on your side with your lower arm bent under your head, your hips vertically stacked, and a weight in your top hand. Bend your knees forward to 45°. Place a folded towel on your waist, rest your elbow on it, and bend your forearm until it is parallel with the floor, palm facing down. Inhale to prepare.

2 As you exhale, slowly raise your forearm to 90°, keeping your top elbow on the towel. Your palm should end up facing forward. Hold for a couple of seconds, then inhale as you lower your arm again. Once you have completed the exercise on one side, turn onto your other side and repeat.

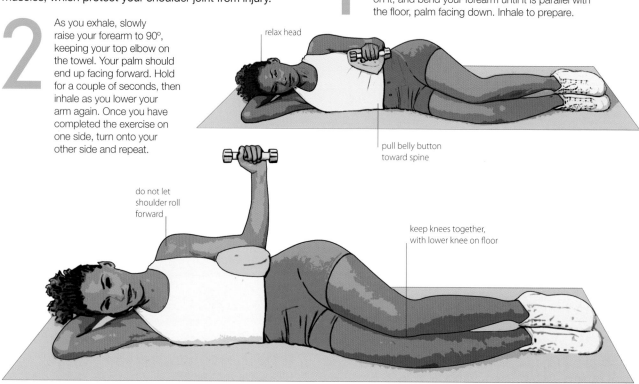

relax head

pull belly button toward spine

do not let shoulder roll forward

keep knees together, with lower knee on floor

Double Arm and Leg Lift

This exercise is a fantastic total back strengthener and, as a bonus, provides a great workout for your glutes, too. It is also useful for building all-around endurance.

1 Lie down on your front with your feet hip-width apart, and the top of your feet and your forehead resting on the floor. Raise your arms above your head, with your arms bent, palms facing down, and fingertips pointing forward. Let all your muscles sink into the floor. Inhale to prepare.

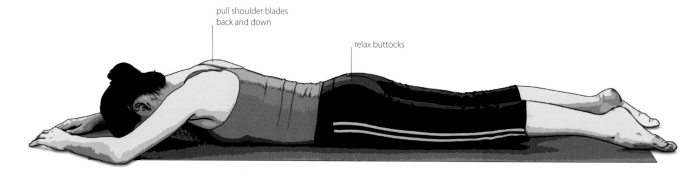

pull shoulder blades back and down

relax buttocks

Reverse Fly on Ball

This exercise strengthens your rhomboids and the often-neglected back parts of your deltoids, so it not only tones your shoulders, but also gives your posture a boost.

1 Kneel on the mat with the exercise ball directly in front of you and bend forward over it. Place your arms vertically down each side of the ball, palms facing in, and with a weight in each hand. Your spine should be in a straight line from your tailbone right up to the base of your head. Inhale to prepare.

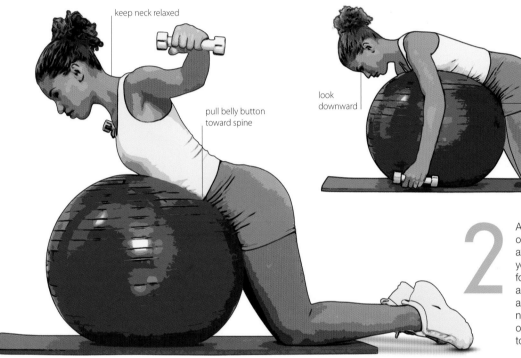

keep neck relaxed

pull belly button toward spine

look downward

ensure contact between exercise ball and upper thighs

2 As you exhale, lift the weights out to the sides until they are at shoulder height, keeping your arms slightly bent. Hold for a few seconds, then inhale as you lower your arms down again. Repeat for the required number of reps, then come off the ball and slowly return to standing.

2 As you exhale, slowly lift your head, shoulders, arms, upper chest, lower legs, and thighs off the floor. Draw your tailbone toward your heels for a sense of extension through your legs, and look down throughout the movement. Hold for a couple of seconds, then inhale as you lower your entire body to the floor.

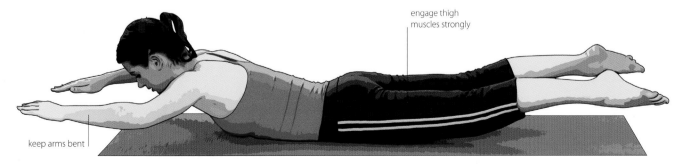

engage thigh muscles strongly

keep arms bent

Your chest

The muscles of your chest can easily become shortened, weakened, and "saggy" as you unintentionally hunch over your desk or steering wheel each day. The following exercises will counteract this by strengthening these muscles, enhancing your posture and giving your bust a healthy "lift": newly toned muscular attachments in this area will act like freshly tightened bra straps!

Mini Push-up

Push-ups, also known as press-ups, are one of the most effective ways to strengthen and tone not only your chest, but also the back of your upper arms (see p.117).

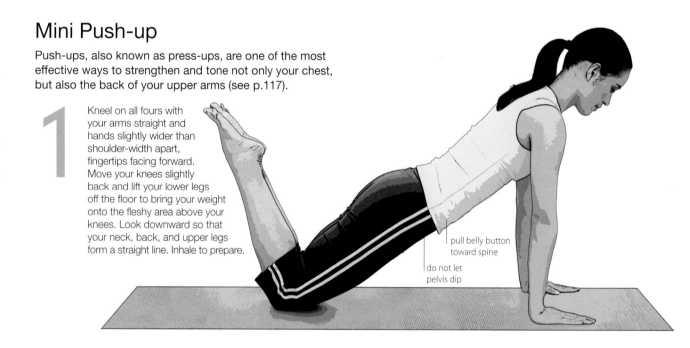

1 Kneel on all fours with your arms straight and hands slightly wider than shoulder-width apart, fingertips facing forward. Move your knees slightly back and lift your lower legs off the floor to bring your weight onto the fleshy area above your knees. Look downward so that your neck, back, and upper legs form a straight line. Inhale to prepare.

pull belly button toward spine

do not let pelvis dip

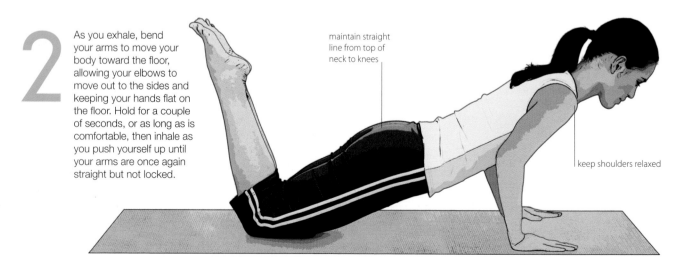

2 As you exhale, bend your arms to move your body toward the floor, allowing your elbows to move out to the sides and keeping your hands flat on the floor. Hold for a couple of seconds, or as long as is comfortable, then inhale as you push yourself up until your arms are once again straight but not locked.

maintain straight line from top of neck to knees

keep shoulders relaxed

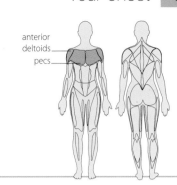

anterior
deltoids
pecs

What am I working?

The pectoralis major muscles, more commonly known as the "pecs," are the main muscles in your chest and are responsible for supporting, protecting, and giving definition to your upper chest; they are also accessory muscles in respiration. The front part of your shoulder muscles, called the anterior deltoids, help your shoulders to flex and rotate.

Full Push-up

Doing push-ups with the body fully extended increases the weight to support when your body is lowered. Only try this when you are fully comfortable with the Mini Push-up, left.

1 Kneel on all fours with your arms straight but not locked and your hands slightly wider than shoulder-width apart, fingertips facing forward. Extend your legs back so that your weight is evenly distributed between your arms and legs. Your body should be in a straight line from your head to your heels. Inhale to prepare.

keep neck relaxed

pull belly button
toward spine

2 As you exhale, slowly bend your arms to lower your body toward the floor. Allow your elbows to go out to the sides and lower yourself only as far as is comfortable. Hold for a couple of seconds, then inhale as you slowly push yourself up again. Repeat for the required number of reps, then slowly lower yourself to the floor and relax.

pull shoulder blades
back and down

look
downward

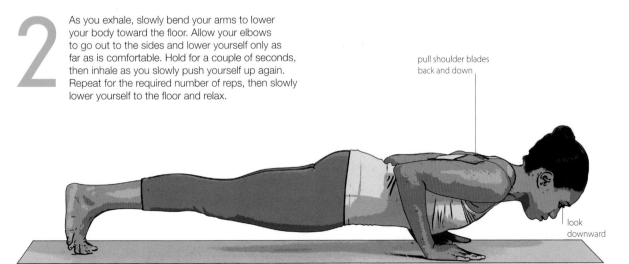

Chest Press

This exercise works your chest, the front of your shoulders, and the back of your upper arms (see p.117). It therefore prevents "bat wings" and creates a firm, lifted bust.

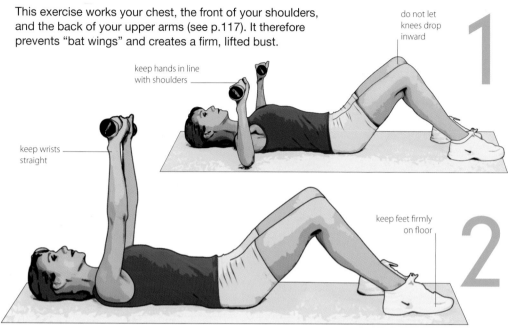

keep hands in line with shoulders

keep wrists straight

do not let knees drop inward

keep feet firmly on floor

1 Lie on your back with your knees bent and your feet flat on the floor, hip-width apart. Extend your arms out to the sides in line with your shoulders, with a weight in each hand. Keeping your upper arms and elbows on the floor, lift your lower arms until they are vertical and your weights are in the air, palms facing forward. Inhale to prepare.

2 As you exhale, slowly push your arms to lift the weights above your chest, straightening your arms without locking them. Slightly direct the weights toward the center as you raise them. Hold for a couple of seconds, then inhale as you slowly bring your elbows back to the floor.

Chest Fly

As well as firming up your bust by working your pecs (the main chest muscles), this exercise targets the front of your shoulders, toning the often flabby area around the armpits.

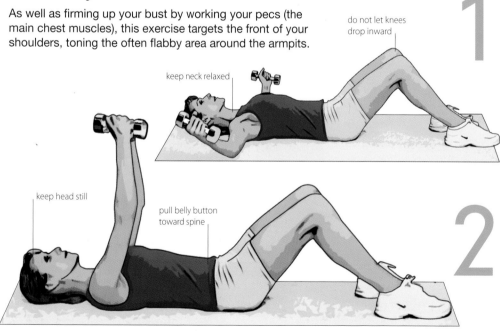

keep neck relaxed

keep head still

pull belly button toward spine

do not let knees drop inward

1 Lie on your back with your knees bent and your feet hip-width apart. Keep your knees in line with your toes and hold a weight in each hand. Maintain a small gap between your lower back and the floor. Bring your arms out to your sides at shoulder level on the floor, then bend your elbows to lift your upper arms slightly off the floor, palms facing up. Inhale to prepare.

2 As you exhale, lift your arms off the floor and slowly raise your hands toward each other above your chest. Your arms should end up straight but not locked and your palms should face each other. Hold for a couple of seconds, then inhale as you slowly lower your arms again.

Chest Expansion

This exercise encourages your shoulders to stay back and down, and lifts and opens your chest, which enhances your posture. It also strengthens your shoulders and arms.

1 Kneel on the floor, knees hip-width apart, and raise your buttocks off your heels so that your body forms a straight line from your knees to the top of your head. Hold a weight in each hand and, as you inhale, raise your arms to 45° in front of you, palms facing your body.

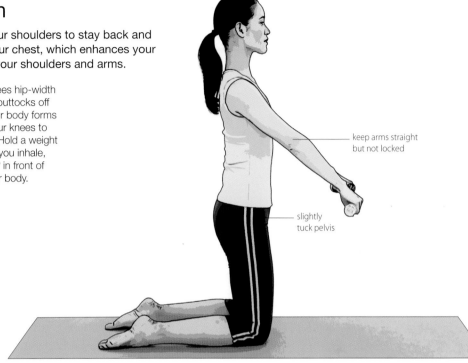

keep arms straight but not locked

slightly tuck pelvis

2 Draw your shoulder blades back and down. As you exhale, move your arms in a slow, controlled manner until they are as far behind you as you can comfortably reach while keeping the rest of your body completely still. Hold for a couple of seconds, then inhale as you sweep your arms forward again. Repeat for the required number of reps, then relax your arms by your sides.

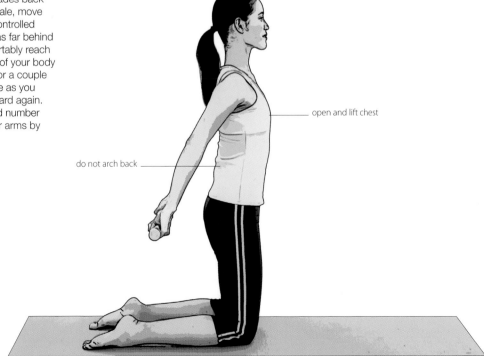

open and lift chest

do not arch back

Your arms

Sometimes we can be so busy focusing on firming up our bottoms and bellies that we overlook our arms. Yet, lean, toned arms can make a big difference to how we look and feel—both in and out of clothes! By regularly doing the exercises that follow, you will soon have beautiful arms that you love, allowing you to go sleeveless with complete confidence.

Biceps Curl

This exercise works your biceps muscles, creating more shapely arms and also developing greater strength for everyday activities such as carrying groceries or luggage.

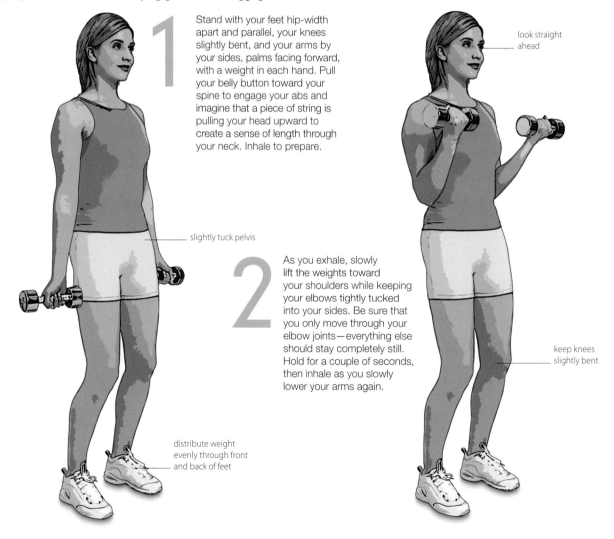

1 Stand with your feet hip-width apart and parallel, your knees slightly bent, and your arms by your sides, palms facing forward, with a weight in each hand. Pull your belly button toward your spine to engage your abs and imagine that a piece of string is pulling your head upward to create a sense of length through your neck. Inhale to prepare.

slightly tuck pelvis

distribute weight evenly through front and back of feet

look straight ahead

2 As you exhale, slowly lift the weights toward your shoulders while keeping your elbows tightly tucked into your sides. Be sure that you only move through your elbow joints—everything else should stay completely still. Hold for a couple of seconds, then inhale as you slowly lower your arms again.

keep knees slightly bent

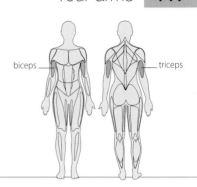

biceps — triceps

What am I working?

The biceps, on the front of your upper arms, are responsible for flexing your arms in everyday actions, such as when you pick up a bag or shake someone's hand. The triceps, on the back of your arms, are, conversely, responsible for extending your arms during such actions. It is therefore important to keep both these sets of muscles in strong working order.

Sitting Side Curl

Working your arms one at a time, this exercise helps you find differences in strength between your two biceps muscles. Once you know your weaker arm, both start and finish with it.

1 Sit on the edge of a chair with your feet flat on the floor, wider than hip-width apart, and a weight in one hand. Lean forward at 45° from your waist and extend the weight-bearing arm toward the floor between your legs, keeping your elbow against the inner knee of the same leg. Then place your other hand on your thigh for support. Inhale to prepare.

2 As you exhale, bend your arm to curl the weight up toward your shoulder, stopping when your forearm is horizontal, with your palm facing up. Hold for a couple of seconds, then inhale as you slowly extend your arm again. Once you have completed the exercise on one side, switch arms and repeat it on the other side.

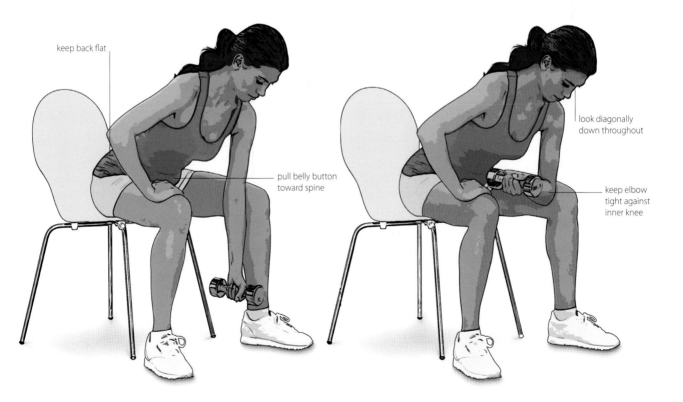

keep back flat

pull belly button toward spine

look diagonally down throughout

keep elbow tight against inner knee

Pull-up

The inward turn of your arms in this exercise targets and tones not only the back of your arms (triceps), but also the front of your shoulders (anterior deltoids, see p.113).

Triceps Lift

This exercise works your triceps in isolation, so is especially effective for firming up the back of your arms and the front of your armpits. Get rid of that flab once and for all!

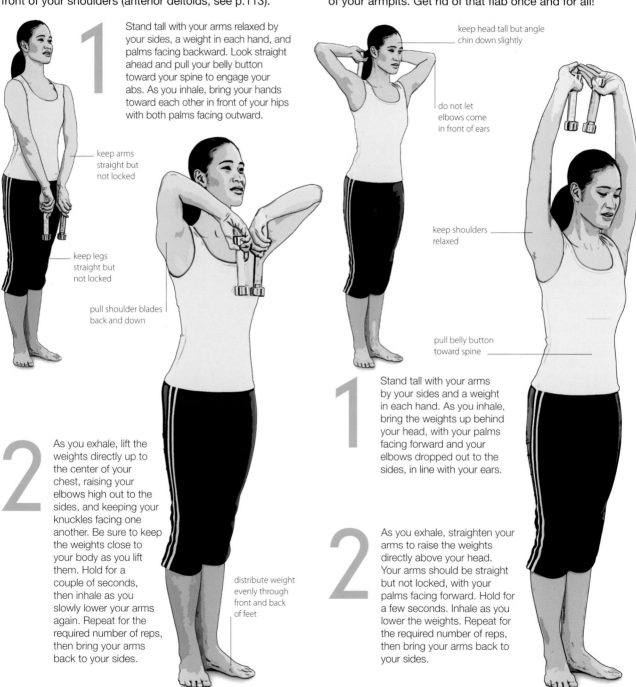

1 Stand tall with your arms relaxed by your sides, a weight in each hand, and palms facing backward. Look straight ahead and pull your belly button toward your spine to engage your abs. As you inhale, bring your hands toward each other in front of your hips with both palms facing outward.

keep arms straight but not locked

keep legs straight but not locked

pull shoulder blades back and down

2 As you exhale, lift the weights directly up to the center of your chest, raising your elbows high out to the sides, and keeping your knuckles facing one another. Be sure to keep the weights close to your body as you lift them. Hold for a couple of seconds, then inhale as you slowly lower your arms again. Repeat for the required number of reps, then bring your arms back to your sides.

distribute weight evenly through front and back of feet

keep head tall but angle chin down slightly

do not let elbows come in front of ears

keep shoulders relaxed

pull belly button toward spine

1 Stand tall with your arms by your sides and a weight in each hand. As you inhale, bring the weights up behind your head, with your palms facing forward and your elbows dropped out to the sides, in line with your ears.

2 As you exhale, straighten your arms to raise the weights directly above your head. Your arms should be straight but not locked, with your palms facing forward. Hold for a few seconds. Inhale as you lower the weights. Repeat for the required number of reps, then bring your arms back to your sides.

Double Punch

An all-around winner for the upper body, this exercise firms up the back of your arms (triceps), your chest (pecs), and the front of your shoulders (anterior deltoids, see p.113).

1 Stand with your feet parallel and slightly wider than hip-width apart. Pull your belly button toward your spine to engage your abs, and bend your knees slightly. As you inhale, make loose fists with your hands and raise them to shoulder height, with your elbows bent out to the sides.

2 As you exhale, slowly move both hands directly forward in a punching movement, keeping your arms at shoulder height, parallel to the floor. Hold for a couple of seconds, then inhale as you slowly bring them back toward your chest. Repeat for the required number of reps, then bring your arms back to your sides.

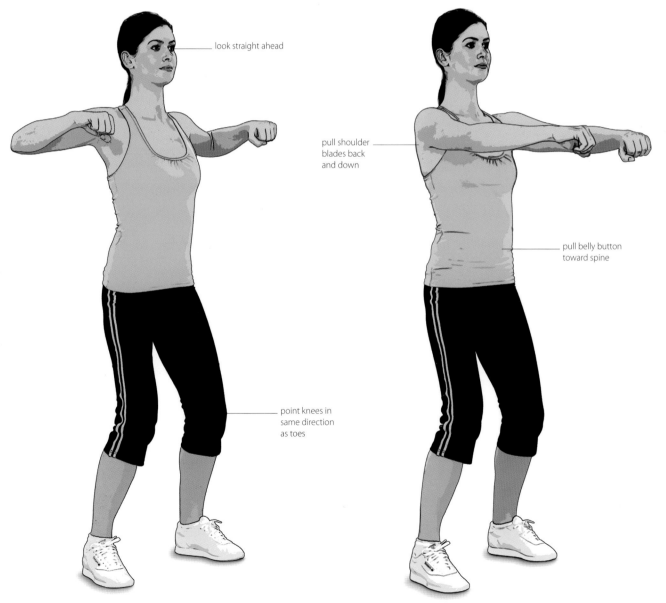

look straight ahead

pull shoulder blades back and down

pull belly button toward spine

point knees in same direction as toes

Triceps Dip

This exercise uses your arms to support your body weight as you move up and down in a sitting position. By targeting your triceps muscles, it strengthens and defines your upper arms.

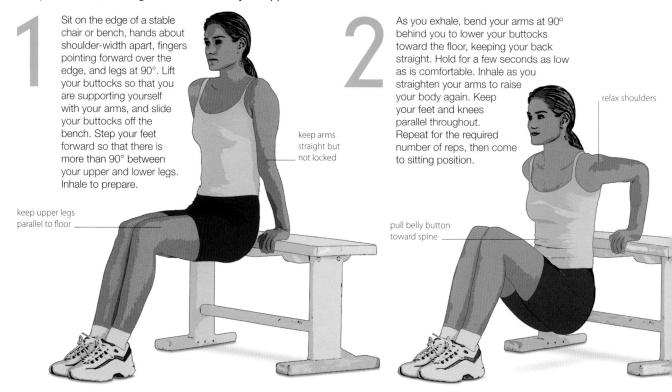

1 Sit on the edge of a stable chair or bench, hands about shoulder-width apart, fingers pointing forward over the edge, and legs at 90°. Lift your buttocks so that you are supporting yourself with your arms, and slide your buttocks off the bench. Step your feet forward so that there is more than 90° between your upper and lower legs. Inhale to prepare.

keep upper legs parallel to floor

keep arms straight but not locked

2 As you exhale, bend your arms at 90° behind you to lower your buttocks toward the floor, keeping your back straight. Hold for a few seconds as low as is comfortable. Inhale as you straighten your arms to raise your body again. Keep your feet and knees parallel throughout. Repeat for the required number of reps, then come to sitting position.

relax shoulders

pull belly button toward spine

Side-lying Triceps Push-up

This challenging exercise uses your own body weight as resistance in a side-lying position, giving first the back of one arm a fantastic workout, then the back of the other.

1 Lie on your side with your shoulders, hips, and feet stacked vertically. Bend your knees forward at 45°, keeping your lower legs angled backward. Place your bottom hand on the top side of your waist and your top hand beside your lower elbow, fingers facing toward your head. Inhale to prepare.

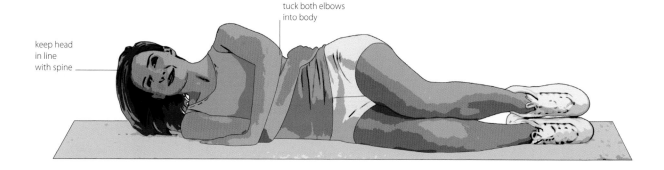

tuck both elbows into body

keep head in line with spine

Triceps Kickback

This classic triceps exercise is a brilliant one for firming up the back of your arms—a problem area for many women. It will get you the lean arms you have always wanted.

1 Stand with your feet hip-width apart, your arms by your sides, a weight in each hand, and your palms facing in. As you inhale, bend your knees, lean 45° forward from the waist, with a flat back, and raise your elbows directly behind you, until your upper arms are parallel to the floor and in line with your shoulders.

pull belly button toward spine

do not let knees bend beyond toes

2 As you exhale, straighten your arms behind you to raise the weights to approximately shoulder height, palms still facing inward. Hold for a couple of seconds, then inhale as you bend your arms to lower the weights again. Continue to engage your abs throughout the movement in order to protect your lower back.

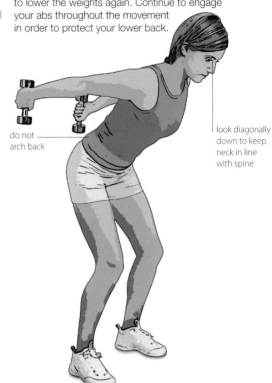

do not arch back

look diagonally down to keep neck in line with spine

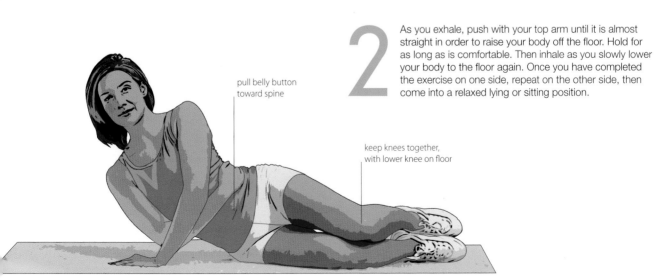

pull belly button toward spine

2 As you exhale, push with your top arm until it is almost straight in order to raise your body off the floor. Hold for as long as is comfortable. Then inhale as you slowly lower your body to the floor again. Once you have completed the exercise on one side, repeat on the other side, then come into a relaxed lying or sitting position.

keep knees together, with lower knee on floor

Your abs

For many women, particularly those with an "apple" body shape (see p.28), excess weight around the middle makes the tummy a real problem area. While healthy eating and cardio training will get rid of any unwanted flab, the following exercises will firm up the mid-section, giving you the flat, toned stomach you've always wanted. Strong, lean abs will also greatly enhance your posture.

Ab Crunch

This basic sit-up is the classic exercise to get your abs in good shape. You don't need to come up far on each crunch to get the results you want.

1 Lie on your back with your knees bent and pointing upward and your feet flat on the floor, hip-width apart. Place your hands behind the base of your head, with your elbows out to the sides, and pull your belly button toward your spine to engage your abs. Inhale to prepare.

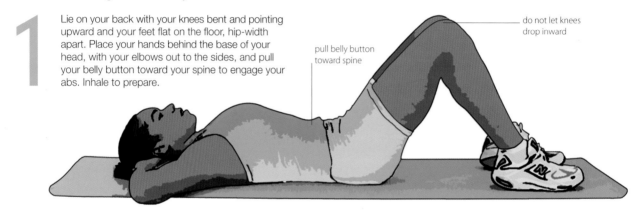

pull belly button toward spine

do not let knees drop inward

2 As you exhale, use your stomach muscles to raise your head and shoulders off the floor as far as is comfortable. Keep your elbows wide as you do so to ensure that you do not force yourself up with your arms. Hold for a couple of seconds, then inhale as you slowly lower yourself to the floor again.

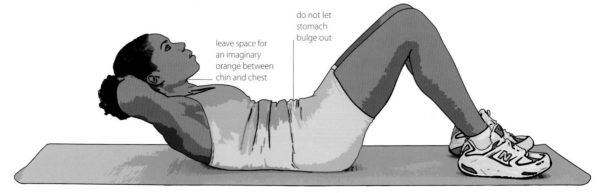

leave space for an imaginary orange between chin and chest

do not let stomach bulge out

What am I working?

The rectus abdominis are two bands of muscle running down the center of your stomach, often referred to as a "six pack" when well defined. These enable you to lean forward and backward, and play a key role in balance and posture. The transversus abdominis wraps horizontally around your lower stomach, providing core strength, and supporting your lower back.

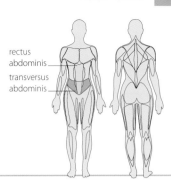

rectus abdominis
transversus abdominis

Ab Stretch and Crunch on Ball

As well as providing an intense workout for your abs, this challenging exercise is a great posture enhancer: it opens up your chest and gives your spine a well-deserved stretch.

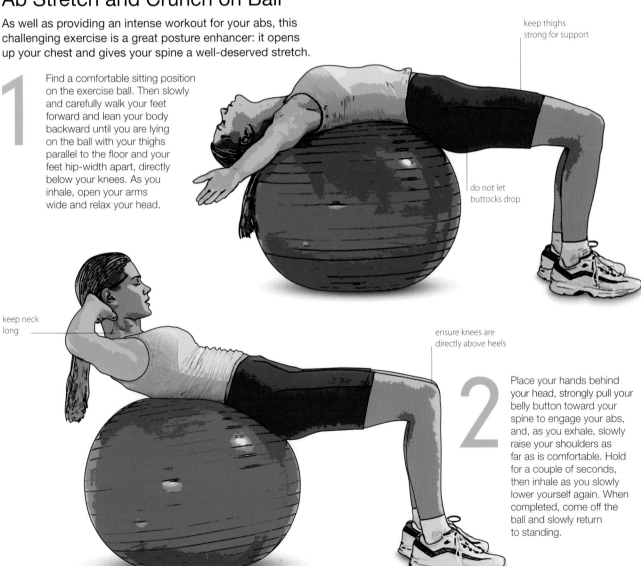

keep thighs strong for support

do not let buttocks drop

keep neck long

ensure knees are directly above heels

1 Find a comfortable sitting position on the exercise ball. Then slowly and carefully walk your feet forward and lean your body backward until you are lying on the ball with your thighs parallel to the floor and your feet hip-width apart, directly below your knees. As you inhale, open your arms wide and relax your head.

2 Place your hands behind your head, strongly pull your belly button toward your spine to engage your abs, and, as you exhale, slowly raise your shoulders as far as is comfortable. Hold for a couple of seconds, then inhale as you slowly lower yourself again. When completed, come off the ball and slowly return to standing.

Alternating Kicks

This exercise sculpts your stomach and waist muscles, enhances hip mobility, and strengthens your back. The lower you take your extended leg, the deeper the challenge.

1 Lie on your back with your knees bent, feet flat on the floor, and a small gap between the floor and your lower back. As you inhale, first lift one knee toward your chest, then the other, stopping when your upper legs are at 90° to the floor and your lower legs are parallel to it—the "90-90" position.

2 As you exhale, bring one knee in toward your chest and straighten the other leg, taking it as low as you can without setting it down. Hold for as long as is comfortable. Inhale as you return to the "90-90" position. Repeat Step 2 with opposing legs.

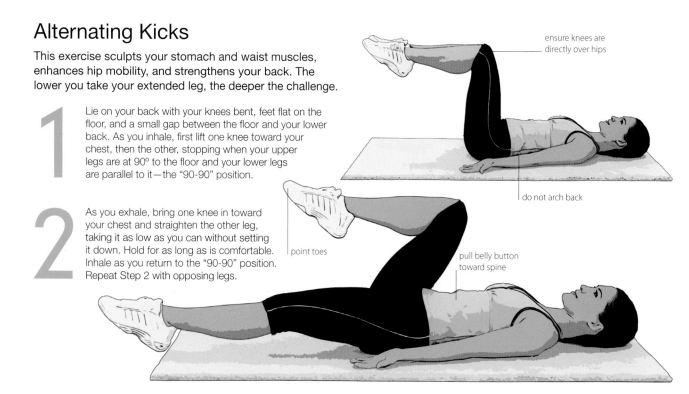

ensure knees are directly over hips

do not arch back

point toes

pull belly button toward spine

Rolling the Ball

This abs exercise is a challenging one, so do it only if you already feel strong in your abs and if you are completely confident using an exercise ball.

1 Kneel upright facing the exercise ball, just far enough away so that your arms are bent at 90° when you rest your hands shoulder-width apart on it. Pull your belly button toward your spine to engage your abs and look diagonally downward to keep your neck relaxed. Inhale to prepare.

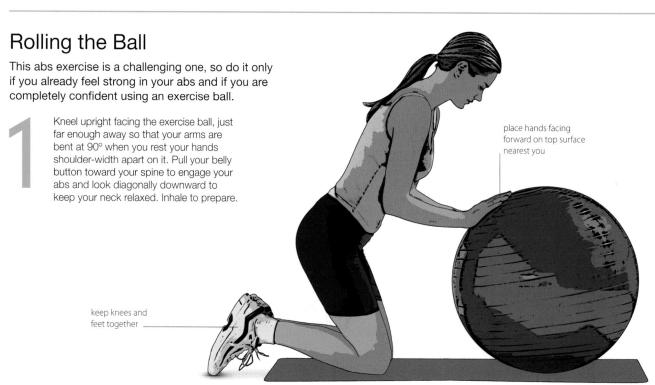

place hands facing forward on top surface nearest you

keep knees and feet together

Double Leg Lowering

This challenging leg-lowering exercise works your deepest abdominal muscles. You can also get a great butt and thigh workout by pressing your legs and buttocks together.

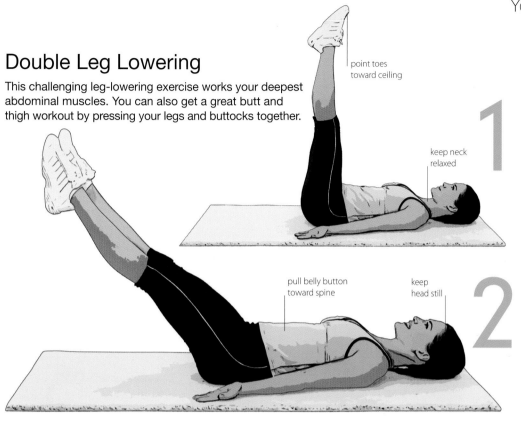

point toes toward ceiling

keep neck relaxed

pull belly button toward spine

keep head still

1 Lie on your back with your knees bent, your feet hip-width apart on the floor, and your arms relaxed by your sides. Pull your belly button toward your spine to engage your abs. As you inhale, slowly extend your legs upward so that they are at 90° to your upper body.

2 As you exhale, slowly lower your legs down as far as is comfortable without your abs shaking or your back arching. Keep your legs straight and firmly pressed together as you move. Hold for a couple of seconds. Inhale as you raise your legs to vertical again.

2 As you exhale, slowly roll the ball forward until your forearms are resting on it and your body forms a straight line from your knees to the base of your neck. Your weight should be evenly distributed between your arms and legs as you balance. Hold for a couple of seconds. Then inhale as you roll back to your starting position.

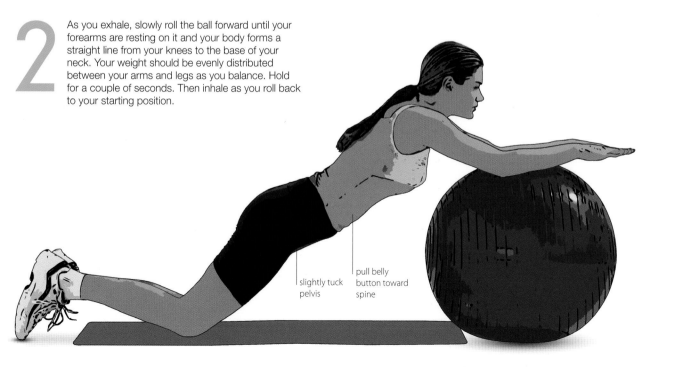

slightly tuck pelvis

pull belly button toward spine

Forearm Plank

This challenging exercise requires you to hold your body in a horizontal line from head to heel like a plank, hence the name. It gives your abs an intense workout.

1 Kneel on all fours. Lower your forearms to the floor and clasp your hands directly under your head, so that your upper arms are more or less vertical and your elbows are angled out at 45° on the floor. Keep your back flat. Pull your belly button toward your spine to engage your abs. Inhale to prepare.

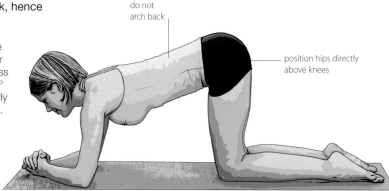

do not arch back

position hips directly above knees

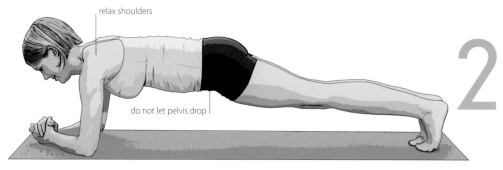

relax shoulders

do not let pelvis drop

2 As you exhale, step one foot back, then the other, until your legs are straight and your body weight is distributed between your forearms and your toes. Continue to engage your abs in order to hold your body in this straight line for as long as possible. Then inhale as you come back onto all fours.

Plank with Leg Lift

This intense abdominal exercise involves starting in the plank position, so only do it once you are completely confident with that position.

1 Kneel on all fours and bend your elbows to lean on your forearms, with your hands held in loose fists beneath your head. As you inhale, engage your abs and walk your legs out behind you to bring your body into a straight line, parallel to the floor.

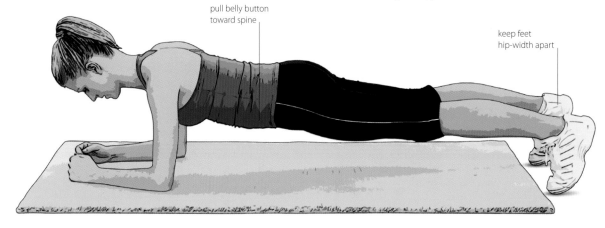

pull belly button toward spine

keep feet hip-width apart

Corkscrew

This tough exercise works all your abdominal muscles at once—obliques (see p.129) as well as core abs. It is therefore great for sculpting both your waist and stomach.

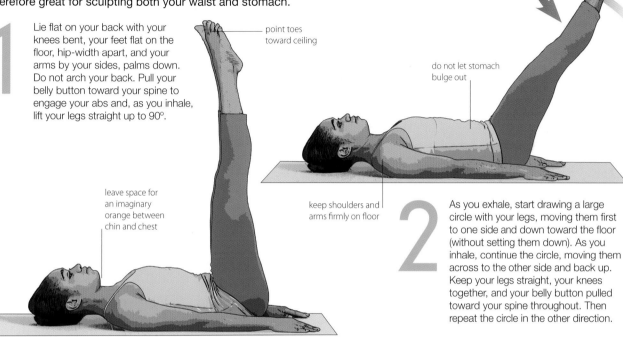

1 Lie flat on your back with your knees bent, your feet flat on the floor, hip-width apart, and your arms by your sides, palms down. Do not arch your back. Pull your belly button toward your spine to engage your abs and, as you inhale, lift your legs straight up to 90°.

point toes toward ceiling

do not let stomach bulge out

leave space for an imaginary orange between chin and chest

keep shoulders and arms firmly on floor

2 As you exhale, start drawing a large circle with your legs, moving them first to one side and down toward the floor (without setting them down). As you inhale, continue the circle, moving them across to the other side and back up. Keep your legs straight, your knees together, and your belly button pulled toward your spine throughout. Then repeat the circle in the other direction.

2 As you exhale, lift one foot off the floor behind you, without twisting your hips. Keep both legs completely straight as you do so and do not move your upper body. Hold for a couple of seconds, then inhale as you lower your foot again. Repeat Step 2 with the other leg.

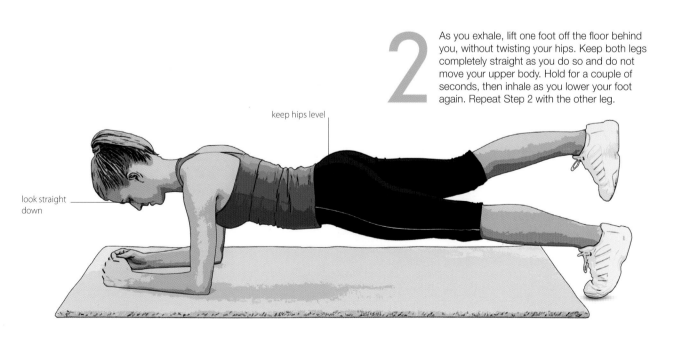

keep hips level

look straight down

Your waist

Your core abdominal muscles (rectus and transversus abdominis, see p.123) are often used in everyday activities such as sitting down and standing up, but your side abs, called your obliques, tend to get a lot less regular use. The exercises that follow will specifically target these side muscles, keeping "love handles" at bay and giving you a slim waist—without a bulge in sight.

Oblique Crunch

This diagonal sit-up requires a twist at the same time as a lift of your upper body, which means it gives both your waist and stomach a great workout.

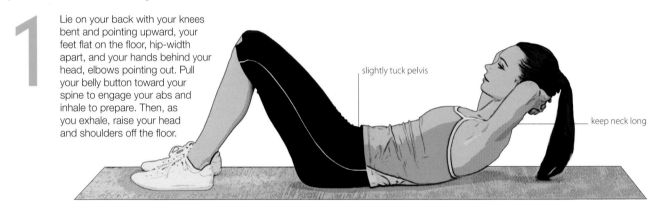

1 Lie on your back with your knees bent and pointing upward, your feet flat on the floor, hip-width apart, and your hands behind your head, elbows pointing out. Pull your belly button toward your spine to engage your abs and inhale to prepare. Then, as you exhale, raise your head and shoulders off the floor.

slightly tuck pelvis

keep neck long

2 As you continue to exhale, twist your upper body so that you move one shoulder toward the opposite knee. Keep your elbows wide as you do so. Hold for a couple of seconds, then inhale as you come back to center. As you exhale, repeat the crunch in the opposite direction. Repeat for the required number of reps, then lower your head and shoulders to the floor.

do not let stomach bulge out

keep hips flat on floor

What am I working?

The oblique muscles (obliquus abdominis) run down the sides of your waist and are responsible for allowing your body to twist and, to a lesser extent, bend sideways. Like all abdominal muscles, they are also accessory muscles in respiration. The external obliques form the outermost layer of muscle, while the internal obliques lie beneath them.

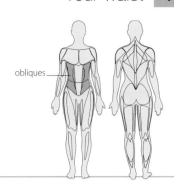

obliques

Criss-cross Leg Extension

This exercise involves lifting and twisting your upper body while alternately extending your legs. It helps to shape your legs as well as firm up your stomach and waist muscles.

1 Lie on your back with your knees bent and your feet flat on the floor. Pull your belly button toward your spine to engage your abs. As you inhale, lift your head and shoulders off the floor. At the same time, raise your legs, aiming to get your thighs at a 90° angle to the floor and your lower legs parallel to it.

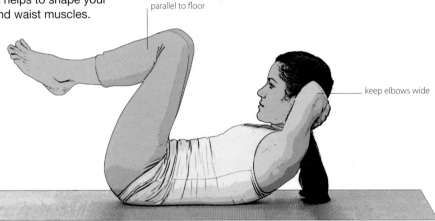

keep lower legs roughly parallel to floor

keep elbows wide

2 As you exhale, extend one leg at 45° to the floor, bend the knee of your other leg toward your chest, and, keeping your head and shoulders raised off the floor, twist your upper body so that your opposite elbow reaches toward your bent knee. Hold for a couple of seconds, then inhale as you come back to center. Repeat with opposite arms and legs.

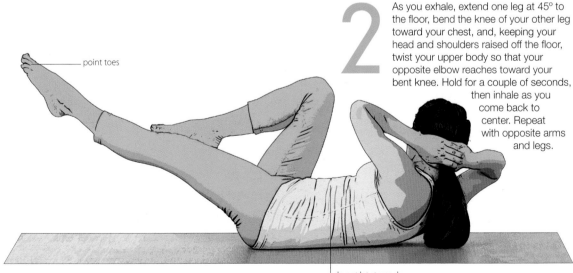

point toes

do not let stomach bulge out

Twist and Reach

This is a great waist exercise since it strengthens and tones your obliques. It also opens up your chest muscles, helping to improve posture and counteract any stiffness.

1 Sit on the floor with your legs straight out in front of you, slightly wider than hip-width apart. Holding a resistance band or towel between your hands, raise your arms above your head so that the band is taut. As you inhale, twist to the side from your waist, imagining your spine spiralling toward the ceiling.

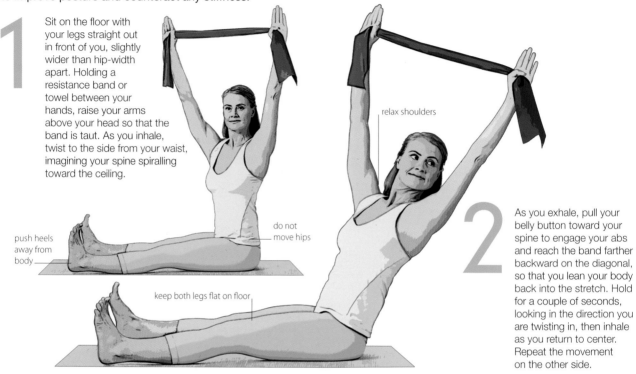

relax shoulders

push heels away from body

do not move hips

keep both legs flat on floor

2 As you exhale, pull your belly button toward your spine to engage your abs and reach the band farther backward on the diagonal, so that you lean your body back into the stretch. Hold for a couple of seconds, looking in the direction you are twisting in, then inhale as you return to center. Repeat the movement on the other side.

Lying Twist with Weight

This exercise involves rotating your upper body to one side and your lower body to the other, which offers a fantastic workout for your obliques, thereby sculpting your waist.

1 Lie on your back with your knees bent and pointing toward the ceiling, your feet together on the floor, your arms relaxed by your sides, and a weight in one hand. As you inhale, raise both arms straight above your chest and hold the weight between your hands.

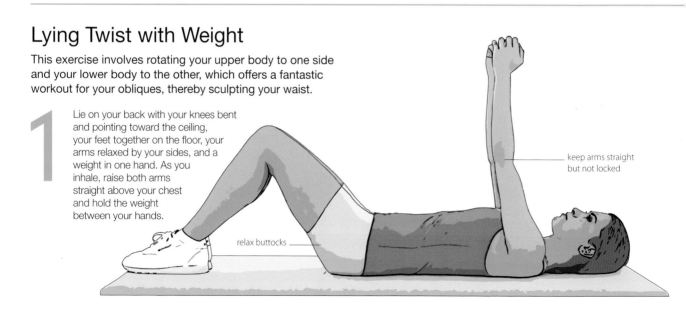

keep arms straight but not locked

relax buttocks

Twist and Bend

The simultaneous twist and forward bend in this exercise means that as you work one side, you enjoy a deep stretch up the other side, as well as a stretch in your legs and back.

1 Sit on the floor with your legs straight out in front of you, slightly wider than hip-width apart, and your feet flexed. As you inhale, raise your arms out to your sides at shoulder height, palms facing down. Engage your abs and twist your upper body as far as you can to one side without moving your lower body.

2 As you exhale, reach your front arm toward the opposite foot, bending your upper body forward and keeping your back arm extended. Allow your head to relax. Hold for a couple of seconds, then come back up to a central sitting position. Repeat the exercise on the other side.

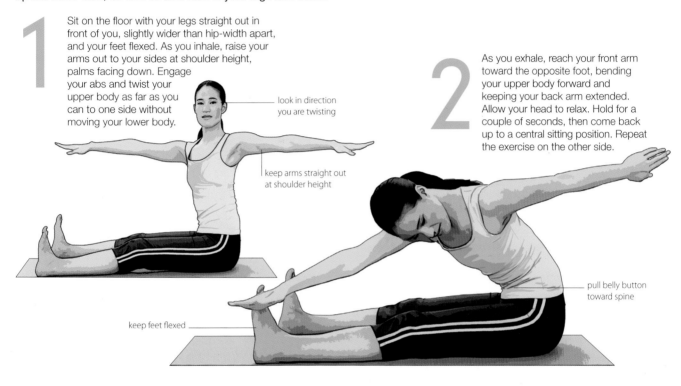

look in direction you are twisting

keep arms straight out at shoulder height

keep feet flexed

pull belly button toward spine

2 As you exhale, slowly lower your knees and feet to one side while twisting your upper body to the other side, lowering the weight toward your shoulder in the direction of your upper body. You will need to extend one arm across your chest and let the other bend to do this. Hold for a couple of seconds, then inhale as you come back to center. Repeat the exercise on the other side.

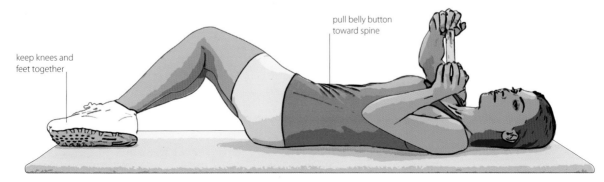

keep knees and feet together

pull belly button toward spine

Your lower back

Your lower back often comes under great strain as you go about your daily activities, so it is particularly important to keep it in healthy working order. Doing the exercises that follow will not only keep it strong, but will also give you a lovely lean and toned look in bikinis and backless dresses. Plus, they will improve your posture, which will allow you to ooze confidence.

Back Extension

This exercise opens up your chest and strengthens your back to alleviate any tension in either. You don't need to raise your upper body far off the floor for an effective workout.

1 Lie on your front, with your feet slightly wider than hip-width apart, and relax all your muscles into the floor. Place your hands, palms facing downward, under your chin so that your elbows are bent out to the sides. Inhale to prepare.

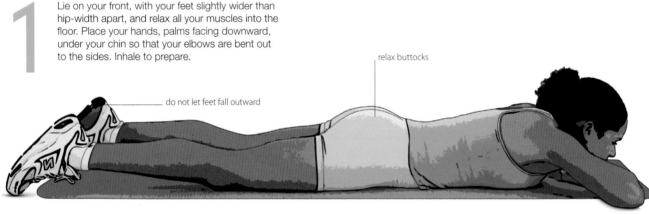

relax buttocks

do not let feet fall outward

2 As you exhale, slowly lift your head, upper chest, and bent arms as far as is comfortable off the floor. Stretch through both the top of your head and your feet as you do so for a sense of extension throughout your body. Hold for a couple of seconds, then inhale as you return to the floor.

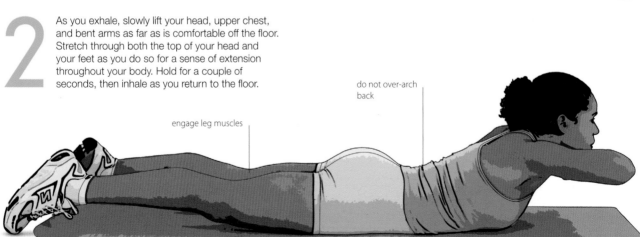

do not over-arch back

engage leg muscles

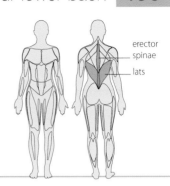

erector
spinae

lats

What am I working?

Your latissimus dorsi, commonly known as "lats," are large, flat triangular muscles on both sides of your mid-back. They are responsible for pushing, pulling, and rotating through the shoulders and arms, and are also accessory muscles in respiration. The erector spinae run down either side of your spine, supporting it and enabling it to move effectively. Both sets of muscles help to protect the spine.

Extended Heel Taps

This exercise strengthens the entire back of your body. The upper body lift works your back muscles, while the leg lift and heel taps give your glutes a great workout.

1 Lie on your front with your hands beneath your forehead, palms facing down, and your elbows bent out to the sides. Rotate your legs so that your heels are together, toes apart. Inhale to prepare. As you exhale, lift your head, shoulders, and legs off the floor, keeping your head facing down.

point toes

pull belly button
toward spine

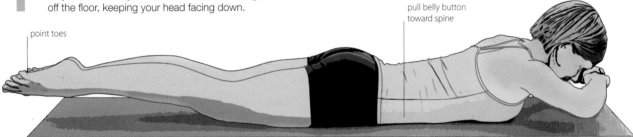

2 With your head, shoulders, and legs still off the floor, slowly open your legs wide and close them again, tapping your heels together. Engage your abs, tuck your pelvis, and look downward throughout the movement. Hold for a couple of seconds, then inhale as you return to the floor.

keep legs as
straight as possible

keep neck long

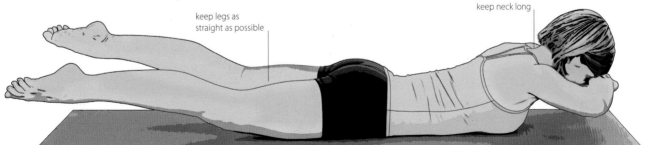

Knee Squeeze

This exercise involves your abs and back muscles working in opposition to keep your body straight as you balance on one leg.

1 Stand with your feet hip-width apart and parallel, with your toes pointing forward. Keep your arms relaxed by your sides and pull your belly button toward your spine to engage your abs. Imagine there is a piece of thread pulling you upward from the top of your head. Inhale to prepare.

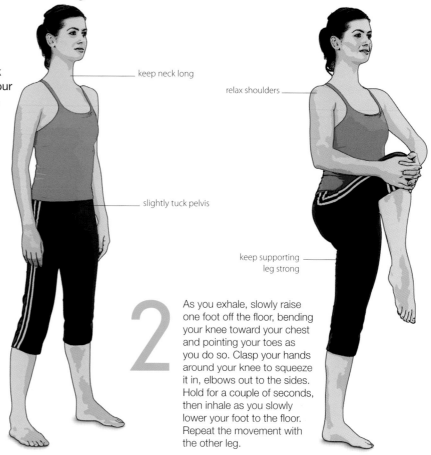

keep neck long

slightly tuck pelvis

relax shoulders

keep supporting leg strong

2 As you exhale, slowly raise one foot off the floor, bending your knee toward your chest and pointing your toes as you do so. Clasp your hands around your knee to squeeze it in, elbows out to the sides. Hold for a couple of seconds, then inhale as you slowly lower your foot to the floor. Repeat the movement with the other leg.

Kneeling Back Extension

This exercise is a great counter-pose to the back bends on pp.132–33, encouraging both length and flexibility through the back and sides of your body.

1 Kneel on the floor, holding a ball between your palms, with your knees slightly wider than hip-width apart and your buttocks resting between your heels. As you exhale, bend forward from your waist, moving your chest toward your knees and your head toward the floor as you stretch your arms with the ball out in front of you.

look straight down toward floor

push buttocks backward

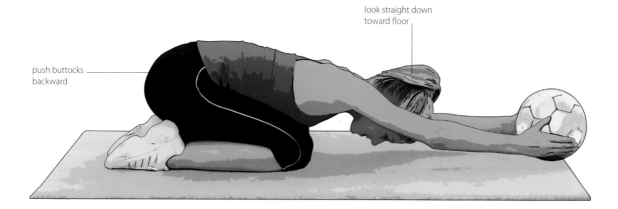

One-arm Lat Row

This exercise works the sides of your back, firming up the area around your armpits and under the back of your bra.

1 Stand, feet hip-width apart, side-on to the back of a chair and rest your nearest hand on it for support. Relax your other arm by your side, with a weight in your hand. Hold the weight in line with your shoulder. As you inhale, take a large step back with your outside leg so that you are in a lunge position, with your back leg straight and your front leg bent. Do not bend your knee beyond your toes.

keep feet facing forward

2 As you exhale, engage your abs and bend your elbow to about 90° behind you, keeping your hand close to your body, palm facing in. Raise the weight to waist height. Hold for a couple of seconds, then inhale as you lower it again. Once you have completed the exercise on one side, turn to face the other way and repeat the movement on the other side. Repeat for the required number of reps, then come up to standing.

keep body in straight line from shoulder to heel

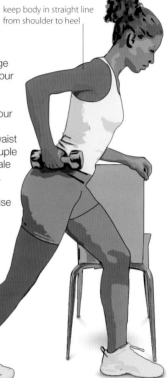

2 Inhale, then as you exhale, move the ball to one side, with your arms still completely extended, your head down, and your back flat. Hold for a couple of seconds, then inhale as you come back to the center. Repeat the movement on the other side. Repeat for the required number of reps, then slowly come up to sitting.

keep hips still

pull shoulders blades back and down

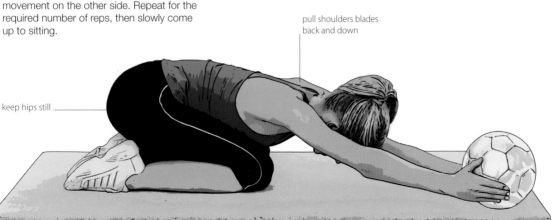

Your glutes and quads

Who doesn't want nice, pert buttocks and firm thighs? Well-conditioned buttock muscles (glutes) and thigh muscles (quads) don't just make you look good; as two of the body's major sets of muscles, they can also help you to manage your weight, as the more active and healthy they are, the more calories they burn. The exercises that follow will help you to achieve all of this.

Squat

This squatting exercise is a classic means of boosting lower body strength and endurance, and of achieving the firm bottom and toned thighs you've always wanted.

1 Stand with your feet hip-width apart and parallel, toes pointing forward and arms relaxed by your sides. Pull your belly button toward your spine to engage your abs, and imagine there is a piece of thread pulling you upward from the top of your head. Inhale to prepare.

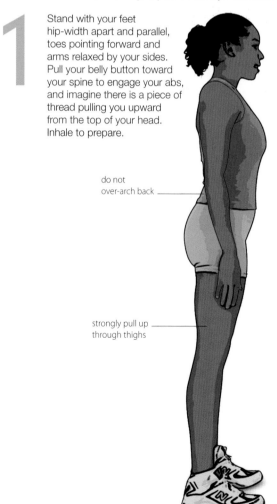

do not over-arch back

strongly pull up through thighs

2 As you exhale, lean your upper body forward at 45°, raise your arms straight out in front of you at shoulder height, and bend your knees into a squatting position, pushing your buttocks downward and backward. Hold for a couple of seconds, then inhale as you come back to standing.

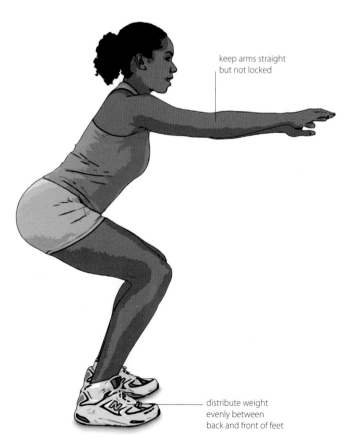

keep arms straight but not locked

distribute weight evenly between back and front of feet

What am I working?

Your glutes are one of the largest and strongest sets of muscles in your body. Together, your gluteus maximus, medius, and minimus give your buttocks their round shape and help to extend your thighs backward. Your quads, or quadriceps, run down the front of each of your thighs and are responsible for straightening your legs.

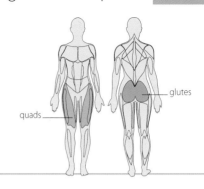

glutes

quads

Wall Squat with Weights

This straight-up-and-down squat tones the front of your thighs. The wall helps to create a deeper squat than otherwise possible and provides resistance as you push back up.

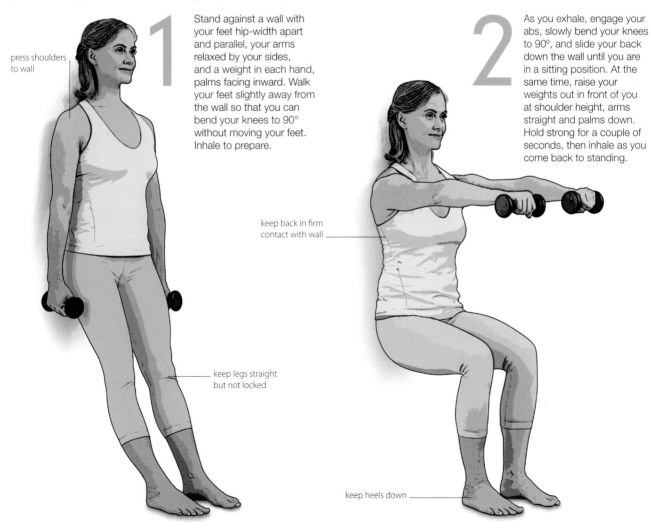

1 Stand against a wall with your feet hip-width apart and parallel, your arms relaxed by your sides, and a weight in each hand, palms facing inward. Walk your feet slightly away from the wall so that you can bend your knees to 90° without moving your feet. Inhale to prepare.

press shoulders to wall

keep legs straight but not locked

2 As you exhale, engage your abs, slowly bend your knees to 90°, and slide your back down the wall until you are in a sitting position. At the same time, raise your weights out in front of you at shoulder height, arms straight and palms down. Hold strong for a couple of seconds, then inhale as you come back to standing.

keep back in firm contact with wall

keep heels down

Curtsy Lunge

The simultaneous lunge and cross-step involved in this clever exercise makes you work both your legs at once, giving your thighs the best workout possible.

1 Stand with your feet hip-width apart and parallel, toes pointing forward. Pull your belly button toward your spine to engage your abs and imagine there is a piece of thread pulling you upward from the top of your head. Lift your arms out to the sides at shoulder height, palms facing down. Inhale to prepare.

2 As you exhale, step one foot diagonally behind the other, bending both legs and lifting the heel of your back foot off the floor so that you are in a curtsy position. Hold for a couple of seconds, then inhale as you come back up to standing. Repeat on the other side.

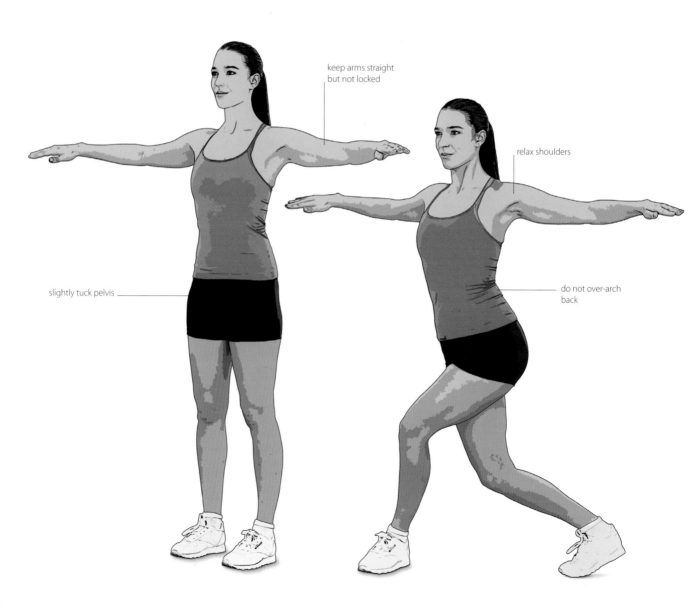

keep arms straight but not locked

relax shoulders

slightly tuck pelvis

do not over-arch back

Side-squat Kick

The muscles at the front of your thighs work particularly hard in this exercise as you alternate between deep squats and leg extensions.

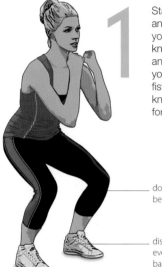

1 Stand with your feet hip-width apart and parallel and your arms relaxed by your sides. As you inhale, bend your knees, push your buttocks backward and downward into a squat, and bend your arms into your chest. Make loose fists, holding them below your chin, knuckles pointing upward and forward, and elbows downward.

do not let knees bend beyond toes

distribute weight evenly between back and front of feet

squeeze buttock

keep supporting leg strong

2 As you exhale, lift one foot off the floor and extend it out to the side. Straighten your supporting leg as you do so and push the heel of your lifted leg away from you to achieve a flexed foot. Hold for a couple of seconds, then inhale and return to the central squat. Repeat with your other leg. When completed, return to standing.

Back Leg Lift

The backward leg lifts in this exercise target not only your glutes, but also your hamstrings (see p.143), strengthening and sculpting your buttocks and the back of your thighs.

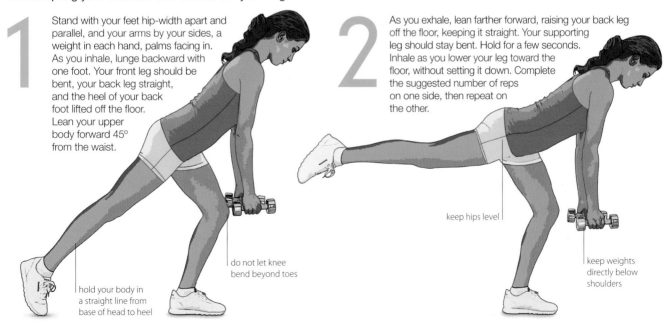

1 Stand with your feet hip-width apart and parallel, and your arms by your sides, a weight in each hand, palms facing in. As you inhale, lunge backward with one foot. Your front leg should be bent, your back leg straight, and the heel of your back foot lifted off the floor. Lean your upper body forward 45° from the waist.

hold your body in a straight line from base of head to heel

do not let knee bend beyond toes

2 As you exhale, lean farther forward, raising your back leg off the floor, keeping it straight. Your supporting leg should stay bent. Hold for a few seconds. Inhale as you lower your leg toward the floor, without setting it down. Complete the suggested number of reps on one side, then repeat on the other.

keep hips level

keep weights directly below shoulders

Kneeling Lean

This backward lean is a great all-around strengthener but provides a particularly good workout for the glutes. It also offers a nice stretch up the front of your thighs—your quads.

1 Kneel on the floor, knees hip-width apart, with a weight in each hand. Raise your buttocks off your heels so that your body forms a straight line from your shoulders to your knees. As you inhale, raise your arms to a 45° angle in front of you, palms facing down.

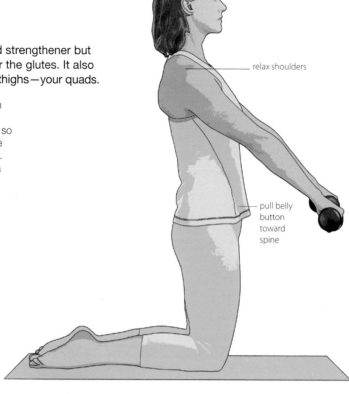

relax shoulders

pull belly button toward spine

2 As you exhale, slowly lean your body backward, keeping your back straight. Simultaneously raise your arms straight out in front of you so that your weights are at shoulder height. Hold for a couple of seconds, then inhale as you bring your arms back down to 45° and your body to the upright position. When finished, relax your arms by your sides.

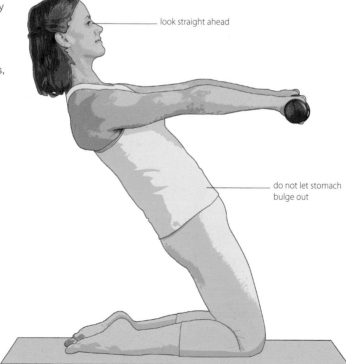

look straight ahead

do not let stomach bulge out

Lunge with Weights

This deep lunge tones and strengthens all your leg muscles at once and also tests your sense of balance.

1 Stand with your feet hip-width apart and parallel. Keep your arms by your sides with a weight in each hand, palms facing inward. Pull your belly button toward your spine to engage your abs. As you inhale, take a large step directly back with one foot and slightly bend your front leg, letting the heel of your back foot come off the floor. Keep your back straight.

let heel lift off floor

ensure feet face directly forward

2 As you exhale, slowly bend your front leg to 90°, lowering your back knee without it touching the floor. Hold for a couple of seconds, then inhale as you straighten your legs and return to standing. Once you have completed the suggested number of reps, repeat on the other side.

do not let knee bend beyond toes

do not let knee rest on floor

Lunge Kick

This deep lunge exercise really puts your glutes and quads to the test to get them in tip-top shape.

1 Stand with your feet hip-width apart and parallel, and your hands on your hips. Pull your belly button toward your spine to engage your abs. As you inhale, lift one leg to hip height in front of you, with your heel pushed forward to flex your foot. Be careful not to lean your body backward as you do so.

relax shoulders

keep supporting leg slightly bent

2 As you exhale, slowly swing your extended leg behind you. Place the toes of that foot on the floor, and bend both legs for a deep lunge. Hold for a couple of seconds, then inhale as you do another forward kick or come up to standing. Repeat the exercise on the other side.

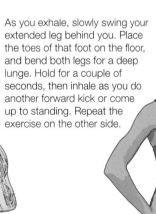

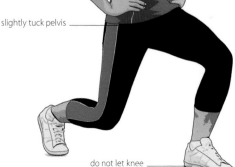

slightly tuck pelvis

do not let knee bend beyond toes

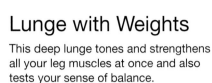

Your hamstrings

The muscles at the backs of your thighs, called hamstrings, may become tight during everyday life, especially if you spend a lot of time sitting at a desk, since the muscles are inactive in this position. The hamstring exercises that follow will not only increase your flexibility and reduce your chances of leg and back injury, but will also help you in your quest for beautiful, sculpted legs.

Hamstring Curl

This classic lower body exercise involves the flexion and extension of each leg from an all-fours position, giving the backs of your thighs a well-deserved workout.

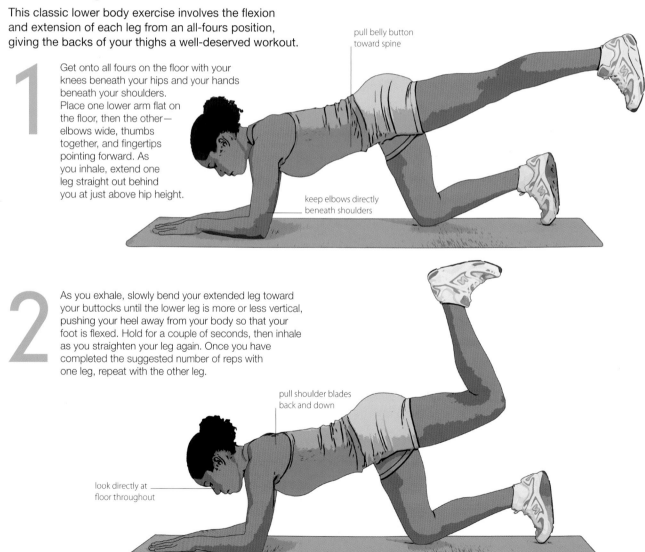

1 Get onto all fours on the floor with your knees beneath your hips and your hands beneath your shoulders. Place one lower arm flat on the floor, then the other— elbows wide, thumbs together, and fingertips pointing forward. As you inhale, extend one leg straight out behind you at just above hip height.

pull belly button toward spine

keep elbows directly beneath shoulders

2 As you exhale, slowly bend your extended leg toward your buttocks until the lower leg is more or less vertical, pushing your heel away from your body so that your foot is flexed. Hold for a couple of seconds, then inhale as you straighten your leg again. Once you have completed the suggested number of reps with one leg, repeat with the other leg.

pull shoulder blades back and down

look directly at floor throughout

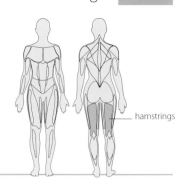

What am I working?

Your hamstrings are the muscles that run from the base of your buttocks to the backs of your knees. They are responsible for moving your legs backward (hip extension) and moving your heels toward your buttocks (knee flexion). They also help your hips to flex during forward bending, taking pressure off your lower back. Keeping them strong will boost your all-around lower body mobility.

hamstrings

Mini Bridge

This mini back bend provides a good stretch for the whole front of your body and a great workout for the whole back of your body, particularly the back of your thighs.

1 Lie flat on your back with your legs and feet together and your arms relaxed by your sides, palms facing down. Push your heels away from your body so that your feet are flexed and press your shoulders and arms into the floor. Look straight ahead to keep your neck long. Inhale to prepare.

pull belly button toward spine

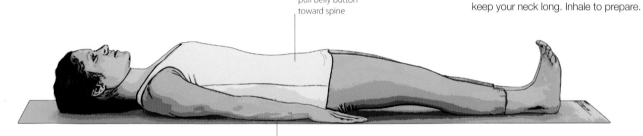

maintain small gap between floor and lower back

2 As you exhale, strongly engage your abs and the backs of your thighs to lift your buttocks off the floor, pressing your shoulders and arms into the floor as you do so. Your entire body weight should now be balanced between your head, shoulders, arms, hands, and feet. Hold for a couple of seconds, then inhale as you lower yourself to the floor.

leave space for an imaginary orange between chin and chest

do not let stomach bulge out

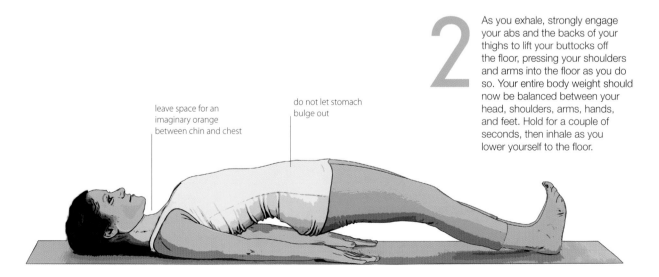

Your inner and outer thighs

While everyday activities such as walking and climbing stairs work the front and back thigh muscles (the quads and hamstrings, see pp.137 and 143), the muscles on the sides of your thighs—called adductors and abductors—often get neglected since they are activated only during sideways leg movement. The following exercises will rectify this, giving amazing definition all over your upper legs.

Plié

This ballet-based exercise is essentially a squat done with turned-out legs and feet: the outward angling works your inner thighs particularly hard during the movement.

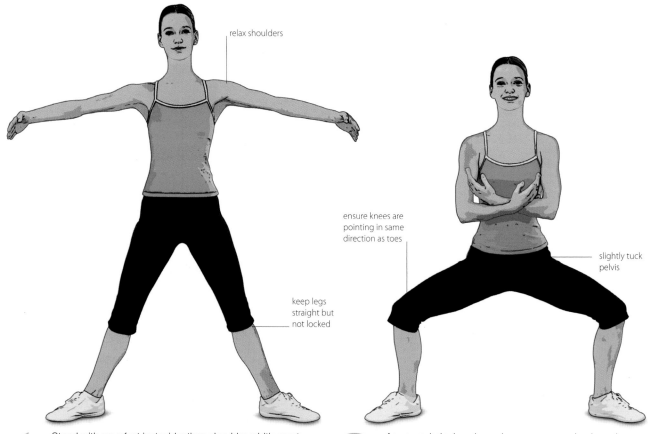

relax shoulders

keep legs straight but not locked

ensure knees are pointing in same direction as toes

slightly tuck pelvis

1 Stand with your feet just wider than shoulder-width apart, toes pointing diagonally outward. Imagine there is a piece of thread pulling you upward from the top of your head. Pull your belly button toward your spine to engage your abs. As you inhale, raise your arms out to the sides and hold them at shoulder height, palms curved forward.

2 As you exhale, bend your knees over your heels and swing your arms inward, across your body, so that your wrists cross at chest height. Keep your back upright throughout. Hold for a couple of seconds, then inhale as you come back up to standing, with arms out. When finished, bring your arms back down to your sides.

What am I working?

Your adductors are the muscles on your inner thighs—from your groin to your knee—that are responsible for moving your legs inward across your body. Your abductors, on your outer thighs, move your legs out to the side, away from your body. It is important to keep these muscles healthy and balanced in order to maintain maximum range of movement through your legs.

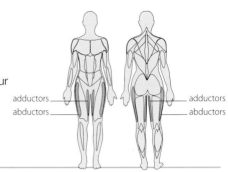

adductors
abductors

adductors
abductors

Ball Squeeze

This exercise is more challenging than the Plié (see left) because the ball adds extra resistance. To get the most from it, squeeze your inner thighs and buttocks throughout.

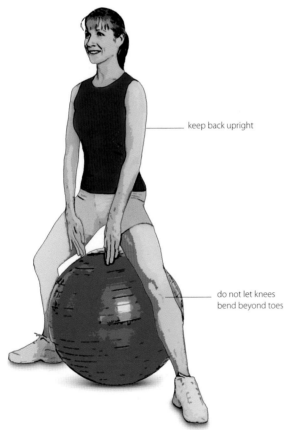

keep back upright

do not let knees bend beyond toes

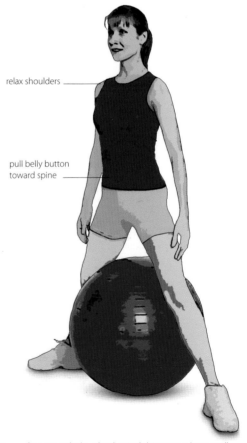

relax shoulders

pull belly button toward spine

1 Straddle the exercise ball with your legs wide enough that you could squeeze your knees against the ball. Point your toes diagonally outward and relax your arms by your sides. As you inhale, bend your knees into the plié position, with both your knees and toes turned outward. Touch the center of the ball with your fingertips for support.

2 As you exhale, slowly straighten your legs until your knees and inner thighs are pressing against the ball—really squeeze them here. Imagine a piece of thread pulling you upward from the top of your head. When you have finished, relax your leg muscles and step away from the ball.

Side-lying Lower Leg Lift

The inner thigh muscles, called the adductors, are particularly difficult to target in isolation but this leg-lifting exercise will really hit the spot.

1 Lie on your side. Bend your lower arm and rest your head on your hand. Place the other hand on the floor in front of your chest for support. As you inhale, bring the foot of your top leg onto the floor in front of the thigh of your lower leg.

2 As you exhale, lift your lower leg off the floor, keeping the rest of your body still. Do not let yourself roll forward or backward as you do so. Hold for a couple of seconds, then inhale as you lower your leg to the floor again. Once you have completed the suggested number of reps on one side, turn onto your other side and repeat.

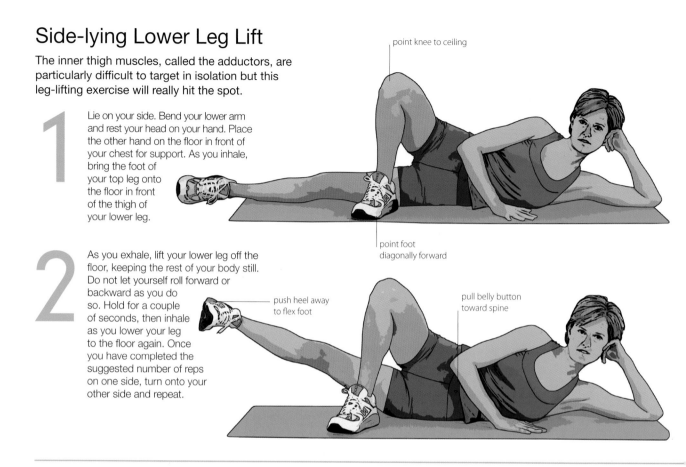

point knee to ceiling

point foot diagonally forward

push heel away to flex foot

pull belly button toward spine

Side-lying Leg Circle

This exercise is a side-lying version of a ballet step called the "rond de jambe," which means "circling of the leg." This large circular movement is an all-around lower body workout.

1 Lie on your side on the floor. Bend your elbows out to the sides, placing your lower elbow on the floor and resting your head in your hand. Point the top elbow to the ceiling, with your hand behind your head. Ensure that your hips, knees, and feet are vertically stacked. As you inhale, bring your legs forward on the diagonal, keeping them straight as you do so, and raise your top leg to hip height.

pull elbow back and up

pull belly button toward spine

Side-lying Upper Leg Lift

This exercise requires lateral leg movement away from the body—a motion that specifically targets your outer thigh muscles, called the abductors. Toned thighs, here we come!

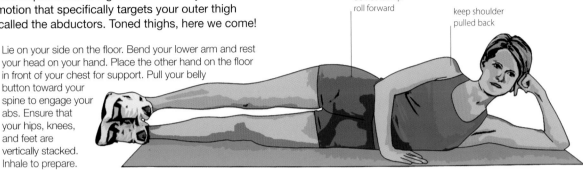

1 Lie on your side on the floor. Bend your lower arm and rest your head on your hand. Place the other hand on the floor in front of your chest for support. Pull your belly button toward your spine to engage your abs. Ensure that your hips, knees, and feet are vertically stacked. Inhale to prepare.

do not let hip roll forward

keep shoulder pulled back

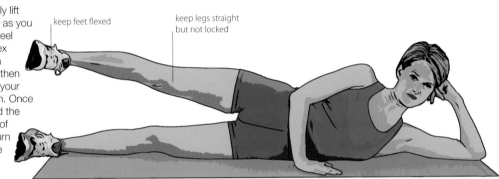

2 As you exhale, slowly lift your top leg as high as you can, pushing your heel away from you to flex your foot. Hold for a couple of seconds, then inhale as you lower your leg to the floor again. Once you have completed the suggested number of reps on one side, turn onto your other side and repeat.

keep feet flexed

keep legs straight but not locked

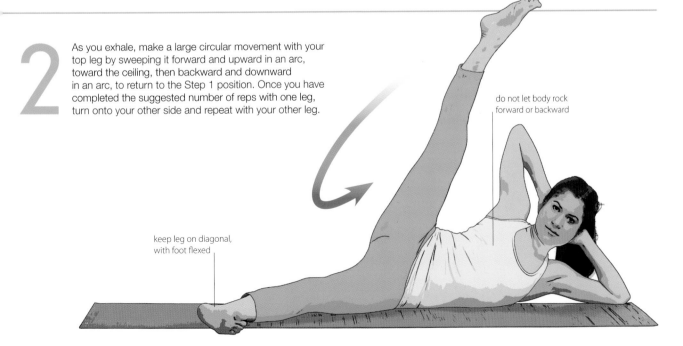

2 As you exhale, make a large circular movement with your top leg by sweeping it forward and upward in an arc, toward the ceiling, then backward and downward in an arc, to return to the Step 1 position. Once you have completed the suggested number of reps with one leg, turn onto your other side and repeat with your other leg.

do not let body rock forward or backward

keep leg on diagonal, with foot flexed

Your lower legs

The muscles on the front and back of your lower legs play an important role in enabling you to carry out activities such as walking and running. They are also key players in promoting lower body balance and alignment, and therefore overall good posture. The exercises that follow will help you to keep your lower legs strong, shapely, and healthy—for optimal daily performance.

Heel Raise against Wall

This exercise increases lower leg strength, boosts foot mobility, and enhances balance. Once you are confident doing it with the wall for support, try it freestanding.

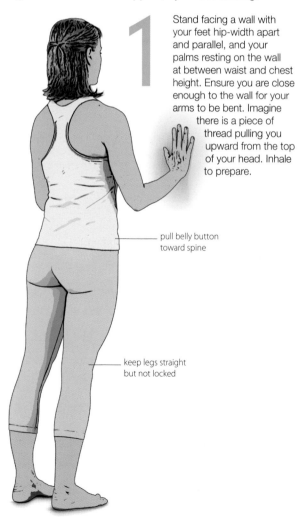

1 Stand facing a wall with your feet hip-width apart and parallel, and your palms resting on the wall at between waist and chest height. Ensure you are close enough to the wall for your arms to be bent. Imagine there is a piece of thread pulling you upward from the top of your head. Inhale to prepare.

pull belly button toward spine

keep legs straight but not locked

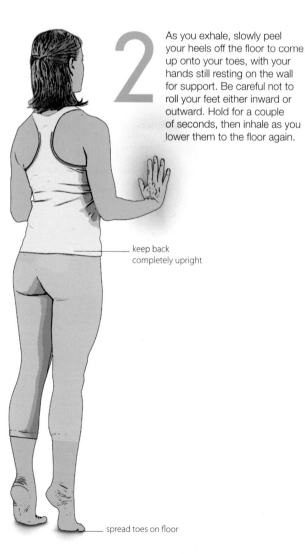

2 As you exhale, slowly peel your heels off the floor to come up onto your toes, with your hands still resting on the wall for support. Be careful not to roll your feet either inward or outward. Hold for a couple of seconds, then inhale as you lower them to the floor again.

keep back completely upright

spread toes on floor

What am I working?

Your gastrocnemius is the main calf muscle, which runs from the back of your knee to your heel, and gives your calf its shape. The soleus is the smaller muscle beneath this. Together, they enable you to lift your heels off the floor. Your tibialis anterior is at the front of your leg, running vertically alongside your shinbone. It enables you to raise the front of your feet off the floor.

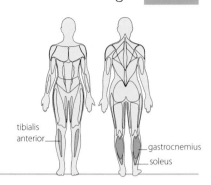

tibialis anterior

gastrocnemius

soleus

Heel–toe Rock

This exercise uses a rocking motion to strengthen not only your calves and ankles but also your shins, all of which come under a lot of pressure every day.

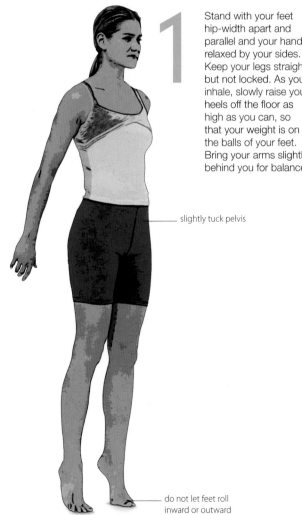

1 Stand with your feet hip-width apart and parallel and your hands relaxed by your sides. Keep your legs straight but not locked. As you inhale, slowly raise your heels off the floor as high as you can, so that your weight is on the balls of your feet. Bring your arms slightly behind you for balance.

slightly tuck pelvis

do not let feet roll inward or outward

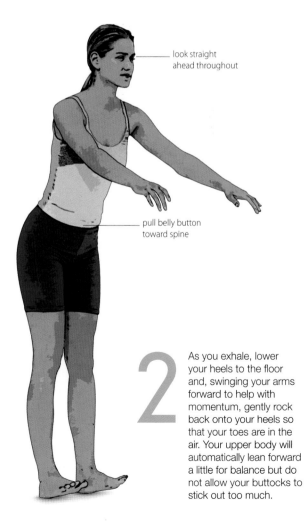

look straight ahead throughout

pull belly button toward spine

2 As you exhale, lower your heels to the floor and, swinging your arms forward to help with momentum, gently rock back onto your heels so that your toes are in the air. Your upper body will automatically lean forward a little for balance but do not allow your buttocks to stick out too much.

Your total body

While exercises that target particular muscles in isolation are enormously useful, it is also helpful to know some exercises that can give you an immediate all-over body blast when desired. Apart from toning more than one area at a time, these compound exercises burn off more calories than isolated exercises and improve your coordination, balance, strength, endurance, and posture.

Twisting Punch

The simultaneous flexion of your legs and feet, along with the extension, flexion, and rotation of your arms, and rotation at the waist make this exercise a fantastic all-over body sculptor.

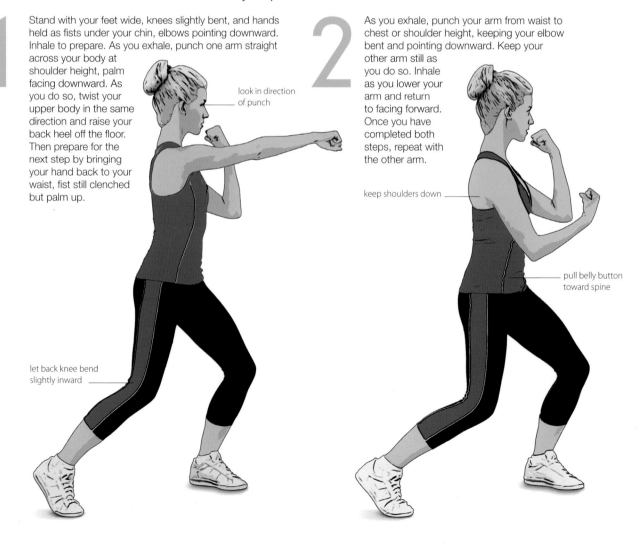

1 Stand with your feet wide, knees slightly bent, and hands held as fists under your chin, elbows pointing downward. Inhale to prepare. As you exhale, punch one arm straight across your body at shoulder height, palm facing downward. As you do so, twist your upper body in the same direction and raise your back heel off the floor. Then prepare for the next step by bringing your hand back to your waist, fist still clenched but palm up.

look in direction of punch

let back knee bend slightly inward

2 As you exhale, punch your arm from waist to chest or shoulder height, keeping your elbow bent and pointing downward. Keep your other arm still as you do so. Inhale as you lower your arm and return to facing forward. Once you have completed both steps, repeat with the other arm.

keep shoulders down

pull belly button toward spine

front upper body

back upper body

front lower body

back lower body

What am I working?

The exercises in this section work as many muscle groups (and in particular as many potential problem areas) as possible at the same time. This involves simultaneous dynamic movements in different planes of motion (see pp.24–25) by different parts of the body—for maximal sculpting. Most exercises will work both your upper and lower body.

Inverted Leg Lift

This exercise is a great total body strengthener—you hold your abs tight against gravity, use your arms and legs for support, and extend your legs backward to work your butt.

1 Get onto all fours on the floor, with your knees beneath your hips and your hands beneath your shoulders. As you inhale, tuck your toes under, lift your knees off the floor, and straighten both your legs and arms so that your body forms an inverted V-shape. Lift one heel off the floor and point the toes of that foot.

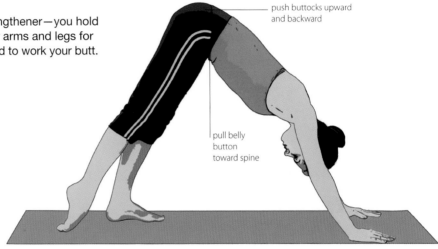

push buttocks upward and backward

pull belly button toward spine

2 As you exhale, slowly lift your leg behind you, keeping the rest of your body still as you do so and pointing the toes of your extended leg. Hold for a couple of seconds, then inhale as you come back to the inverted V-shape. Repeat with your other leg. When completed, return to all fours and slowly come up to standing.

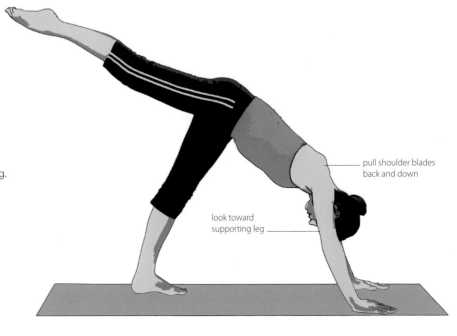

pull shoulder blades back and down

look toward supporting leg

Plié with Lateral Raise

The simultaneous leg bend and lateral arm raise in this exercise mean that both your upper and lower body are worked.

1 Stand with your feet slightly wider than shoulder-width apart and turned diagonally outward, your arms relaxed by your sides, and a weight in each hand, palms facing inward. Imagine there is a piece of thread pulling you upward from the top of your head. Pull your belly button toward your spine to engage your abs. Inhale to prepare.

slightly tuck pelvis

keep legs straight but not locked

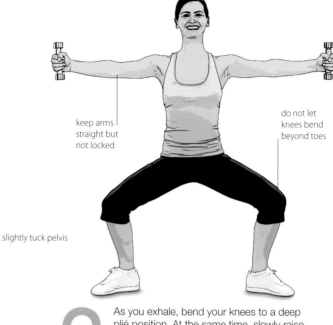

keep arms straight but not locked

do not let knees bend beyond toes

2 As you exhale, bend your knees to a deep plié position. At the same time, slowly raise the weights to the sides until your arms are at shoulder height, palms facing forward. Hold for a few seconds, then inhale as you come back up to standing.

Lunge and Twist

This high diagonal arm stretch, followed by a deep lunge, gives not only your legs and arms a great workout, but also your back and waist.

1 Stand with your feet hip-width apart, holding a weight between your hands at hip height in front of you. Inhale to prepare. As you exhale, stride your right foot forward, raise your weight above your head, and twist your body and arms to your left and backward, while keeping both your hips and gaze pointing forward. Hold for a couple of seconds, ending in an inhalation.

pull belly button toward spine

keep legs straight but not locked

keep knee in line with heel

aim to have lower leg parallel with floor

2 Bring your hands down to waist-height, and as you exhale, bend your legs into a deep lunge, raising your back heel off the floor. Then twist your body to the right and lower the weight toward the little toe of your front foot. Hold for a couple of seconds, then inhale as you straighten your legs and return to upright. Complete both steps on one side, then repeat on the other side.

Lateral Lift

This exercise has lateral arm and leg lifts, which define your shoulders and thighs. It also targets your core as you work to stop your body from leaning sideways during the movement.

1 Stand with your feet hip-width apart and parallel, and your arms relaxed by your sides, with a weight in each hand. Imagine there is a piece of thread pulling you upward from the top of your head. Pull your belly button toward your spine to engage your abs. Inhale to prepare.

2 As you exhale, lift one leg sideways, straightening and pulling up through your supporting leg to stay upright. At the same time, raise your arms out to the sides until they are at shoulder height—straight but not locked. Hold for a few seconds. As you inhale, lower your arms and leg to return to standing. Repeat on the other side.

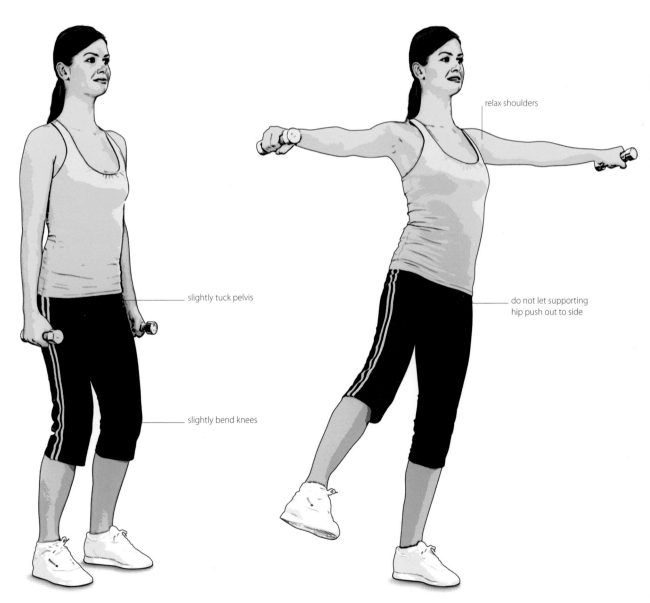

slightly tuck pelvis

slightly bend knees

relax shoulders

do not let supporting hip push out to side

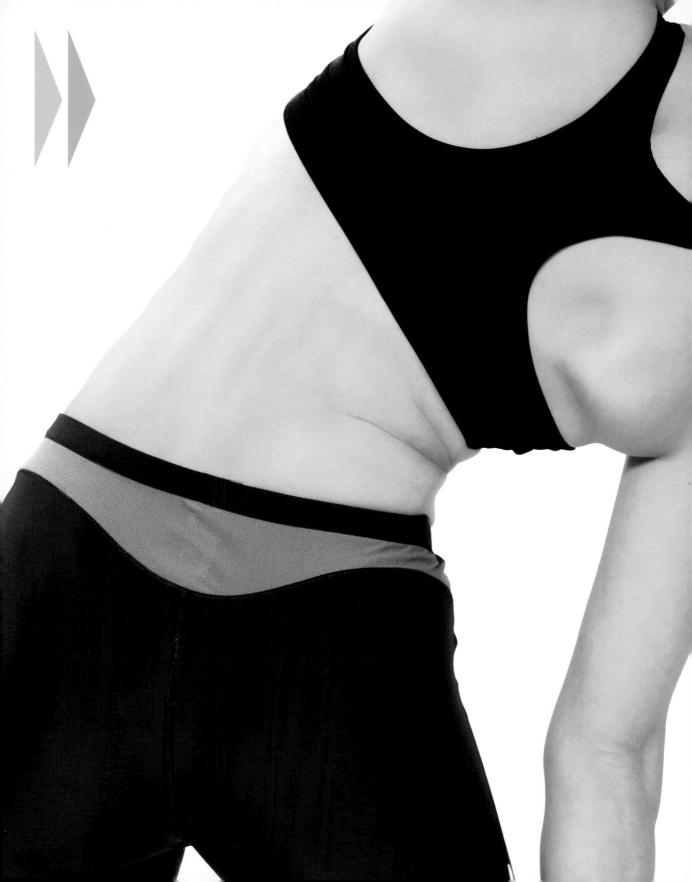

Stretching

Regular stretching lengthens your muscles to keep them healthy and supple, counteracting the wear and tear of everyday actions, which can make them tight and sore. Some people think that you have to be super fit and flexible to enjoy and benefit from stretching, but this is simply not the case. No matter how athletic (or not) you are, the exercises that follow will:

- relax and energize your body

- release any tension held in your hardworking muscles

- maintain optimal mobility, which ensures maximal fat-burning capacity, too

- increase flexibility, making everyday activities easier

- address any muscular imbalances to restore a sense of healthy alignment

- improve your posture, preventing the shoulder-hunching that aging can cause

- create fluidity of movement throughout your body, enhancing elegance

- reduce the chance of injuries due to muscle tightness

Why stretch?

As you focus on trying to get in better shape, stretching can often be overlooked in favor of cardio and resistance exercises. However, stretching plays a vital role in helping to sculpt your body and keep it in optimal working order. Not only does it help to keep you as flexible as possible, but it also keeps you in good natural alignment with a strong, elegant, and balanced posture.

Maximize your range of safe movement

Flexibility refers to the range of motion at your joints as a result of the action of your muscles. Stretching increases this range of motion, making actions of all kinds easier, whether reaching for a top shelf, bending to pick something up, or sitting cross-legged. However, in addition to increasing your flexibility, stretching exercises will help to stabilize your joints, providing a stronger base from which your bones can move and reducing the risk of injury during all other movement. The older you get, the more important stretching becomes, since you naturally start losing elasticity in the connective tissues around your muscles—the very tissue that enables your flexibility in the first place.

Enhance your youthful elegance

The nature of stretching means that it creates length through your muscles, counteracting the natural impact of gravity. Stretching exercises can therefore help to make you look taller, leaner, and more elegant—think of the grace and poise of a ballerina. Believe it or not, they can also help to prevent or smooth out wrinkles in certain areas, such as across the chest. They therefore help to keep you feeling and looking youthful for longer.

Balance your body and mind

As we go about our daily actions, we each tend to carry out certain types of movement more than others (see pp.24–25), especially sitting and standing. This means

that not all our muscles get used on a regular basis and certain ones can become short and tight, while others become loose and weak. Stretching allows you to correct this imbalance: as you stretch to lengthen one muscle, its opposing muscle automatically shortens.

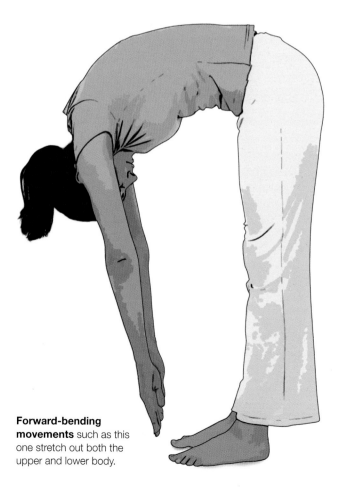

Forward-bending movements such as this one stretch out both the upper and lower body.

For example, if you stretch your hamstring (on the back of your thigh), your quadriceps (on the front of your thigh) shortens. Other sets of opposing muscles include:

- Upper back/Chest
- Lower back/Abdominals
- Biceps/Triceps

It's important to stretch both sides until they feel in balance. Using long, slow stretching exercises to balance out your body also encourages your mind to come more into balance, leaving you feeling more relaxed.

Is stretching for everyone?

Some people are naturally more flexible than others due to the genetic architecture of their bones and joints. But whatever your starting point of flexibility, there is always progress to be made, since stretching exercises can be done at different intensities to suit absolutely anyone. It's not about being super-athletic or becoming ultra-flexible; it's simply about doing movements that will make your daily actions easier to perform and will keep your body supple and mobile for longer. If a position seems too strong or challenging at first, just do it with whatever minimal movement you can. It's how well you do a stretch that matters, not how far you can reach in that stretch, so never sacrifice good form and alignment for what you perceive as more of a stretch.

The effect of tight muscles

No matter where muscle tightness occurs, it limits your range of movement. Below are some of the specific consequences of tension in your main muscles. The stretching exercises that follow will help to avoid these problems, enhancing your overall well-being:

Tight neck = jutting chin, tension headaches
Tight shoulders = restricted arm movement, hunched posture, short-looking neck
Tight lower back = bulging stomach, compressed vertebrae and nerves, possible sciatica
Tight chest = collapsed (and wrinkled) chest, hunched posture, possible sore shoulders and arms
Tight arms = stiffness or soreness in hands and arms, possible repetitive strain injury
Tight waist and front hips = difficulty doing twisting actions, lower body stiffness, possible knee problems
Tight hamstrings = pressure on lower back
Tight quads = difficulty kneeling
Tight inner thighs = difficulty sitting cross-legged
Tight calves = possible Achilles tendon injuries.

Lateral stretches such as this one open up the whole side of your body, while the wide-legged position stretches your inner thighs.

How to stretch

Stretching is a simple way to enhance your posture, balance, and flexibility. But it's important to choose the exercises most relevant to your needs at any given time, depending on where in your body there are areas of tension, stiffness, or imbalance. It's also essential to know the fundamentals of stretching so that you can do your chosen exercises as safely and effectively as possible.

Types of stretching

Ballistic: where you adopt a certain position and bounce to encourage a deeper stretch, but this can be difficult to do safely without expert guidance.

Dynamic: where you continuously move your joints through their range of motion, such as Shoulder Circling and Elbow Circling (see p.164).

Static or active: where you adopt a position and simply hold it for a certain number of seconds so that you can relax into it, such as the Calf Lunge (see p.190) and many of the other exercises in this section.

Passive: a type of static stretching where you adopt a certain position and apply some form of resistance in order to deepen the stretch by increasing the range of movement through which the joint moves. The "resistance" can come in the form of an external object, such as a towel, a step, or a resistance band (see p.107) or from pressure being applied by a second person or by another part of your own body, such as in Triceps Overhead (see p.180), where you use one hand to ease your other hand farther down your back.

Isometric: a type of static stretching where you once again adopt a certain position and apply a form of resistance in order to intensify the stretch, but this time by creating tension in the muscle that is being stretched, such as in the Corner Press (see p.174), where you use a wall as resistance.

How far should I stretch?

Whatever form of stretching you do, it's crucial to work at a level that is safe and comfortable for you. This means stretching to a point where you feel a healthy amount of tension within the target muscle(s), without any pain. If you feel any discomfort, lessen the stretch position a little.

It's best to hold static stretches for at least 8 seconds, maintaining correct alignment throughout; we suggest 10 seconds for most of the exercises in the pages that follow to be sure that your muscle fibers are given enough time to adapt to the lengthening. However, feel free to hold for longer. With regular practice, you'll probably soon achieve a greater range of motion within the same time.

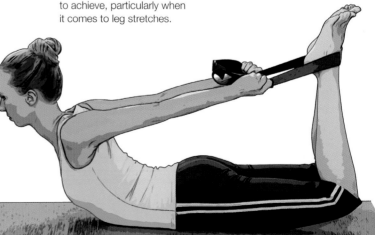

Using a resistance band can help you to get into certain positions that you otherwise might not be able to achieve, particularly when it comes to leg stretches.

Top tips for stretching

- Choose stretching exercises that target the areas of your body where you feel the most tightness, stiffness, or imbalance.
- Aim for a balanced body. You may find that you are more flexible on one side than the other, or on the front or back of your body, so vary the frequency and intensity of your exercises on each side as you need to.
- Be willing to adapt. Accept that you'll be less flexible on some days than on others and respect this—never overstep what your body is instinctively telling you. If you need to decrease the intensity, lessen the range of movement through which you are putting the joint(s) in question; if you don't feel adequate tension, try increasing the range of motion on your next exhalation.
- Work in a slow, controlled manner. Avoid any jerky, unstable movements that could damage your joints.
- Hold each stretch steadily. This will bring both your body and mind into stillness, which is of benefit to your nervous system (see p.22), as well as your muscles.

- Remember to breathe! Always prepare on an inhalation, and move into, or deepen, your position on an exhalation. After all, your muscles need oxygen in order to operate.
- Use stretching as a chance to relax. Doing some stretching exercises at the end of a long workout or a long day can be a lovely (and healthy!) way to unwind.

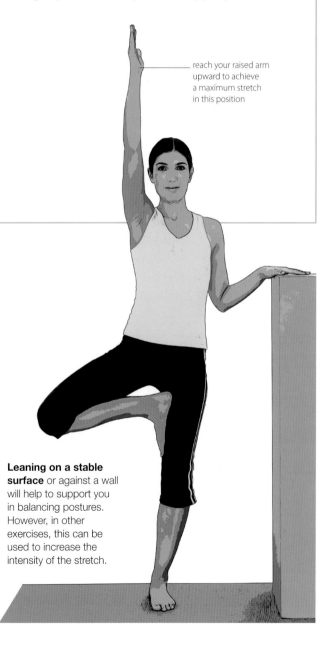

reach your raised arm upward to achieve a maximum stretch in this position

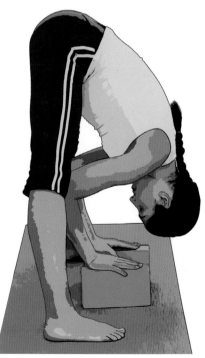

Using a block can help you to get into positions that you might otherwise find hard to achieve, particularly when it comes to forward bends.

Leaning on a stable surface or against a wall will help to support you in balancing postures. However, in other exercises, this can be used to increase the intensity of the stretch.

Your head and neck

Your neck muscles come under great pressure supporting the substantial weight of your head. As a result, they can become stiff and sore. The neck exercises that follow will ease tension and restore healthy movement to your neck and head. Meanwhile, the eye exercises will work your eye muscles through their full range of movement, helping to keep your eyes feeling refreshed and vibrant.

Eye Exercises

These simple eye movements are both relaxing and strengthening, helping to give your eyes a boost if they feel tired from the everyday pressures placed on them.

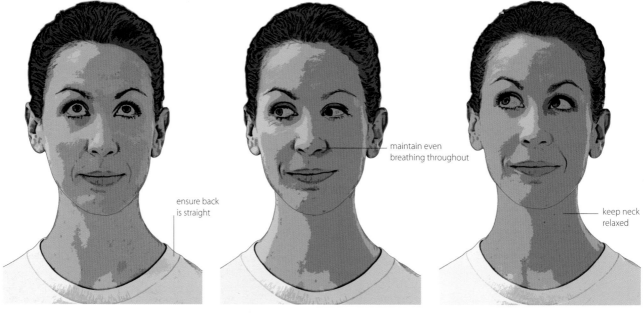

maintain even breathing throughout

ensure back is straight

keep neck relaxed

1 Roll your eyes directly upward and hold for 5 seconds, without moving your neck or head. Then slowly roll your eyes to look directly downward and hold for 5 seconds, before returning them to the center. Do this 5 times, then close your eyes for about 30 seconds to relax them.

2 Roll your eyes as far as you can to one side and hold for 5 seconds without moving your neck or head. Then slowly roll your eyes to the other side and hold for 5 seconds, before returning them to the center. Do this 5 times, then close your eyes for about 30 seconds to relax them.

3 Roll your eyes diagonally upward and hold for 5 seconds. Then roll your eyes to the diagonally opposite corner and hold for 5 seconds, before returning them to the center. Repeat on the other diagonal axis. Do this 5 times, then close your eyes for about 30 seconds to relax them.

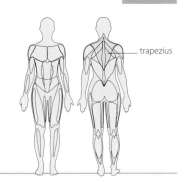

trapezius

What am I working?

Forming a large diamond shape on your back, the two triangular trapezius muscles (one on each side) cover your upper back, shoulders, and neck, and are involved in all head movements. The sternocleidomastoid muscle (not shown), runs diagonally down each side of your neck and is responsible for moving your head from side to side.

Head Turn

This simple exercise rotates your head from side to side, giving your neck a much-deserved stretch and enhancing its mobility. It can easily be done anywhere, any time.

Sit or stand comfortably. Imagine there is a piece of thread pulling you upward from the top of your head. Inhale to prepare. Then exhale as you slowly turn your head as far as possible to one side, leading with your chin. Hold for 4 seconds, then inhale as you return to center. Repeat on the other side.

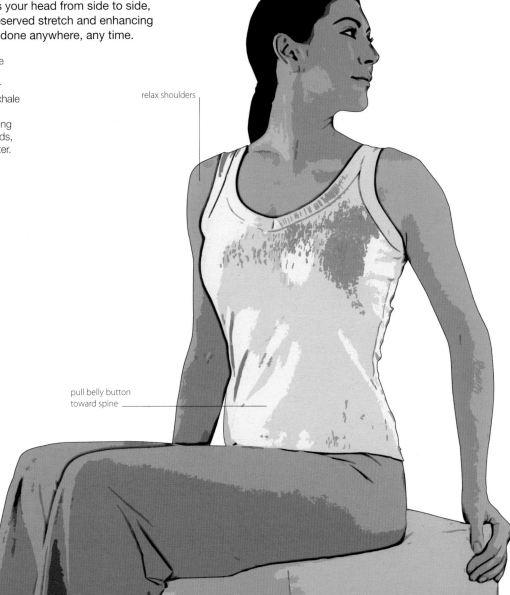

relax shoulders

pull belly button toward spine

Stretch and Roll-down

This exercise involves first a chest-opening movement, stretching the front of your neck, then a deep stretch down the back of your neck and upper back.

1 Sit comfortably. Imagine there is a piece of thread pulling you upward from the top of your head, and pull your belly button toward your spine to engage your abs. As you inhale, bend your arms and lightly clasp your hands behind your head, with your elbows out to the sides.

2 As you inhale, open and lift your chest, tilt your head slightly backward, and look upward. Your elbows should now be pushed slightly backward and your back ever so slightly arched. Be sure that you keep your abs engaged for support. Hold for 10 seconds.

3 As you exhale, gently tuck your chin into your neck, let your elbows come forward, and roll your head down as far as is comfortable so that you are looking toward your chest. Hold for 10 seconds, then inhale as you come up to sit tall.

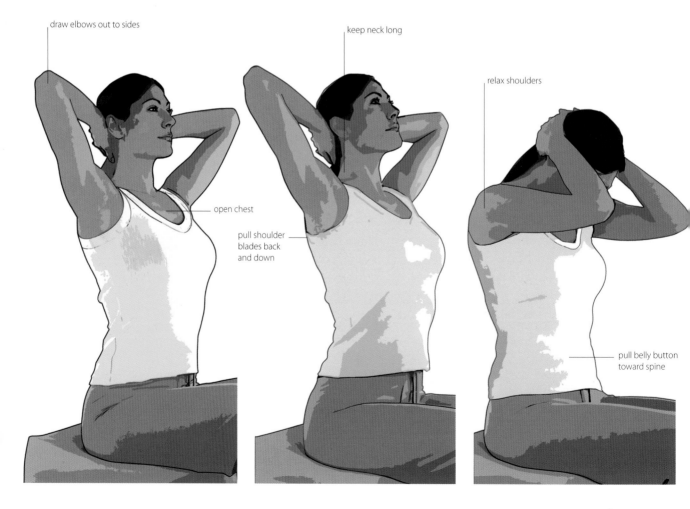

draw elbows out to sides

keep neck long

relax shoulders

open chest

pull shoulder blades back and down

pull belly button toward spine

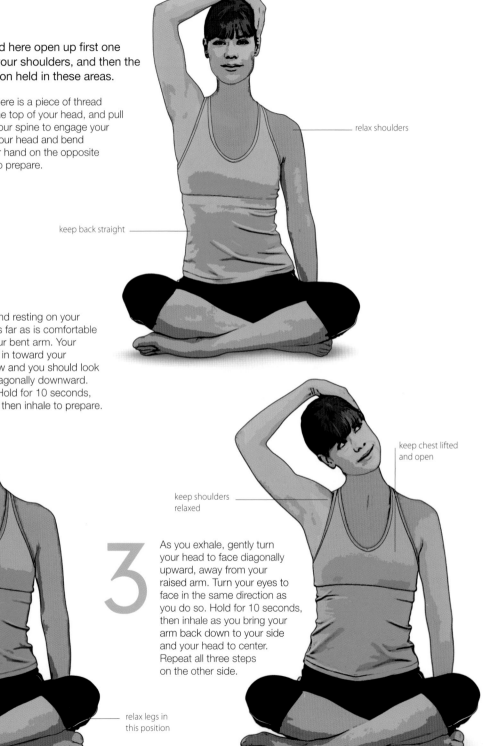

Neck Side Bend

The lateral neck stretches involved here open up first one side of your neck and the top of your shoulders, and then the other, helping to release any tension held in these areas.

1 Sit comfortably. Imagine there is a piece of thread pulling you upward from the top of your head, and pull your belly button toward your spine to engage your abs. Raise one arm over your head and bend it to place the palm of your hand on the opposite side of your head. Inhale to prepare.

relax shoulders

keep back straight

2 As you exhale, use the hand resting on your head to ease your head as far as is comfortable toward the shoulder of your bent arm. Your head should now be tilted in toward your elbow and you should look diagonally downward. Hold for 10 seconds, then inhale to prepare.

do not let elbow fall forward

relax legs in this position

3 As you exhale, gently turn your head to face diagonally upward, away from your raised arm. Turn your eyes to face in the same direction as you do so. Hold for 10 seconds, then inhale as you bring your arm back down to your side and your head to center. Repeat all three steps on the other side.

keep chest lifted and open

keep shoulders relaxed

Your shoulders

Our shoulders can become rounded and stiff as we hunch over our desks, laptops, and cell phones each day. The stretching exercises that follow will counteract this, helping to release any tension in this area. The exercises will also increase your range of upper body movement and help to prevent any shoulder injuries—particularly helpful if you play sports such as tennis or golf.

Shoulder Circling

This simple rotation mobilizes your shoulder muscles and limbers up your shoulder joints, strengthening these areas and eliminating stiffness. It can also be done sitting down.

Stand tall, with your arms relaxed by your sides. Imagine there is a piece of thread pulling you upward from the top of your |head, and inhale to prepare. Then exhale as you start to circle your shoulders backward. Do this 8 times, then circle them forward 8 times.

open and
lift chest

keep legs straight
but not locked

Elbow Circling

Using your bent arms as levers during this rotation exercise provides a deeper stretch for your shoulders than Shoulder Circling (see left). It also gives your triceps a little workout.

Stand tall, imagining there is a piece of thread pulling you upward from the top of your head. Place your palms loosely on your shoulders, fingertips facing backward and elbows forward. Inhale to prepare. Then exhale as you circle your elbows backward. Do this 8 times, then circle them forward 8 times.

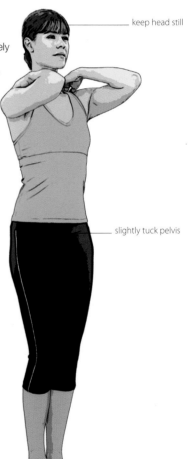

keep head still

slightly tuck pelvis

What am I working?

The front and back deltoids are the main muscles in your shoulders and are responsible for the overall mobility of your shoulder joints (see also p.109). The rotator cuff muscles (not shown) are a set of four muscles on each shoulder that help to stabilize the joint, particularly when it is being moved in isolation, such as when throwing a ball or serving during a game of tennis.

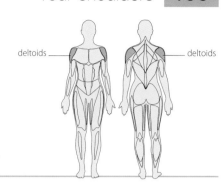

deltoids

deltoids

Arm Cross

This exercise provides a deep stretch for your shoulders and upper arms. It is important to keep your shoulders down during the movement in order to get the most from it.

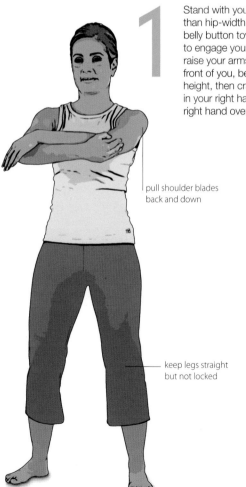

1 Stand with your feet slightly wider than hip-width apart. Pull your belly button toward your spine to engage your abs. As you inhale, raise your arms out horizontally in front of you, bend them in at chest height, then cradle your left elbow in your right hand and rest your right hand over your left elbow.

pull shoulder blades back and down

keep legs straight but not locked

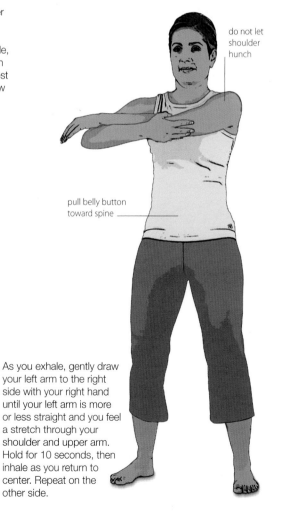

do not let shoulder hunch

pull belly button toward spine

2 As you exhale, gently draw your left arm to the right side with your right hand until your left arm is more or less straight and you feel a stretch through your shoulder and upper arm. Hold for 10 seconds, then inhale as you return to center. Repeat on the other side.

Backward Arm Raise

This exercise provides a workout for your core abs as well as offering a good strong stretch through your shoulders and arms.

1 Stand with your feet hip-width apart and parallel. Clasp your hands behind your back, arms straight and relaxed, and palms facing inward. Imagine there is a piece of thread pulling you upward from the top of your head. Pull your belly button toward your spine to engage your abs. As you inhale, raise your clasped hands slightly upward, away from your body.

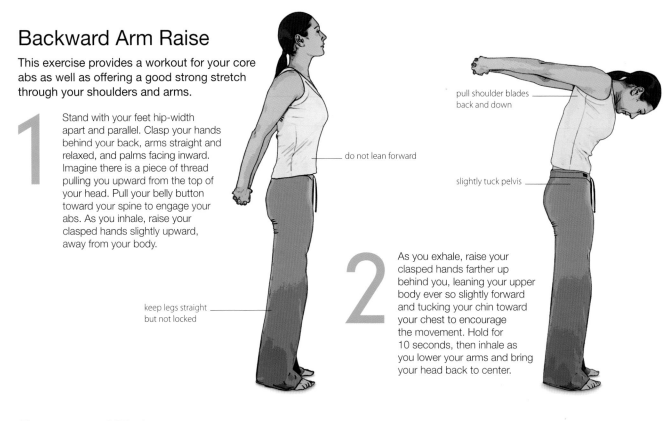

do not lean forward

keep legs straight but not locked

pull shoulder blades back and down

slightly tuck pelvis

2 As you exhale, raise your clasped hands farther up behind you, leaning your upper body ever so slightly forward and tucking your chin toward your chest to encourage the movement. Hold for 10 seconds, then inhale as you lower your arms and bring your head back to center.

Press and Twist

This exercise stretches first the front of your shoulders, upper arms, and chest; then, one side at a time, the back of your shoulders, upper arms, and neck.

1 Stand with your feet hip-width apart in front of a horizontal surface of hip height. Place your hands shoulder-width apart on the surface, fingertips facing inward. Inhale to prepare. As you exhale, bend your elbows to the sides to lower your upper body. Keep your abs engaged as you do so. Hold for 10 seconds, then inhale to prepare.

2 As you exhale, twist your upper body to press one shoulder diagonally downward, toward the opposite hand. Keep your elbows wide when you do so and look in the direction that you are twisting. Hold for 10 seconds, then inhale as you come back to center and exhale as you repeat on the other side. Then slowly come up to standing.

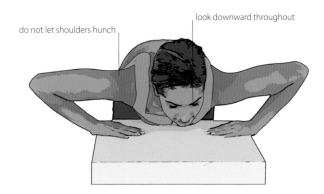

do not let shoulders hunch

look downward throughout

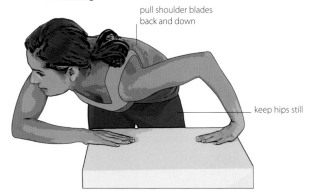

pull shoulder blades back and down

keep hips still

Sideways Lean

This lateral bend gives one side of your body, especially your shoulder, a rewarding stretch, while giving the muscles on the other side of your upper body a good workout.

1 Stand with your feet hip-width apart and parallel. Imagine there is a piece of thread pulling you upward from the top of your head. Pull your belly button toward your spine to engage your abs. As you inhale, raise your arms above your head and clasp your left wrist with your right hand.

2 As you exhale, bend your upper body to the right, keeping your lower body absolutely still and being careful to lean neither forward nor backward. Your left arm should now be straight, while your right one is slightly bent. Hold for 10 seconds, then inhale as you return to center. Repeat on the other side.

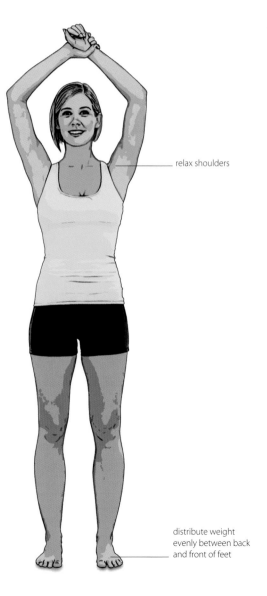

relax shoulders

distribute weight evenly between back and front of feet

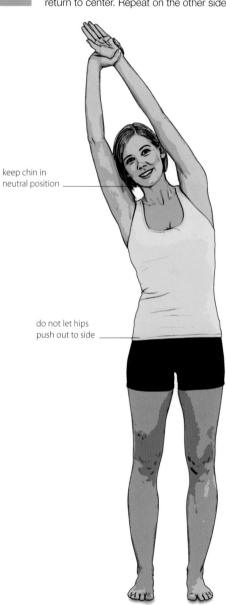

keep chin in neutral position

do not let hips push out to side

Your back

Together with the muscles in the front of your body, the muscles in your back support you in all sitting and standing positions, and also protect your spine. They can therefore end up feeling tired and tight at times. The stretches that follow will help to release any tension in your back, re-energize the area, and also greatly enhance your posture, strength, balance, and flexibility.

Knees to Chest

This exercise stretches out your whole back but lengthens your lower back in particular—an area that often becomes compressed during daily life.

1 Lie on your back on the floor with your knees bent and pointing toward the ceiling, and your feet flat on the floor, hip-width apart. Pull your belly button toward your spine to engage your abs. As you inhale, lift your bent legs toward your chest and place your hands on the back of your upper thighs.

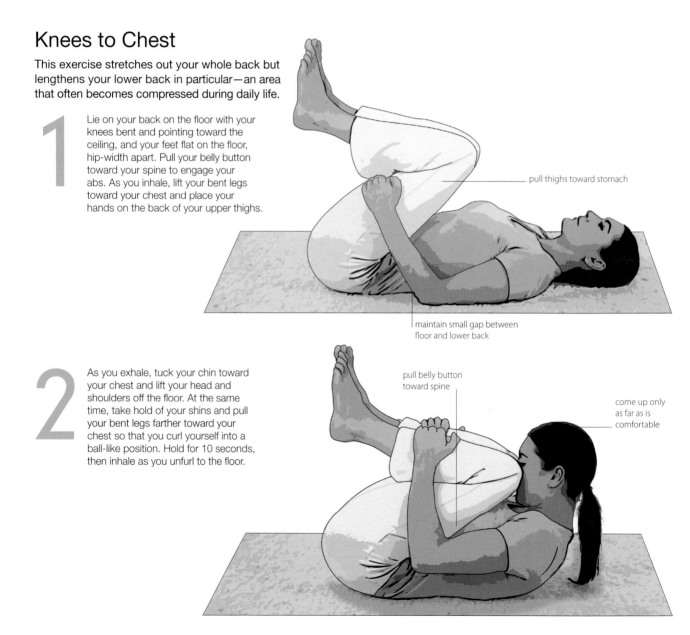

pull thighs toward stomach

maintain small gap between floor and lower back

pull belly button toward spine

come up only as far as is comfortable

2 As you exhale, tuck your chin toward your chest and lift your head and shoulders off the floor. At the same time, take hold of your shins and pull your bent legs farther toward your chest so that you curl yourself into a ball-like position. Hold for 10 seconds, then inhale as you unfurl to the floor.

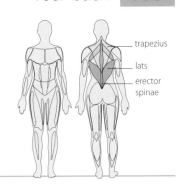

What am I working?

The trapezius is the large muscle that covers your upper and middle back. The lats (latissimus dorsi) are on either side of the middle back, and the erector spinae are the muscles that run down either side of your spine. All of these support and protect your spine as well as enable movement through your back and arms.

Lying Arm Twist

This lying upper body and extended arm rotation gives a nourishing stretch through each side of your body and into your middle back. It is also a fantastic chest opener.

1 Lie on your side on the floor, with your hips, knees, and feet vertically stacked. Reach your arms straight out in front of you, one on top of the other, palms together, and bend your upper legs to 90° in front of you, with your lower legs pointing slightly backward. Inhale to prepare.

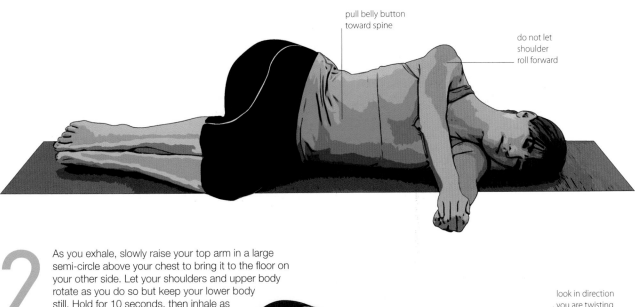

pull belly button toward spine

do not let shoulder roll forward

2 As you exhale, slowly raise your top arm in a large semi-circle above your chest to bring it to the floor on your other side. Let your shoulders and upper body rotate as you do so but keep your lower body still. Hold for 10 seconds, then inhale as you return to the start position. Then turn onto your other side and repeat both steps.

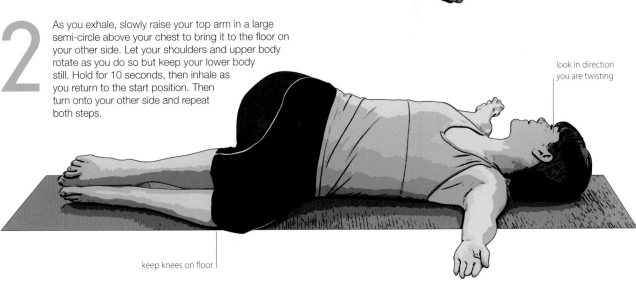

look in direction you are twisting

keep knees on floor

Rounding and Arching

The rounding and arching movements in this exercise give you a fantastic stretch throughout the whole of your back, releasing any tension in the rhomboids in particular.

1 Get onto all fours on the floor with your knees beneath your hips, your hands beneath your shoulders, and your lower legs about hip-width apart and parallel. As you inhale, strongly pull your belly button toward your spine to engage your abs and round your back by tucking both your tailbone and your chin inward. Hold for 10 seconds.

2 As you exhale, untuck your tailbone and head so that your back is once again flat. Continue to lift your tailbone and your head in order to gently arch your back and look diagonally upward, keeping your abs firmly engaged. Hold for 10 seconds, then inhale as you return your back to flat again. Once you have completed the suggested number of reps of both steps, slowly return to sitting or standing.

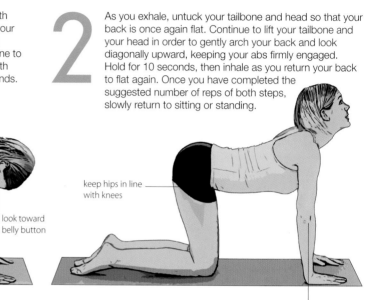

look toward belly button

press hands firmly into floor

keep hips in line with knees

keep arms straight but not locked

All-fours Twist

This nifty exercise curves your spine first to one side, then to the other. It therefore creates a great stretch down each side of your back and enhances general spine mobility.

1 Get onto all fours on the floor with your knees beneath your hips and your hands beneath your shoulders. Pull your belly button toward your spine to engage your abs. Inhale to prepare. As you exhale, swing your hips to one side and turn your head and shoulders to look back toward it. Hold for 10 seconds, ending in an inhalation.

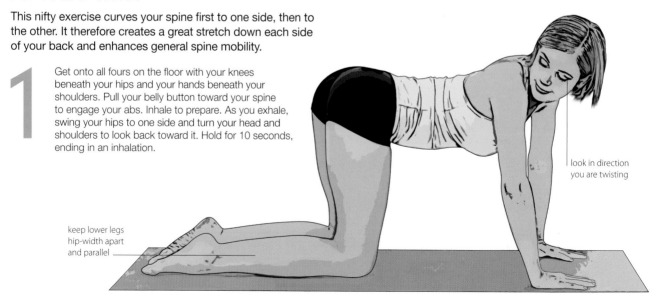

keep lower legs hip-width apart and parallel

look in direction you are twisting

Squat Twist

As well as giving you a fantastic stretch through the middle and top of your back, this squatting and twisting exercise provides a great workout for both your thighs and your waist.

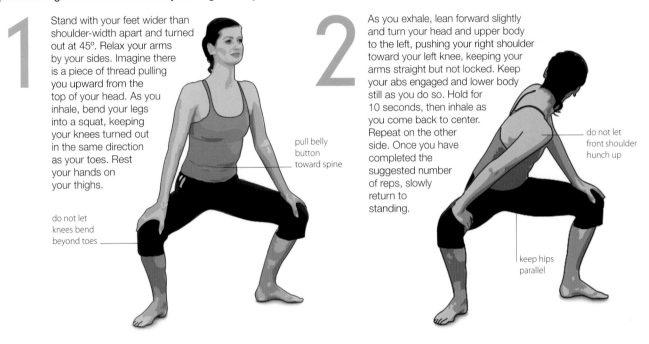

1 Stand with your feet wider than shoulder-width apart and turned out at 45°. Relax your arms by your sides. Imagine there is a piece of thread pulling you upward from the top of your head. As you inhale, bend your legs into a squat, keeping your knees turned out in the same direction as your toes. Rest your hands on your thighs.

pull belly button toward spine

do not let knees bend beyond toes

2 As you exhale, lean forward slightly and turn your head and upper body to the left, pushing your right shoulder toward your left knee, keeping your arms straight but not locked. Keep your abs engaged and lower body still as you do so. Hold for 10 seconds, then inhale as you come back to center. Repeat on the other side. Once you have completed the suggested number of reps, slowly return to standing.

do not let front shoulder hunch up

keep hips parallel

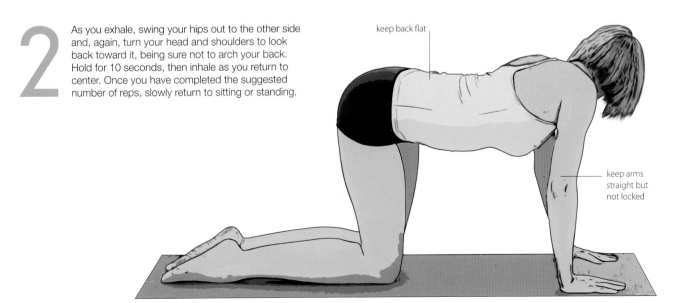

2 As you exhale, swing your hips out to the other side and, again, turn your head and shoulders to look back toward it, being sure not to arch your back. Hold for 10 seconds, then inhale as you return to center. Once you have completed the suggested number of reps, slowly return to sitting or standing.

keep back flat

keep arms straight but not locked

Kneeling Forward Bend

This intense exercise gives your entire back a lovely stretch but is particularly good for your upper back, which is trickier to target and can therefore often feel stiff and "stuck."

1 Kneel on the floor with your knees slightly wider than hip-width apart and your buttocks resting between your heels. Place a towel under your knees for comfort. As you inhale, tuck your toes under and lift your heels off the floor. As you exhale, hold your heels with your hands, tuck your chin to your chest, and lean forward, bending your head toward the floor.

2 Continue to lean forward from this position, aiming to rest the top of your head on the floor, if possible. Continue to pull gently with your hands. Keep your abs engaged and be sure not to overly tuck your head. Hold for 10 seconds, then inhale as you return to the starting position.

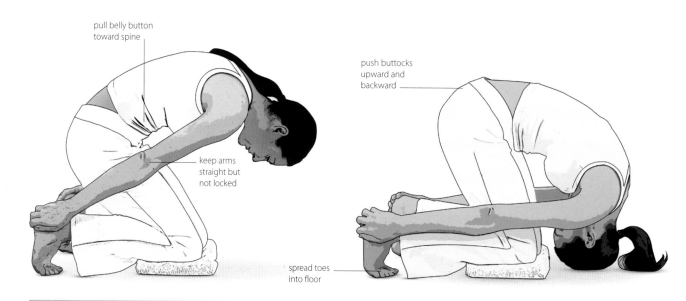

pull belly button toward spine

keep arms straight but not locked

push buttocks upward and backward

spread toes into floor

Front-lying Back Bend

This exercise is a modified version of the Cobra (see p.232). Placing your hands in front of you, rather than at waist level, creates a deeper stretch through your back.

1 Lie down on your front with your legs hip-width apart, your toes touching the floor, and your head facing downward. Extend your arms above your head with palms facing down. As you inhale, reach as far as you can with your fingertips and toes to get a maximal sense of length throughout your body.

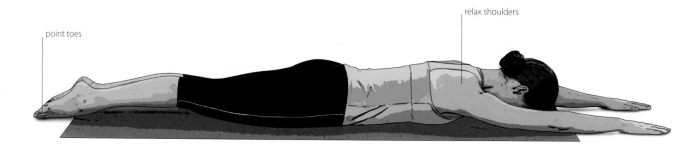

relax shoulders

point toes

Knee to Shoulder

This lying knee-lift stretches and relaxes your lower back and your buttocks, which makes it useful to do any time your back is feeling tired or stiff.

1 Lie on your back with your knees bent and pointing upward. Keep your feet flat on the floor, hip-width apart, and your arms relaxed by your sides. Look straight ahead. Be sure to pull your shoulders down, away from your ears. Inhale to prepare.

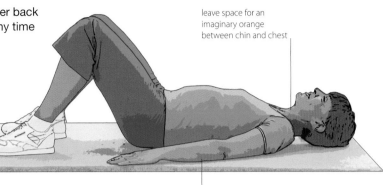

leave space for an imaginary orange between chin and chest

maintain small gap between floor and lower back

2 As you exhale, raise one foot off the floor, bending your leg toward your chest and clasping both hands behind your thigh to bring it closer to your body. Hold for 10 seconds, then inhale as you return your foot to the floor. Repeat with the other leg.

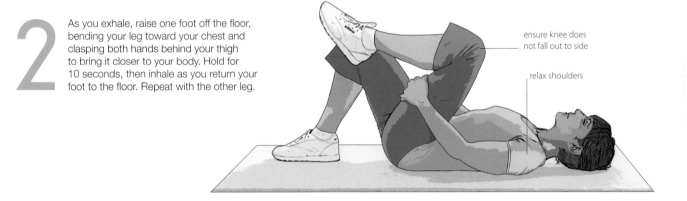

ensure knee does not fall out to side

relax shoulders

2 As you exhale, bring your arms slightly back toward your shoulders and press your hands into the floor for support. Slowly raise your head and upper body off the floor as far as is comfortable. Be sure to engage your legs and abs as you do so. Hold for 10 seconds, then inhale as you return to the starting position.

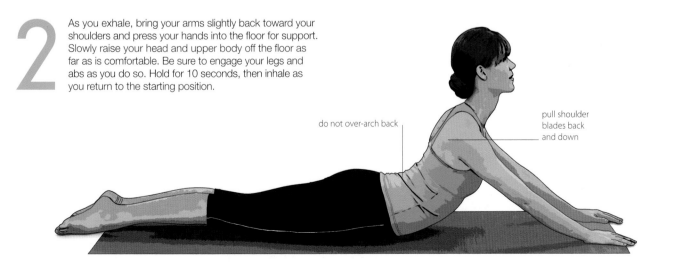

do not over-arch back

pull shoulder blades back and down

Your chest

Everyday activities such as sitting at a desk, working at a computer, or leaning over a sink or stovetop can, over time, cause your back and shoulders to become a little hunched, which, in turn, shortens and tightens the muscles in your chest. The stretches that follow will lengthen and open this area, both correcting your posture and helping to smooth out any wrinkles in your upper chest.

Backward Arm Raise

This double arm lift creates a sense of release through both sides of your chest—very useful if you have rounded shoulders due to sitting hunched over a desk all day.

Stand with your feet hip-width apart and parallel. As you inhale, clasp your hands behind your lower back, with your arms straight, shoulder blades pulled back and down, and palms facing inward. As you exhale, slowly raise your arms as far as you can behind you. Hold for 10 seconds, then inhale to lower them again.

Corner Press

This standing push-up exercise, which requires you to use two walls as resistance for your arms, provides a deep, liberating stretch through your entire chest area.

Stand facing a corner of a room. As you inhale, raise your arms out to the sides and bend them to 90° so that they remain parallel to the floor at shoulder height, with your palms facing forward. As you exhale, place one hand on each wall and lean your body weight into the corner. Hold for 10 seconds, then return to standing tall.

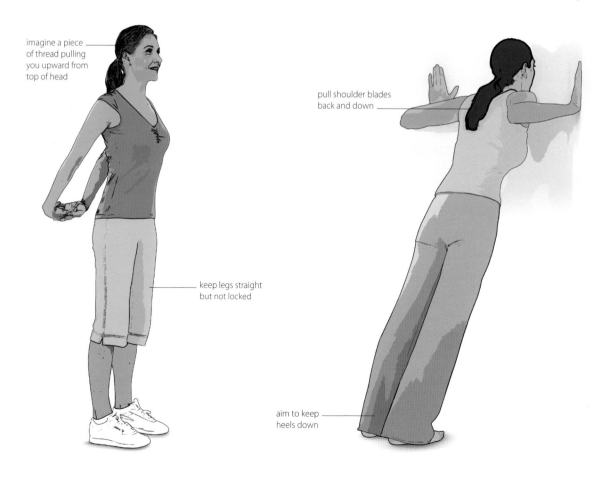

imagine a piece of thread pulling you upward from top of head

keep legs straight but not locked

pull shoulder blades back and down

aim to keep heels down

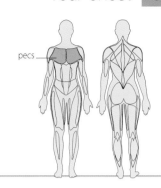

pecs

What am I working?

The pecs (or pectorals) consist of the pectoralis major—large, fan-shaped muscles that cover the front of each side of your rib cage—and the smaller, thinner pectoralis minor, which lie under each side of the pectoralis major. These muscles are responsible for moving your arms across your chest (adduction), moving your shoulder area forward, and rotating your shoulders.

Opposing Arm Extension

This simple arm extension provides a stretch through each side of your chest and armpits, and into your shoulders—areas that are often under-stretched and tight.

1 Stand with your feet hip-width apart and parallel, and your arms relaxed by your sides. Imagine there is a piece of thread pulling you upward from the top of your head. Pull your belly button toward your spine to engage your abs. As you inhale, lift one arm straight in the air.

relax shoulders

slightly tuck pelvis

2 As you exhale, lean slightly to the opposite side from your raised arm. Then gently pull your relaxed arm toward the floor, and stretch your raised arm as high as you can in the air. Hold for 10 seconds, then inhale as you relax your arms back down to your sides. Repeat both steps on the other side.

tilt head in same direction as body

pull belly button toward spine

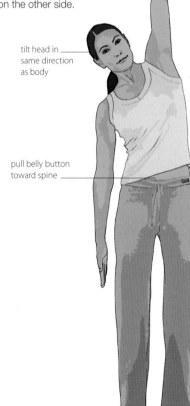

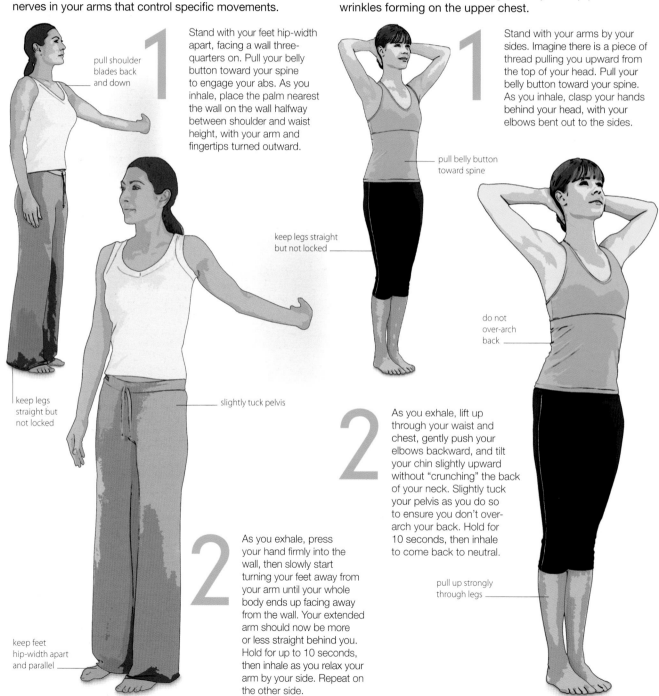

Single Arm Press

This exercise creates a sense of opening in your shoulders, upper arms, and the sides of your chest, and energizes the nerves in your arms that control specific movements.

pull shoulder blades back and down

1 Stand with your feet hip-width apart, facing a wall three-quarters on. Pull your belly button toward your spine to engage your abs. As you inhale, place the palm nearest the wall on the wall halfway between shoulder and waist height, with your arm and fingertips turned outward.

keep legs straight but not locked

slightly tuck pelvis

keep legs straight but not locked

keep feet hip-width apart and parallel

2 As you exhale, press your hand firmly into the wall, then slowly start turning your feet away from your arm until your whole body ends up facing away from the wall. Your extended arm should now be more or less straight behind you. Hold for up to 10 seconds, then inhale as you relax your arm by your side. Repeat on the other side.

Elbow Push Back

This exercise gives a real sense of opening through your armpits and chest. It is also a great way to help prevent wrinkles forming on the upper chest.

1 Stand with your arms by your sides. Imagine there is a piece of thread pulling you upward from the top of your head. Pull your belly button toward your spine. As you inhale, clasp your hands behind your head, with your elbows bent out to the sides.

pull belly button toward spine

keep legs straight but not locked

do not over-arch back

2 As you exhale, lift up through your waist and chest, gently push your elbows backward, and tilt your chin slightly upward without "crunching" the back of your neck. Slightly tuck your pelvis as you do so to ensure you don't over-arch your back. Hold for 10 seconds, then inhale to come back to neutral.

pull up strongly through legs

Sitting Rotation

The combination of seated twist and arm extension in this exercise decompresses your waist area and provides a good stretch across your chest and down each arm.

1 Sit on the edge of a chair or other flat surface, with your feet flat on the floor, hip-width apart. As you inhale, lean your upper body forward and take hold of your lower right calf with your left hand. As you exhale, pull your left shoulder downward and your right one upward and backward to twist your body to the right. Hold for 10 seconds, ending on an inhalation.

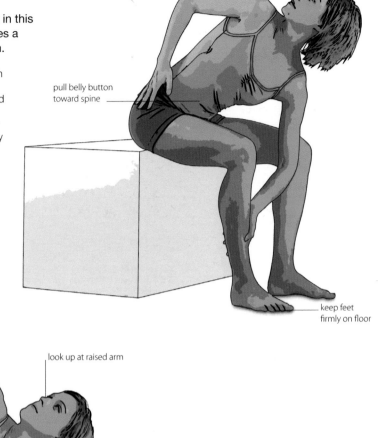

pull belly button toward spine

keep feet firmly on floor

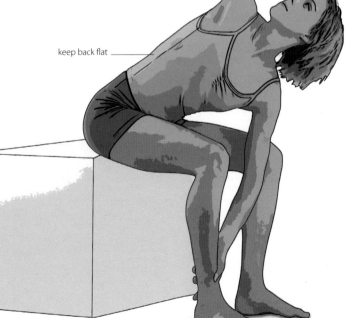

look up at raised arm

keep back flat

2 As you exhale, raise your right arm straight in the air. As you do so, continue to push your top shoulder backward and press your lower elbow against the inside of your left knee, in order to encourage the extension through the side of your body. Hold for 10 seconds, then inhale as you return to center. Repeat on the other side, then come back up to sitting.

Your arms and hands

We use our arm and hand muscles for the majority of our activities during our daily lives, whether brushing our teeth or typing on the computer. This puts them under a lot of strain. It is therefore vital to keep them as strong and flexible as possible. The following exercises will counteract everyday exertions, leaving your arms and hands ready to respond more effectively to your daily needs.

Wrist Press

This wrist exercise gives the muscles right down the back of your arms a much-deserved stretch as well as limbering your overworked wrists and fingers.

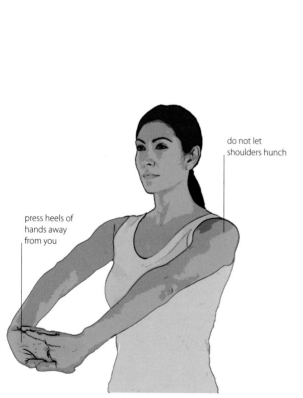

do not let shoulders hunch

press heels of hands away from you

Sit or stand comfortably. As you inhale, clasp your hands together in front of you. As you exhale, turn the palms of your clasped hands to face away from you, straighten your arms at between waist and chest height, and push your hands away from you. Hold for 10 seconds, then relax your arms by your sides.

Arm Reach and Palm Press

As well as stretching your wrist joints, lower arms, and the often-neglected areas under your arms, this exercise opens up the sides of your waist from your hips to your ribs.

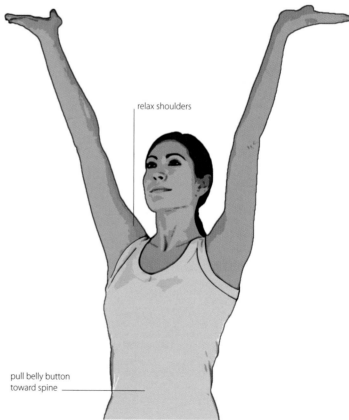

relax shoulders

pull belly button toward spine

Stand with your feet hip-width apart and parallel. As you inhale, reach both arms upward and drop your fingers out to the sides, palms facing upward. As you exhale, push the heels of your hands directly upward and pull your fingertips down toward the floor. Hold for 10 seconds, then relax your arms and lower them to your sides.

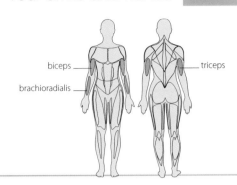

biceps

triceps

brachioradialis

What am I working?

The biceps muscles, on the front of your upper arms, allow you to flex your arms, such as when lifting or pushing objects, while the triceps, on the back of your upper arms, enable you to extend your arms. The brachioradialis, a muscle in your forearms, enables you to open and close your hands, as well as to flex your arms at the elbow.

Forearm Extend and Flex

This exercise, which requires a horizontal surface for resistance, stretches the muscles in the front and back of your forearms. It also helps to keep your wrists flexible.

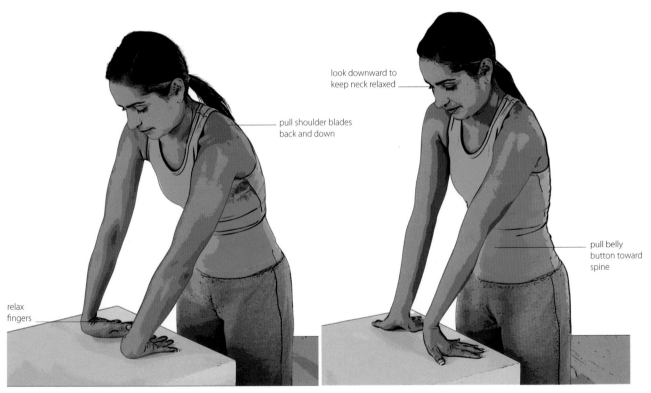

pull shoulder blades back and down

look downward to keep neck relaxed

pull belly button toward spine

relax fingers

1 Stand in front of a stable, horizontal surface and place both your hands on it. As you inhale, slowly turn your hands onto the other side, leading with your fingertips, so that they are now knuckles down, fingertips facing toward you. As you exhale, lean your weight gently forward onto your wrists. Hold for 10 seconds.

2 As you inhale, turn your hands over so that your palms face downward and your fingertips point diagonally toward your body. As you exhale, lean your weight gently forward onto your palms and pull back slightly with your body to increase the stretch. Hold for 10 seconds, then inhale as you relax your arms by your sides.

Triceps Overhead

This classic arm exercise stretches the muscles on the back of your upper arms (triceps), which are often not given the attention they deserve in order to stay in good shape.

Sit or stand comfortably. As you inhale, reach one arm up in the air, then bend it and reach the hand of this arm down the middle of your back. As you exhale, use your other hand to gently push your raised elbow backward and downward. Hold for 10 seconds, then relax your arms. Repeat with the other arm.

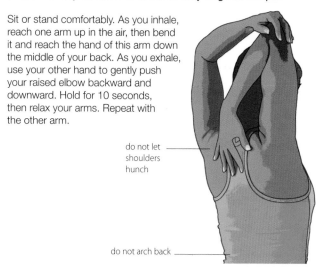

do not let shoulders hunch

do not arch back

Bent Arm Reach

The arm position adopted in this exercise, known as "cow face" in yoga, gives the back of your arms a fantastic stretch, while opening up your chest.

Sit or stand comfortably. As you inhale, reach one arm up in the air, then bend it and reach the hand of this arm down the middle of your back. As you exhale, bring your other hand behind your waist and reach it up, palm facing outward. Clasp both hands together if you can and keep your top elbow pushed back throughout. Hold for 10 seconds. Inhale and relax your arms by your sides. Repeat with the other arm.

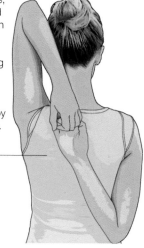

pull shoulder blades back and down

Hand Swim

This flowing arm exercise provides a stretch from your shoulders down to your wrists and through your hands to your fingertips, enhancing overall arm and hand mobility.

Sit or stand comfortably. As you inhale, raise your elbows to chest height and press your palms together in front of you. As you exhale, move them in a horizontal figure 8: first down to one side and up, then diagonally back through center, down to the other side, up, and back to center. Do this 8 times.

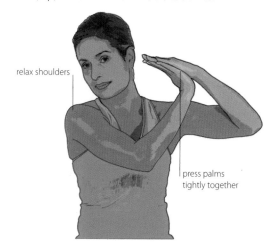

relax shoulders

press palms tightly together

Wrist Mobilizer

This exercise stretches your forearms and keeps your wrists flexible—particularly helpful if your daily life involves repetitive hand activities such as typing.

Sit or stand comfortably. As you inhale, bend your arms behind your lower to middle back. As you exhale, reach the palms of your hands toward one another, pulling your shoulders back and down. If your palms touch, press them together; if not, reach them toward each other. Hold for 10 seconds, then relax your arms by your sides.

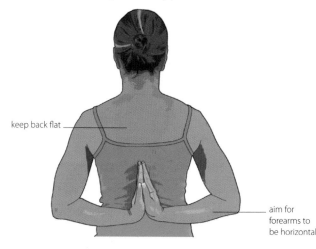

keep back flat

aim for forearms to be horizontal

Hand Rotations

These exercises are great to do when your arms or hands feel stiff or tired. They encourage maximal mobility through your wrists and fingers, and stretch up through your arms, too.

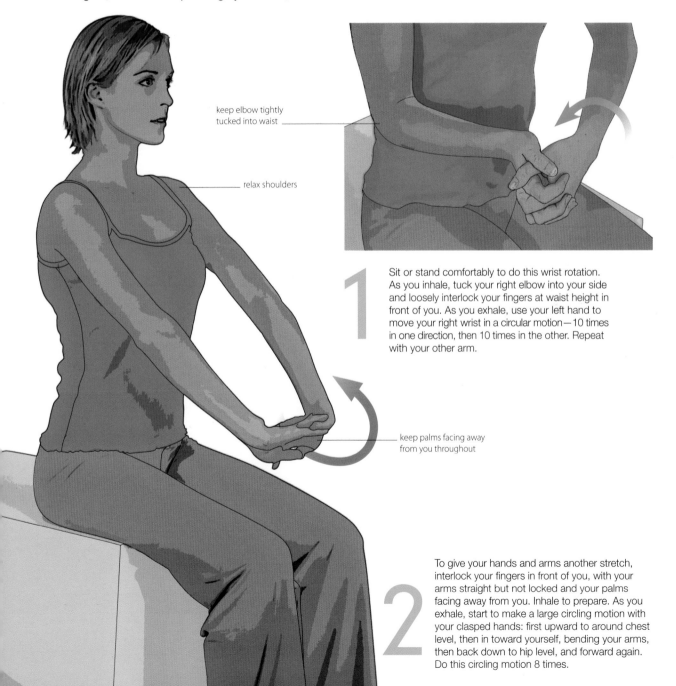

keep elbow tightly tucked into waist

relax shoulders

keep palms facing away from you throughout

1 Sit or stand comfortably to do this wrist rotation. As you inhale, tuck your right elbow into your side and loosely interlock your fingers at waist height in front of you. As you exhale, use your left hand to move your right wrist in a circular motion—10 times in one direction, then 10 times in the other. Repeat with your other arm.

2 To give your hands and arms another stretch, interlock your fingers in front of you, with your arms straight but not locked and your palms facing away from you. Inhale to prepare. As you exhale, start to make a large circling motion with your clasped hands: first upward to around chest level, then in toward yourself, bending your arms, then back down to hip level, and forward again. Do this circling motion 8 times.

Your waist and hips

Your stomach and waist muscles constantly work hard to hold your body in a balanced posture, while your hip muscles are pivotal in fundamental actions such as sitting and walking. The following exercises will keep tightness at bay in these areas to ensure that your muscles can perform their essential tasks to the maximum of their ability. The result: enhanced posture and increased mobility.

Standing Waist Twist

This simultaneous arm extension and upper body rotation opens up the sides of your body, from hip to armpit, lengthening and strengthening your waist area and improving your posture.

Stand with your feet hip-width apart and parallel. As you inhale, place your left hand, fingers pointing downward, on the side of your lower back so that your elbow is pointing backward. As you exhale, twist your body to the left and raise your right arm diagonally above your head, looking in the direction that you are twisting. Hold for 10 seconds, then inhale as you return to the front. Repeat on the other side.

Lying Waist Twist

This twisting exercise stretches the whole middle section of your body, one side at a time, as well as really opening up through the buttock and hip of your twisting leg.

Lie flat on your back. As you inhale, bend your right leg so that your knee points toward the ceiling. As you exhale, use your left hand to pull your raised knee across your body, toward the floor on the left side, keeping your foot behind your opposite knee. As you do so, reach your right arm out at shoulder height on the floor and turn your head to look at this hand. Hold for 10 seconds, then inhale as you come back to center. Repeat on the other side.

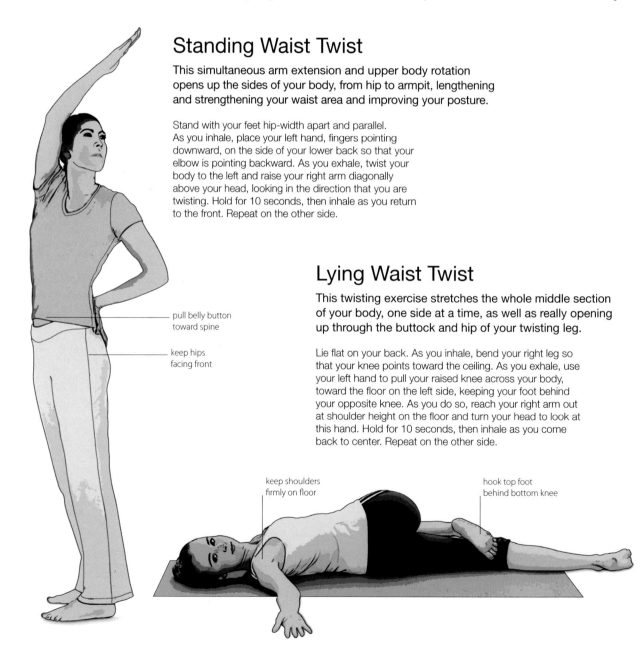

pull belly button
toward spine

keep hips
facing front

keep shoulders
firmly on floor

hook top foot
behind bottom knee

What am I working?

The obliques (obliquus abdominis) are the muscles down the sides of your body that enable you to twist and bend sideways. The rectus abdominis and transversus abdominis are the central abdominal muscles, which provide you with core support. And the hip flexors (not shown) are a group of muscles that allow your legs to bend up toward your stomach and down again.

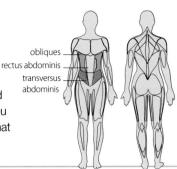

obliques
rectus abdominis
transversus abdominis

Seated Side Bend

While the arm extension and lateral bend in this stretch release the tension in your waist and side, the leg position provides a stretch through the hip and thigh of your back leg.

Sit with your legs bent upward in front of you. As you inhale, gently lower your knees down to the right and swing your feet to the left, so that your left heel ends up near your left buttock and your right foot beside your left knee. As you exhale, reach your right arm in the air and lean both it and your upper body to the left. Hold for 10 seconds, then inhale as you return to center. Swing your legs to the other side and repeat in the opposite direction.

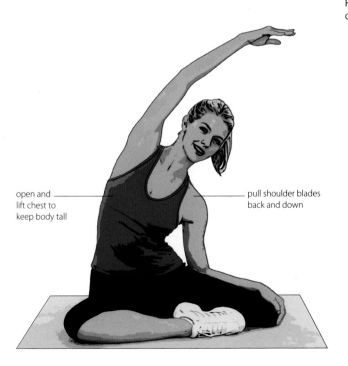

open and lift chest to keep body tall

pull shoulder blades back and down

Cross-legged Side Stretch

This standing cross-legged side bend provides a satisfying stretch through the hip of your back leg and up the rest of the side of your body.

Stand with your hands on your hips and cross your left leg in front of your right one so that your feet are parallel and your left leg is bent, with its heel raised. As you inhale, raise your right arm toward the ceiling. As you exhale, lean to the left, stretching your raised arm across. Hold for 10 seconds, then inhale as you relax to standing. Repeat on the other side.

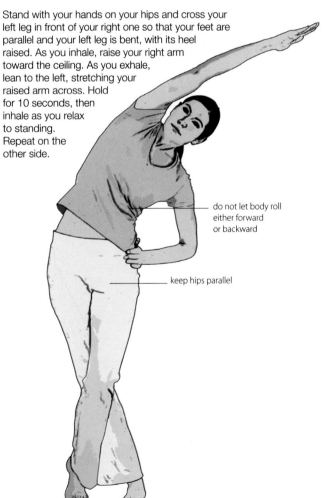

do not let body roll either forward or backward

keep hips parallel

Front Hip Stretch

This stretch works the hip flexor muscles, releasing stiffness in the front of your hips. Try it if you spend a lot of time sitting.

Stand with your feet hip-width apart and parallel, and your hands on your hips. Pull your belly button toward your spine to engage your abs. As you inhale, step one foot forward. As you exhale, lift your back heel off the floor and lean your weight onto the toes of your back foot, pushing your hips forward. Hold for 10 seconds, then inhale as you come back to neutral. Repeat on the other side.

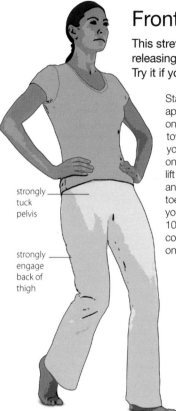

strongly tuck pelvis

strongly engage back of thigh

Foot on Knee

The leg position here gives the glutes and hips of your raised leg an intense stretch, reducing stress on the back caused by tight upper leg muscles.

Sit with your legs in front of you and hands resting on the floor behind you, fingers pointing backward. As you inhale, bend your knees to point upward. As you exhale, raise the side of one foot onto the opposite thigh, opening the knee of your lifted leg out to the side. Hold for 10 seconds, then inhale as you lower your leg. Repeat on the other side.

gently press raised knee away from you

keep arms straight but not locked

Lying Foot on Knee

This version of the Foot on Knee exercise (see above) requires less initial flexibility but still gives an intense stretch to your glutes and thighs. It is also a welcome release for your back.

1

Lie flat on your back and bend both knees to point upward. As you inhale, raise your right foot onto your left thigh, opening your right knee to the side. Then place your left hand on the back of your left thigh and your right hand on the knee of the crossed leg and start to lift your left leg off the floor.

keep neck relaxed

maintain small gap between floor and lower back

Hip Rocking

The leg position in this exercise provides a super stretch through your glutes and the back of your thighs, while the flowing movement makes it a great overall tension reliever.

1 Lie flat on your back and bend both knees so that they point upward. As you inhale, raise both legs toward your chest, keeping your knees bent. Push your heels away to flex your feet and reach your hands in the air to take hold of the soles of your feet (or your lower legs if you can't reach your feet).

2 As you exhale, gently rock your whole body to one side so that one knee lowers toward the floor while the opposite buttock raises off the floor, then do the same on the other side. Keep your belly button pulled toward your spine to engage your abs throughout. Rock for a total of 10 times.

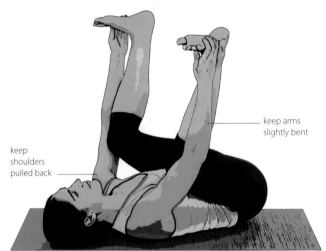

keep arms slightly bent

keep shoulders pulled back

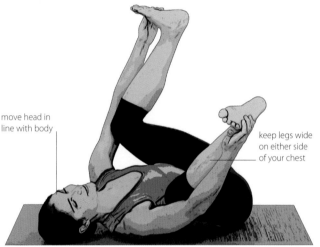

move head in line with body

keep legs wide on either side of your chest

2 Pull your belly button toward your spine to engage your abs. As you exhale, use your left hand to pull your legs toward your chest, keeping your head on the floor. At the same time, gently press your hand on your right knee to increase the stretch. Hold for 10 seconds, then inhale as you lower your legs. Repeat both steps on the other side.

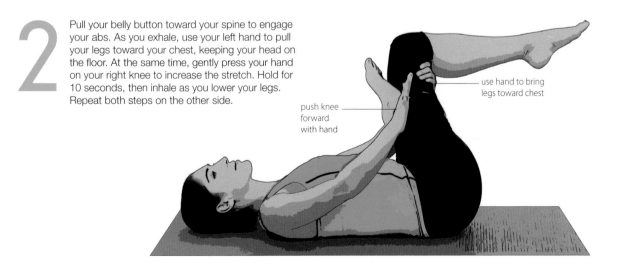

push knee forward with hand

use hand to bring legs toward chest

Your upper legs

The muscles in your upper legs work hard each day, whether you're standing, walking, running, or dancing. Depending on the ratio of different activities you do, certain muscles may become out of balance, causing tightness and misalignment. The exercises that follow will help to relieve any such problems, leaving your legs feeling strong, balanced, and once again raring to go.

Quad Stretch

This classic quad exercise really stretches the front thigh of your lifted leg while giving the muscles in your supporting leg an effective workout. It is also a great balance enhancer.

Stand with your feet hip-width apart and parallel. Lift one foot behind you, take hold of it with the hand on the same side, and pull your foot toward your buttocks, keeping your knees together and your supporting leg straight but not locked. Hold for 10 seconds, then inhale as you come back to standing. Repeat on the other side.

Deep Lunge

This lunge stretches the quads (front thighs) of your back leg and sculpts the quads of your front leg. It also targets your hip flexors, enhancing overall lower body mobility.

Stand with your feet hip-width apart and parallel. As you inhale, take a large stride forward with one foot. As you exhale, slowly bend your front leg to 90°, allowing your back knee to lower to the floor. Hold for 10 seconds, then inhale as you straighten your legs and return to upright. Repeat on the other leg.

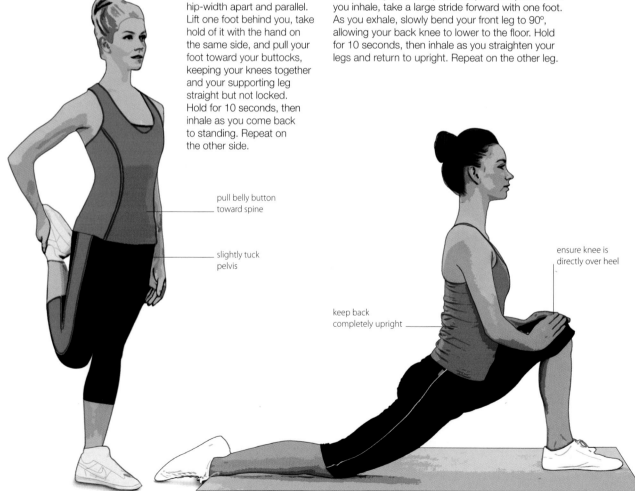

pull belly button toward spine

slightly tuck pelvis

ensure knee is directly over heel

keep back completely upright

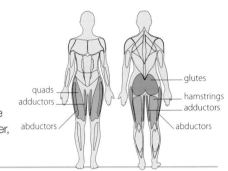

What am I working?

The glutes are the large muscles in your buttocks; the quads, are located in the front of your thighs; the hamstrings run up the back of your thighs; the adductors are on the insides of your thighs; the abductors are on the outside of your thighs; and the hip flexors (not shown) run through your thighs. Together, these muscles work to move your legs through their full range of movement.

Standing Hamstring Stretch

This classic exercise is the perfect way to stretch the back of your thigh if it feels tight or sluggish—particularly useful after a long day of sitting stationary at a desk.

Stand with your feet hip-width apart and parallel. As you inhale, bend one leg and place the heel of your other foot out in front of you, toes in the air. As you exhale, lean your upper body forward, rest your hands on the thigh of your bent leg, and push your buttocks in the air. Hold for 10 seconds, then inhale as you return to standing. Repeat on the other side.

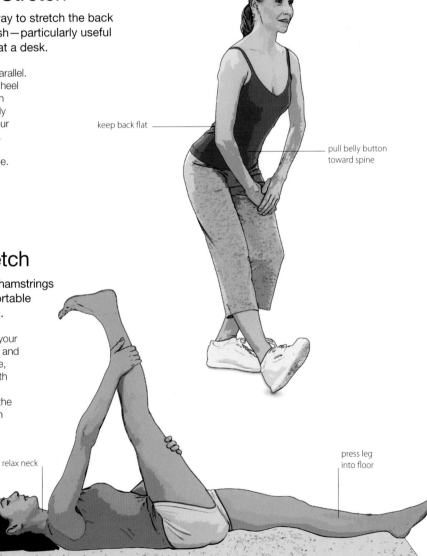

keep back flat

pull belly button toward spine

Lying Hamstring Stretch

Try this more intense stretch for your hamstrings and calves only when you are comfortable with the Standing Hamstring Stretch.

Lie flat on your back. As you inhale, bend your legs so that your knees point to the ceiling and your feet are flat on the floor. As you exhale, raise one leg off the floor, take hold of it with both hands, and gently pull it toward your chest. Aim to straighten both this leg and the one on the floor. Hold for 10 seconds, then inhale as you lower your leg. Repeat with opposite legs.

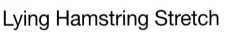

relax neck

press leg into floor

Cross-knee Forward Bend

This exercise creates a sense of lengthening through your buttocks and outer thighs. If it feels too intense, try sitting on a large book or yoga block to lessen the stretch.

1 Sit comfortably with your legs out in front of you. As you inhale, bend one leg to place your foot beneath the opposite buttock, then bend your other leg on top of the first leg, bringing the foot toward the opposite buttock. Take hold of your feet with your hands.

2 As you exhale, gently pull your feet upward and backward, lean your upper body forward, allowing your back to round slightly, and tuck your head toward your knee. Push down through your buttocks at the same time as extending through your neck and head. Hold for 10 seconds, then return to upright and slowly uncross your legs.

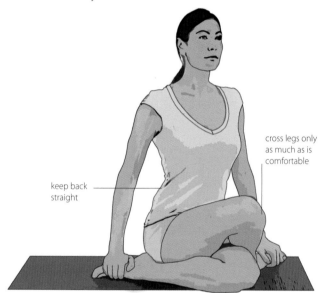

keep back straight

cross legs only as much as is comfortable

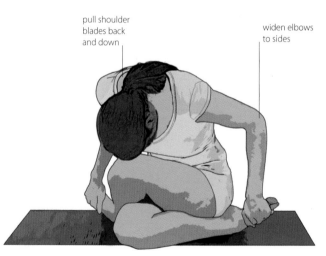

pull shoulder blades back and down

widen elbows to sides

Rolling Leg Lift

This exercise provides a fantastic stretch for your thighs. Keeping your raised leg still as you roll your body onto the side targets the inner thigh of your raised leg in particular.

1 Lie flat on your back. As you inhale, extend your right arm above your head on the floor. As you exhale, lift your left leg off the floor, take hold of it with your left hand, and gently pull it toward your chest until it is as straight as you can manage. Hold for 10 seconds.

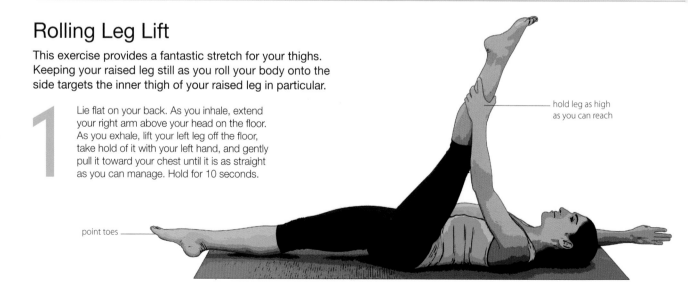

hold leg as high as you can reach

point toes

Straddle Side Bend

This exercise stretches the inside of your thighs, boosting lower body mobility. The arm raise opens your chest and arms, and the bend opens your waist.

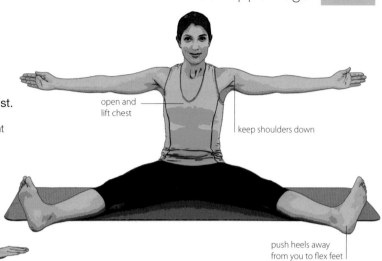

open and lift chest

keep shoulders down

push heels away from you to flex feet

1 Sit on the floor with your legs straight out in front of you. Pull your belly button toward your spine to engage your abs. As you inhale, widen your legs out to 45° and raise your arms out to the sides at shoulder height. As you exhale, reach out through your head, hands, and feet. Hold for 10 seconds, ending on an inhalation.

relax shoulders

press lower legs to floor

2 As you exhale, slowly lean your upper body to one side, using the hand on that side for support on the floor and raising your other arm up and over your head. Hold for 10 seconds, then inhale as you return to center. Repeat this step on the other side.

2 As you exhale, strongly engage your abs and slowly roll onto your right side without changing the angle of your raised leg. Your front thigh should therefore still face toward your waist rather than toward the front, as your face does now. Your extended arm should now be beneath your head. Hold for 10 seconds, then inhale as you lower your leg. Repeat both steps on the other side.

keep lower leg firmly on floor

do not let yourself roll forward or backward

Your calves

The muscles in your calves and feet come under a lot of pressure every day as they work to keep you upright and mobile. They can therefore easily become tight, stiff, or sore. The stretching exercises that follow will lengthen and strengthen these muscles, reduce any tension, and improve your balance and posture, as well as lessen your chance of lower leg injury.

Calf Lunge

This classic exercise stretches your calf muscles. It provides particularly effective relief after wearing high heels, which can shorten your calf muscles and tendons.

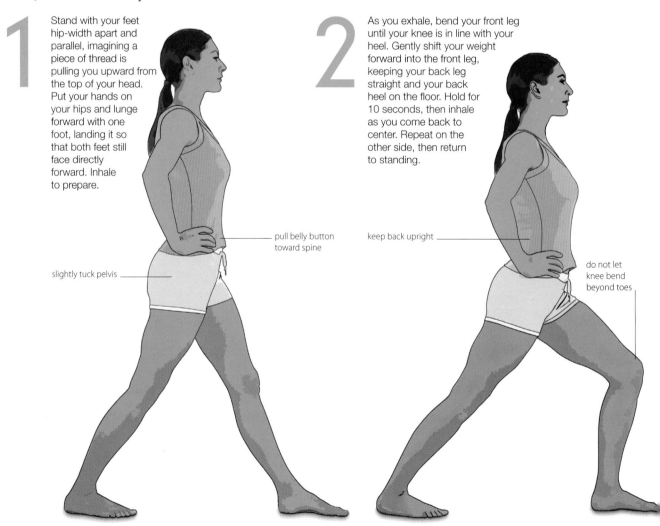

1 Stand with your feet hip-width apart and parallel, imagining a piece of thread is pulling you upward from the top of your head. Put your hands on your hips and lunge forward with one foot, landing it so that both feet still face directly forward. Inhale to prepare.

pull belly button toward spine

slightly tuck pelvis

2 As you exhale, bend your front leg until your knee is in line with your heel. Gently shift your weight forward into the front leg, keeping your back leg straight and your back heel on the floor. Hold for 10 seconds, then inhale as you come back to center. Repeat on the other side, then return to standing.

keep back upright

do not let knee bend beyond toes

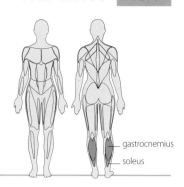

What am I working?

The gastrocnemius and soleus are the muscles in your calf that enable movement of your lower leg and foot. The gastrocnemius, on the upper calf, is larger and dictates how rounded (or not) your calves are, while the soleus lies in the lower half of each calf. The Achilles tendon (not shown) is the thickest, strongest tendon in your body and attaches your calf muscles to your heels.

gastrocnemius

soleus

Step Drop

This exercise stretches your lower calves, your Achilles tendons, and the soles of your feet. It is particularly useful for runners, who can be prone to Achilles injuries.

1 Stand on the edge of a step or any other slightly raised, stable surface, with your feet hip-width apart and parallel. As you inhale, slowly rise onto your toes, making sure that your feet roll neither inward nor outward. If you are unable to balance, hold on to a firm surface in front of you for stability. Hold for 10 seconds.

2 As you exhale, slowly lower your heels again. Allow the back halves of your feet to hang off the back of the step, keeping your toes flat on the step. As before, hold onto a firm surface in front of you to help with stability and control if required. Hold for 10 seconds, then inhale as you come back to standing.

pull belly button toward spine

slightly tuck pelvis

keep legs straight but not locked

aim to keep feet steady

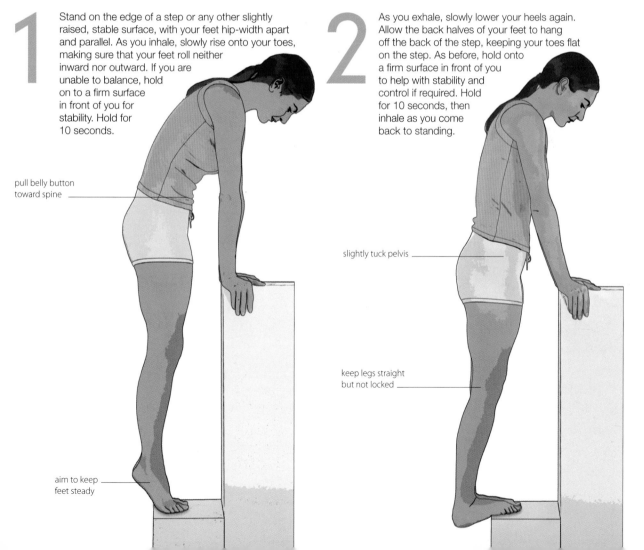

Your total body

Most of the stretching exercises so far target particular muscles in isolation. While these are useful for opening and lengthening specific areas, it is also helpful to know a few exercises that will give you more of an all-over body stretch when needed. Apart from releasing tension and tightness, these compound exercises will help to improve your coordination, balance, alignment, and posture.

Lunge with Extended Arms

The lunges in this exercise create a deep calf stretch, and the arm and head movements release first the muscles in your upper back and neck, then those in your chest and arms.

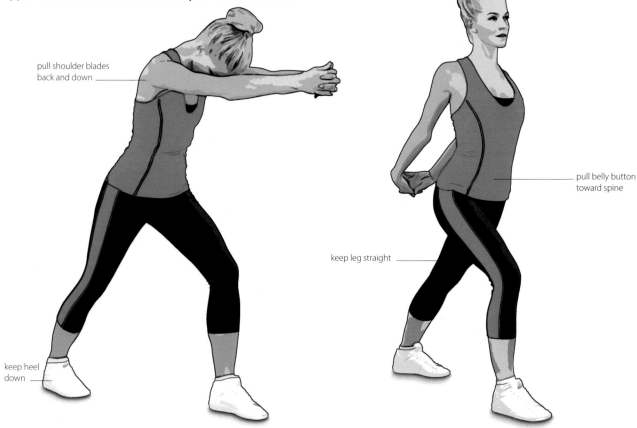

pull shoulder blades back and down

pull belly button toward spine

keep leg straight

keep heel down

1 Stand with your feet hip-width apart and parallel. Inhale to prepare. As you exhale, lunge forward with one leg, bending your front leg until your knee is in line with your heel. At the same time, clasp your hands straight in front of you at shoulder height, tilt your head forward, and press your knuckles away from you. Hold for 10 seconds, then inhale as you return to center.

2 As you exhale, lunge forward with the opposite leg, again bending your front leg until your knee is in line with your heel. This time, clasp your hands behind your back, arms straight but not locked, and raise them as high as you can. Hold for 10 seconds, then inhale as you return to center.

What am I working?

The exercises in this section have been especially selected to stretch as many muscle groups as possible at the same time. The lunges target your lower body as well as your core ab and back muscles, which provide balance and alignment throughout the movements. The arm raises lengthen and open the muscles of your upper body, and the twisting stretches your mid-section.

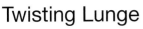

front upper body

back upper body

front lower body

back lower body

Twisting Lunge

The lunges in this exercise stretch your upper leg muscles, the twist opens up your obliques, and the arm raise provides release through your shoulders, arms, and hands.

1 Stand with your feet hip-width apart and parallel. As you inhale, take a large stride forward with one foot. As you exhale, slowly bend your front leg to 90°. Keeping your back leg straight but not locked, allow your heel to come off the floor and rest your hands on your front thigh for support. Hold for 10 seconds. Inhale to prepare.

keep back upright

keep knee directly above heel

2 As you exhale, slowly raise your hands straight out in front of you at shoulder height, being careful to maintain balance. Then twist your upper body in the direction of your bent leg and swing your leading arm horizontally out to the other side of your body. Your arms should now be spread wide at shoulder height. Hold for 10 seconds, then slowly come back to standing, with your arms by your sides. Repeat both steps on the other side.

look in direction you are twisting

keep back leg straight

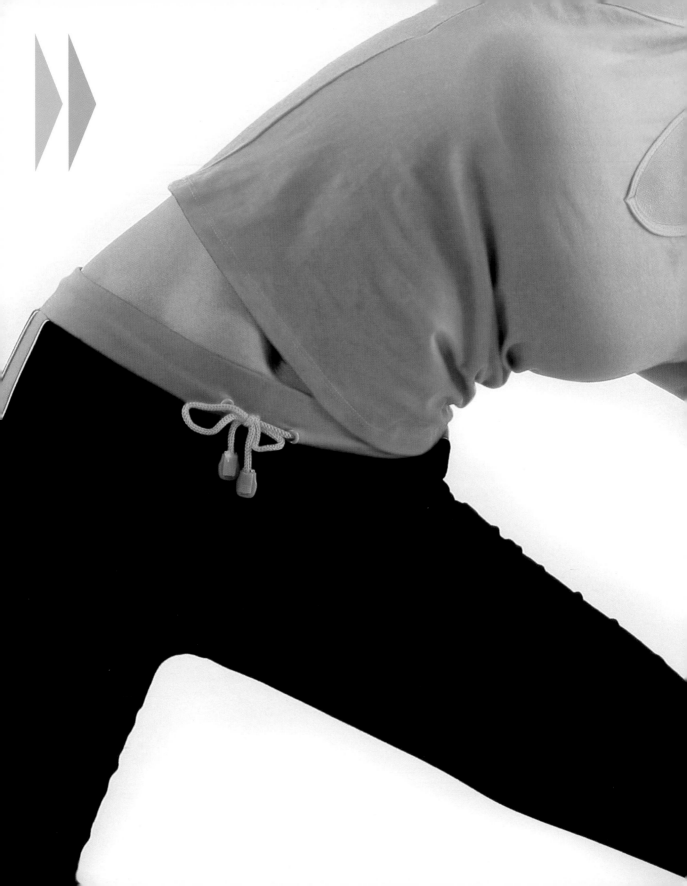

Pilates

Pilates is a low-impact but highly effective approach to fitness that will challenge your entire body from the inside out. Initially called "Contrology" by its creator Joseph Pilates, the aim is to do every movement with complete awareness, focus, and precision so that you can develop subtle control over your body rather than being at its mercy. If you try it, you will love the results, which include:

- fantastic core strength, allowing more efficient movement throughout your body

- enhanced mobility throughout your spine, and indeed your whole body

- strong, toned abs, buttocks, and legs

- great posture that will help you to appear instantly taller and slimmer

- heightened body awareness due to a stronger mind-body connection

- increased ease and grace in all movements

- improved coordination skills

- greater stability and balance

What is Pilates?

Pilates combines the precision of gymnastics, the elegance of dancing, and the deep, flowing breathing of yoga to provide a mind-body fusion of strength and concentration. Although it originated at the start of the 1900s, it has only really gained mainstream popularity over the last 15 years, and classes can now be found on timetables of almost every gym across the country.

The origins of Pilates

Pilates is a series of exercises performed slowly and deliberately that focus on core stability, in order to maintain good posture and increase strength and flexibility. The name comes from Joseph Pilates, who was born in Germany in 1883. Joseph's father was a gymnast and his mother, a naturopath; both influenced his approach. As a child, Pilates had been stricken by sickness which led him on a lifetime quest to build his own—and other's—physical strength and fitness.

Like many of his modern-day fitness counterparts, Pilates' passion and a desire to learn led him in many different directions, and over his lifetime of 83 years, he worked as a circus performer, an anatomical model, a gymnast, a boxer, an author, and an inventor of fantastic fitness machines. He developed his system and workout regimen in the US, where he founded a fitness studio in a building that was shared with dancers. He took no mercy on his clients, many of whom were dancers. He became known as a hard taskmaster—and a perfectionist.

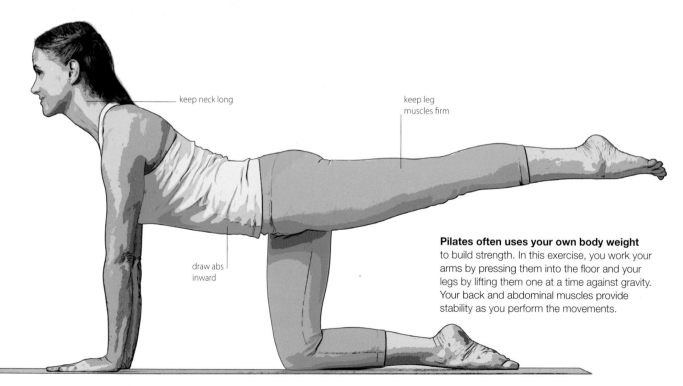

keep neck long

keep leg muscles firm

draw abs inward

Pilates often uses your own body weight to build strength. In this exercise, you work your arms by pressing them into the floor and your legs by lifting them one at a time against gravity. Your back and abdominal muscles provide stability as you perform the movements.

How Pilates builds strength

To become stronger, muscles need to work against some form of resistance. In Pilates, resistance can be provided by your body's own weight and in this book we focus on this type of mat-based exercise. However, if you go to a Pilates studio, you may encounter special equipment with springs that provide resistance. Pilates does not rely on heavy weights to build strength, but is able to achieve results through low-resistance training. Key to this is the 3D nature of Pilates exercises, with each movement designed to work particular muscles from several different directions. When performing Pilates exercises, you are encouraged to link movements together, building

your own rhythm, so that muscles strengthen as you move. At the heart of Pilates' ability to build strength without strain is its emphasis on developing a strong, stable core (see box on p.199).

How Pilates increases flexibility

Flexibility is the range of motion of your joints, and is largely determined by the ability of the surrounding muscles to stretch, or elongate. In Pilates, muscles are often elongated by dynamic stretching, in which you move your body into a stretch and then release repeatedly. In static stretching, you stretch a muscle to its maximum and then hold. Some static exercises may be included in a Pilates routine to help relax you or as part of your cool-down.

Is Pilates for you?

Pilates is a low-impact form of exercise that is suitable and beneficial for everyone, from exercise newcomers to elite athletes. The mind-body coordination required is likely to appeal to "Take-it-easy" personalities (see p.34), the dynamic movements will probably appeal to "Get-up-and-go" personalities, while the fantastic core strength that it builds within just weeks of regular practice is likely to appeal to "Let's-do-it!" types since this will enhance performance in all other activities, too.

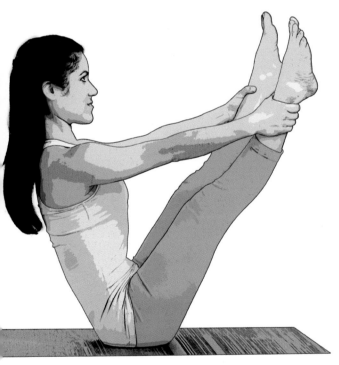

Challenging exercises like this one require a lot of strength, control, and balance so you may not be able to do them at first but, with regular practice of the Pilates basics, you will soon build up the physical skills required.

*Pilates does not rely on heavy weights to build strength, but is able to achieve results through **low-resistance training**. Each Pilates movement is designed to work particular muscles from several different directions.*

Principles of Pilates

The underlying principles of Pilates make this form of exercise unique. There's no fixed number of principles—instructors tend to list anything up to nine—but the concepts below communicate the main messages that founder Joseph Pilates wanted to get across to his pupils about how to make the most of every movement in every exercise and get maximum value from a workout.

Things to consider

Thinking about the six principles below as you do any of the Pilates exercises in the pages that follow or the Core Pilates workout on pp.274–75 means that your body can benefit in a variety of ways from each exercise.

Control

Joseph Pilates initially called his fitness method "Contrology," which means that control is, of course, one of the key concepts of his approach. Exercising with control means moving slowly and gradually, without any jerky movements. It also means staying relaxed yet fully alert and strong. Without control, Pilates is not as effective and there is a chance of injuring yourself. With control, on the other hand, and observing the correct form throughout each movement, you can do a safe and highly effective movement each time.

Concentration

To get the best out of any exercise, you need to dedicate 100% concentration to what you're doing. Spend time really focusing your mind on every aspect of each Pilates exercise to ensure that one body area doesn't fall out of alignment when you correct another. Check in with your body now and then to see how it's responding to whatever exercise you're doing and adapt your position as required. In this way, you will become your own trainer, get to know your body better, and also demand the best from yourself.

Centering

Absolutely key to the Pilates method, and arguably its most distinguishing feature, is centering. This requires you to use the core of your body (see right) as the driving force of all your movements. Before you start any exercise, engage all the muscles in the mid-section

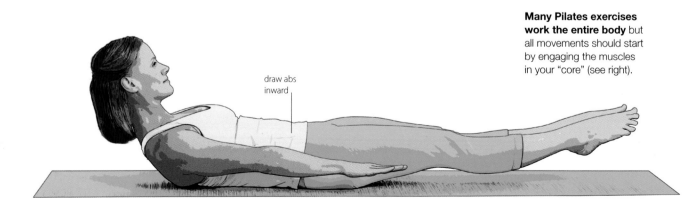

Many Pilates exercises work the entire body but all movements should start by engaging the muscles in your "core" (see right).

draw abs inward

of your body—your abs, back, glutes, and hips. Then when you are mid-movement, check that you can feel them working and that your abs are drawn in and up—there's never any reason for a bulging stomach in Pilates.

Precision

Precision was paramount for Joseph Pilates. In practice, the key to this is ensuring that each part of your body is in precisely the right place at the right time during each exercise. This involves paying close attention to the step-by-step guidance on the pages that follow and checking in with yourself to make sure everything remains in alignment. It also involves repeating or holding each exercise for an appropriate amount of time for your body, since no two bodies are the same. Use the instructions on the pages that follow as approximate guidance for this. However, never do the suggested amount if the movement is causing you any discomfort or pain.

Breath

Good breathing is key to all exercise. In Pilates, the idea is to breathe slowly and deeply, coordinating your movements with the flow of your breath so that there is a sense of ease and harmony. When you breathe fully and correctly, your lungs will be emptied of stale air on each exhalation and rejuvenated with fresh oxygen for your muscles on each inhalation. A simple Pilates breathing rule to remember is: inhale to prepare for a movement and exhale to perform it.

Flow

The aim in Pilates is to make any sequence of movements as flowing and seamless as possible, like a well-choreographed dance routine. One exercise should flow into the next without rest in between, and without any unnecessary or jerky movements. It's also good to aim to maintain a steady pace throughout your workout.

Getting to the core of it

The "core" of your body, also called the powerhouse in Pilates, consists of the muscles in the mid-section of the body, mainly the abdominal and back muscles, but also the hips and buttocks, since we often need to work the whole middle area as one. It's essential to build strength in these "core" muscles in order to provide a solid foundation from which all movements can be done safely, effectively, and with stability. A strong, stable core will not only improve posture, enhance athletic performance, and help to prevent back pain, but it will also make day-to-day functional movements easier since you will do them more efficiently, and less strain will be placed on the rest of your body.

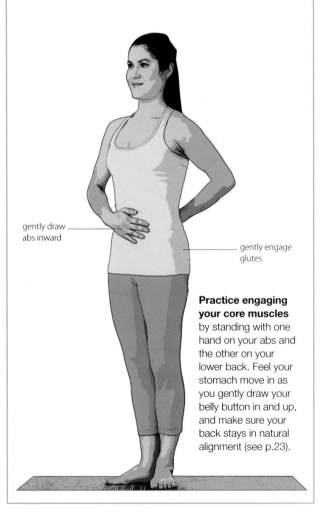

gently draw abs inward

gently engage glutes

Practice engaging your core muscles by standing with one hand on your abs and the other on your lower back. Feel your stomach move in as you gently draw your belly button in and up, and make sure your back stays in natural alignment (see p.23).

Essential alignment

Perfecting your basic body position when standing and lying down is the starting point for most of the mat-based exercises you'll do in Pilates, so below is some guidance on how to do this. Using your core muscles to keep you in correct alignment means that you will work from a safe, steady base and put minimal pressure on the rest of your muscles and joints as you exercise.

Standing posture

Ensure that your head is in the center of your body, neither tilted to one side nor the other. It can be useful to imagine a thread attached from the crown of your head to the ceiling, drawing you directly upward, and lengthening your spine and neck. This should lift your head without lifting your chin so that your neck doesn't become "crunched." Relax your shoulders by gliding your shoulder blades back and down. It can help to hunch your shoulders up to your ears and release them down once or twice to feel the difference between the two positions. It can also help to coordinate this with your

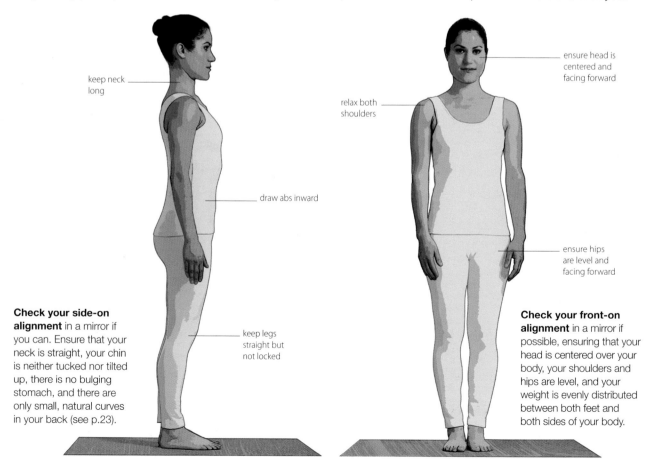

keep neck long

draw abs inward

keep legs straight but not locked

ensure head is centered and facing forward

relax both shoulders

ensure hips are level and facing forward

Check your side-on alignment in a mirror if you can. Ensure that your neck is straight, your chin is neither tucked nor tilted up, there is no bulging stomach, and there are only small, natural curves in your back (see p.23).

Check your front-on alignment in a mirror if possible, ensuring that your head is centered over your body, your shoulders and hips are level, and your weight is evenly distributed between both feet and both sides of your body.

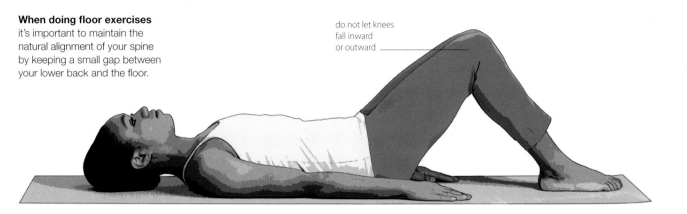

When doing floor exercises it's important to maintain the natural alignment of your spine by keeping a small gap between your lower back and the floor.

do not let knees fall inward or outward

breathing: inhale as you lift your shoulders, exhale as you relax them down. It's important to open your chest too, without pushing it out or over-arching your back. Find your neutral spine by placing one hand on your abs and one on your lower back: first scoop your belly button inward and upward, toward your spine, so that you feel your belly sucking in and your spine becoming more supported; second, tilt your pelvis forward and backward, then find the mid-point between these two movements and keep it here since this will dictate the curvature of the rest of your spine. Third, imagine that your torso is in a box from your shoulders to your hips— this should ensure even, front-facing shoulders and hips. Aim to keep your legs straight but don't lock your knees. In some instances, keep your feet together, toes facing forward. In others, turn your thighs out slightly so that your knees point directly forward, but your feet point slightly outward (see below left). Spread your toes out on the floor for stability, and focus on lifting the arches of your feet upward to create a small dome in each foot.

Lying posture

In order to get the most from Pilates floor exercises, it's important to know the neutral position from which to start. Lie on your back on the floor with your arms by your sides. As you inhale, bend your legs so that your knees point upward and your feet are flat on the floor, hip-width apart, facing forward. As you exhale, let your body weight sink into the floor, keeping your head, neck, and jaw relaxed, and avoiding crunching the vertebrae of your neck or tightening your throat. Gently press your shoulders back and down to sink farther into the floor. Next, find your neutral pelvis position. Gently rock your pelvis up and down: as you push it up, your back will flatten into the floor, and as you push it down, your back will arch and a gap will form between your lower back and the floor. "Neutral" lies between these two points, with just a small gap between your lower back and the floor. When you find this, take a few breaths here: as you inhale, feel your rib cage opening and expanding; as you exhale, engage your abdominal muscles by pulling your belly button inward and upward, toward your spine. Re-check this alignment now and then as you do each exercise so that you work with strength and stability.

Pilates stance
Many standing Pilates exercises are done with your heels touching and toes apart. To get into this stance, stand with your feet together, turn your hip joints slightly outward, and move the toes of one foot outward, then the other.

The basics

These basic movements form the foundation of many of the exercises in Pilates. You'll learn how to master working from the torso, using your powerhouse, or core, (see right) to drive the movement in your limbs, and familiarize yourself with the intricacies of your spine and the deep muscles around your spinal column. These slow, simple movements will also help to develop alignment and control.

Centering

Centering is the ability to move your limbs from your core. This movement, which is the basis for many other Pilates exercises, will reinforce this ability.

Lie on the floor with your knees bent and feet flat on the floor, facing forward. Inhale to prepare. As you exhale, stretch one arm behind your head and the opposite leg out along the floor. As you move your limbs, focus on keeping your abs in and spine long. As you inhale, slide your arm and leg back to the start position. Do up to 10 times, alternating sides between each repetition.

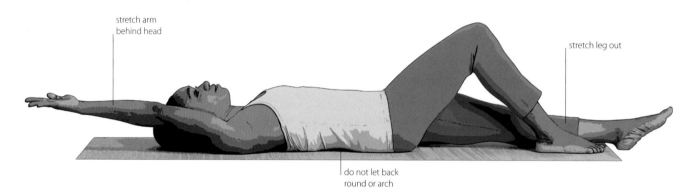

stretch arm behind head

stretch leg out

do not let back round or arch

Box Position

Precision is central to Pilates movements. To keep your shoulders and hips aligned and level, it is useful to visualize a square, and the box position helps you to do this.

Get onto all fours on the floor, keeping your hands in line with your shoulders and your knees in line with your hips. Visualize your hands and knees connected by four lines that create a box. Imagine a central line going from the crown of your head through to your tailbone and ensure all your muscles and bodyweight are evenly balanced on both sides of this line, with your abs drawn in. Hold for up to 5 breaths.

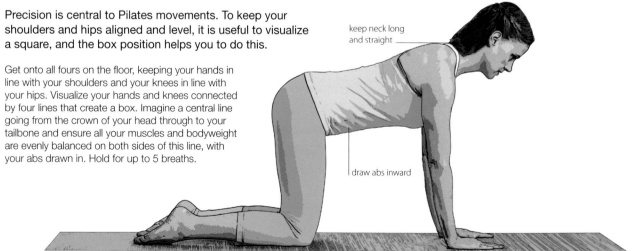

keep neck long and straight

draw abs inward

Centering: a core principle

Centering correctly takes practice and requires you to feel and activate your abs, glutes, and pelvic floor—the muscles that make up your core. Imagine scooping your abs up and in. To hold them in place, draw in an imaginary belt and let it release to a notch that holds a little tension, but isn't too tight.

Pelvic Curl

This curl teaches you how to move your spine, vertebra by vertebra. Called spine articulation, this technique is used in many Pilates exercises and helps to release a tight spine.

Lie on your back with your knees bent and legs apart, feet flat on the floor facing forward. Keeping your head and arms down, lengthen your lower back, feeling the vertebrae separate. Exhale as you lift your hips, curl your pelvis up 4–6in (10–15cm) off the mat, and draw your belly button toward your spine. Inhale as you lower your spine onto the floor, vertebra by vertebra, with control. Do up to 10 repetitions.

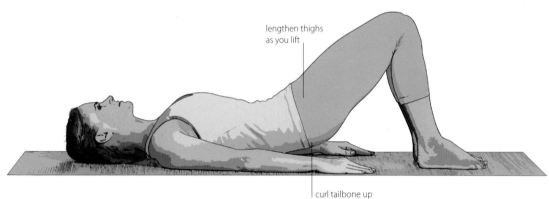

lengthen thighs as you lift

curl tailbone up

C-curve

The C-curve, a Pilates basic, curves each vertebra with control, which helps to improve spinal mobility.

Sit with your knees bent and feet hip-width apart. Place your hands behind your knees and round your back forward to make a "C" shape. Inhale deeply into your core. As you exhale, scoop your abs up higher and lift your rib cage to stretch the sides of your waist. Hold for 3–5 breaths, scooping your abs farther up with each exhalation. Then relax into a normal sitting position.

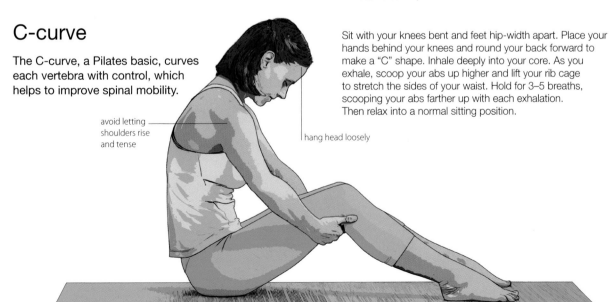

avoid letting shoulders rise and tense

hang head loosely

Upper body stability

Day-to-day work at desks, driving, lifting, and carrying can create tension in your upper body and impair posture. These exercises will strengthen and relax key postural muscles and help you to walk tall all day long, as well as relieve any tension. Both exercises use key principles of control and precision (see pp.198–99), ensuring that your body is aligned and moving as a whole.

Swan Prep

Your skeleton works hard all day keeping you upright and fighting gravity. This exercise will release the pressure that builds up and strengthen the muscles that keep you upright.

1 Lie on your front with your toes pointing long. Draw your belly button toward your spine and lengthen through your torso. Place your palms flat on the floor beneath your shoulders, fingers pointing forward, and bent elbows close to your body. Keep your neck in line with your spine and your face down. Inhale to prepare.

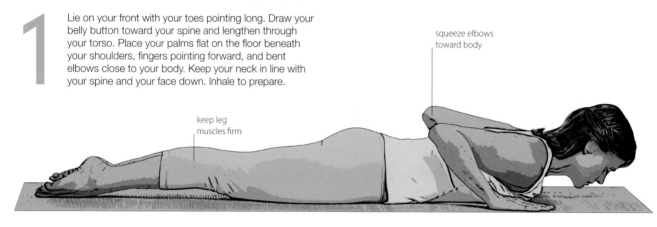

squeeze elbows toward body

keep leg muscles firm

2 As you exhale, lift up your chest and head with control and precision and look forward. Hold this position for 5 breaths, pulling your abs up and in, and squeeze your shoulder blades together to contract your upper back. As you inhale, lower yourself slowly and with control. Do up to 10 repetitions.

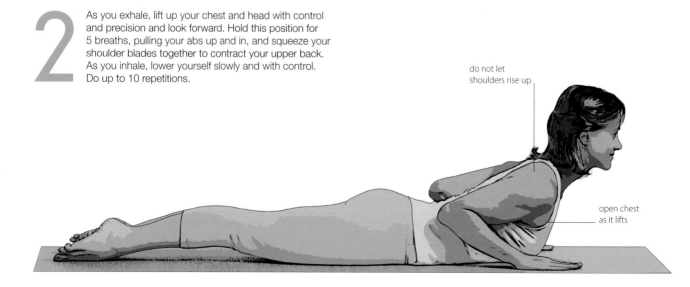

do not let shoulders rise up

open chest as it lifts

Focus on control and precision

Keeping movements slow, controlled, and within a range of motion that allows for stability and accuracy means that, with repetition, Pilates exercises become imprinted onto your brain, enabling you to flow through the movements like a dancer. Postural strength then naturally becomes part of all your daily movements.

Letter T

As you inhale and exhale through these movements, focus your attention on the muscles that you are working in your upper body to ensure that you get the maximum benefit.

1 Lie on your front with your legs together and inhale to prepare. As you exhale, raise your arms out to your sides, like the wings of a plane, raising your chest slightly off the floor as you do so. (Hold weights if you wish to work harder.) Do not drop your head, but do look slightly downward. Inhale to prepare for the next movement.

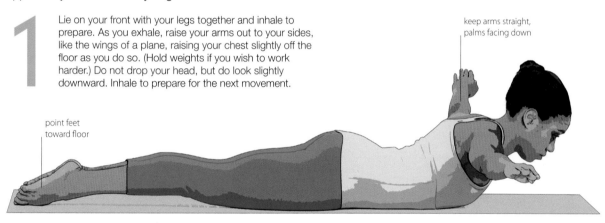

keep arms straight, palms facing down

point feet toward floor

2 As you exhale, lift your chest and head farther off the floor and look forward. At the same time, sweep your arms behind your shoulders, keeping them straight, with fingers reaching behind as if trying to touch your heels. Do not let your arms rise above shoulder height. Squeeze your shoulder blades together to contract the muscles in your upper body. Inhale as you release. Do up to 10 repetitions. Then relax into the floor.

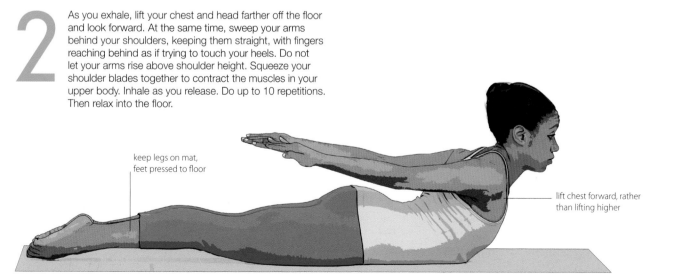

keep legs on mat, feet pressed to floor

lift chest forward, rather than lifting higher

Spine mobilization

The spine is so important—it keeps you upright and supports your limbs as you go about your daily life. These exercises will help to mobilize your spine, creating space between each vertebra, transforming it from what one teacher described as a "stiff rod" to a "string of pearls," allowing you to move freely, stand tall and relaxed, and move gracefully throughout the day.

Roll-down

This exercise helps you to become aware of your spine's mechanism as you curl your back slowly forward, vertebra by vertebra, and then curl slowly back up.

1 Stand with your feet slightly apart and let your toes splay out. Ensure that your abs are drawn in and up, and that your back is straight but retains its natural curve. Inhale to prepare. As you exhale, bend your neck forward and start the roll-down.

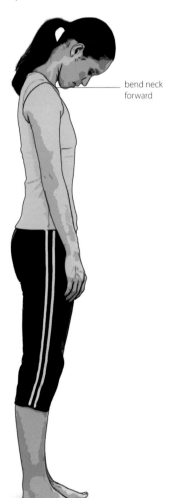

bend neck forward

keep weight centered through your feet

2 Continue to exhale as you fold forward, one vertebra at a time, until your whole spine is curled forward. Let your arms and head hang loosely toward the floor. Inhale to hold at the bottom of the roll-down, then exhale as you roll back up to the erect standing position. Repeat both steps 3–5 times.

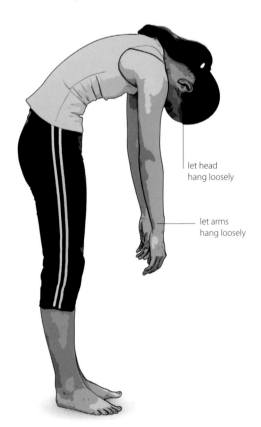

let head hang loosely

let arms hang loosely

Control your body and flow

Let the movement from your spine—which is made up of many individual but connected parts—unite to become one flowing movement by breathing in a controlled and rhythmic pattern. Learn to control your core (see pp.198–99) with precise exercises. By combining control with flowing movements, you will become more mobile in everyday life, whatever your age.

Spine Twist

This twist helps you to focus on control through your torso and precise movements that can strengthen and stretch your spine. Learn to make the movements flow.

1 Sit tall with your abs drawn in, your spine lengthened, and your chest open and expanded. Clasp your hands behind your head, with elbows bent and opened wide. Make your legs long and flex your toes, keeping the muscles in your legs taut. Inhale to prepare.

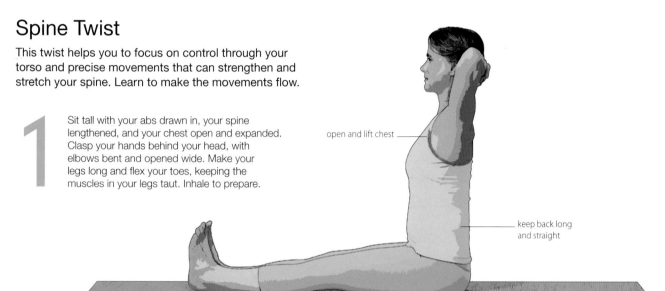

open and lift chest

keep back long and straight

2 As you exhale, twist to the right without moving your hips, legs, or feet. Keep your lower body solid by maintaining tension in the belt of muscles around your middle. Make the movement fluid, and grow tall as you twist. Inhale to return to center and then twist to the left. Continue to twist from side to side, and when you feel you've mastered the rhythm, do two pulses on each side. Do up to 10 times in total, alternating sides between each repetition.

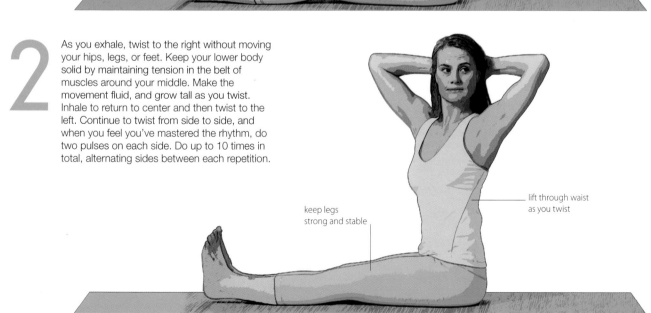

keep legs strong and stable

lift through waist as you twist

Core abdominals

Pilates is known for its emphasis on the core (see p.199), and these exercises are fantastic for creating strong abs, glutes, and lower back muscles, which will help you get a flat tummy and will enable you to perform all your other exercises more effectively.

Hundred Prep

This exercise encourages you to engage your deep abdominal muscles by using controlled breathing. As you pump your arms, you'll raise your heart rate and work your core abs hard.

1 Sit evenly on your sit bones, with your knees bent and hands placed behind your knees. Make sure you maintain a neutral spine and good alignment. Inhale to prepare.

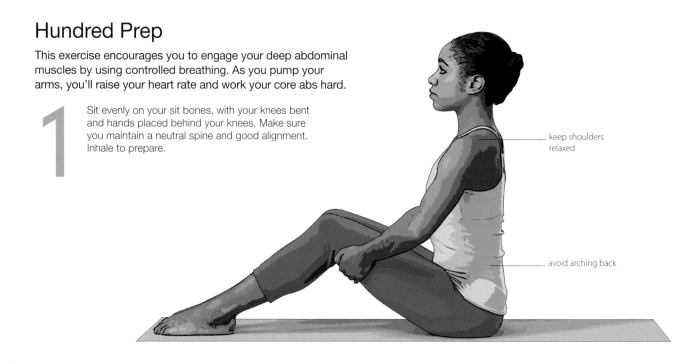

keep shoulders relaxed

avoid arching back

2 As you exhale, curl your back toward the floor, going as low as you can. Tuck your hips under you as you let your lower back touch the floor. At the same time, release your arms so that your palms are face-down by your thighs. Pump your arms up and down up to 100 times, inhaling for 5 pumps, then exhaling for 5 pumps. When you've completed your set, take hold of your legs. Exhale as you return to the starting position by rounding through your spine.

straighten arms to pump up and down

keep legs strong and stable

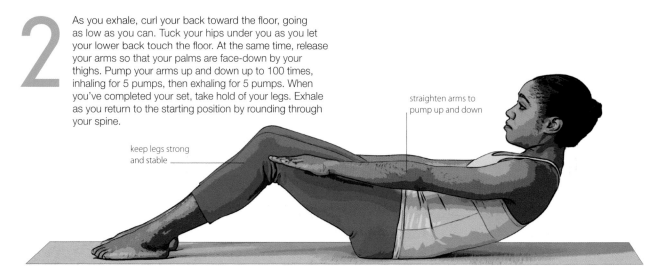

Work your core right

You need to remind yourself of the key movements of the C-curve (see p.203) before embarking on these roll-back and roll-up exercises. With all of these exercises it's vital that you are working your abdominal core effectively. A good check point is to make sure that your belly doesn't pop up, so that you don't see bulging.

Supported Abdominal Prep

This exercise helps you to avoid a sore neck while toning your abs. As you peel your neck off the floor one vertebra at a time, focus on the precise and controlled movement.

1 Lie on your back with a towel or band firmly placed under your upper back and head. Bend your knees, keeping your feet flat on the floor and your abs drawn in. Hold the band in your hands with your arms extended out above your head.
Inhale to prepare.

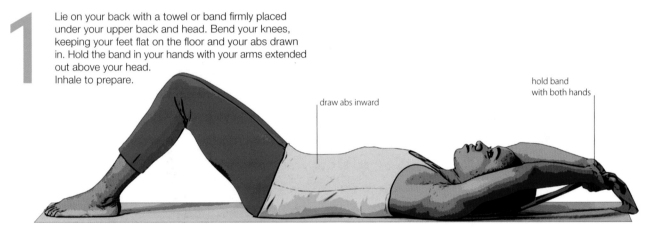

draw abs inward

hold band
with both hands

2 As you exhale, lift your head and shoulders off the floor, using the band for support. Allow your head to be heavy and focus on the precise movement of peeling your neck off the floor, letting your abs do the work. Inhale as you hold the pose at the top. Exhale as you return to the starting position, slowly melting your spine back into the floor. Do up to 10 repetitions.

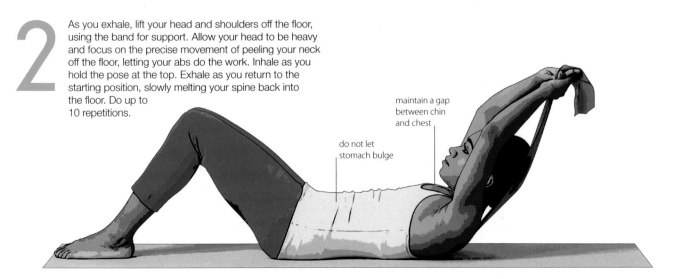

maintain a gap
between chin
and chest

do not let
stomach bulge

Single Leg Stretch

This exercise tones your abdominal muscles as you move from your center. Because your legs are in motion, there is some coordination involved.

1 Lie on your back with your abs drawn in so that your belly isn't bulging. Inhale to prepare. As you exhale, lift your head and shoulders off the floor and draw one knee toward your chest, holding onto it with your hands. At the same time, contract your glutes and stretch your opposite leg out and up with your toes pointed. Inhale as you prepare to switch legs.

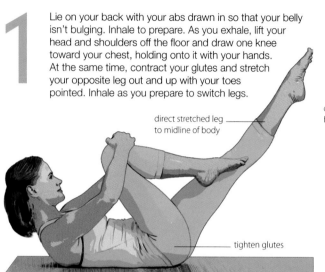

direct stretched leg to midline of body

tighten glutes

2 Exhale as you switch legs, keeping your head and shoulders off the floor. To maintain alignment, think of an imaginary line running down the center of your body lengthwise. Alternate the legs, breathing and building up to a faster tempo, but be sure to maintain control throughout. Do up to 10 times in total, alternating legs between each repetition.

do not let head drop

hold hands softly over knee

Tick-tock

For this exercise, imagine your body is like a well-tuned grandfather clock—all parts working in unison to get the tick-tock (side-to-side) motion with absolute precision.

1 Lie on your back and extend your legs at 90°. Visualize the muscles in your legs stretching out to lengthen them, and make a small V-shape with your feet. Anchor your torso by tightening an imaginary belt and spread your arms out to the sides with your palms flat on the floor. Inhale to prepare.

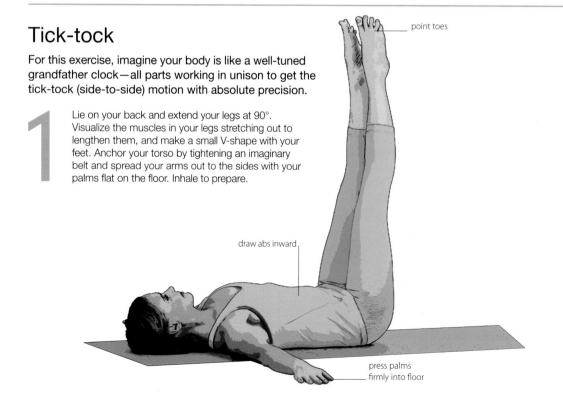
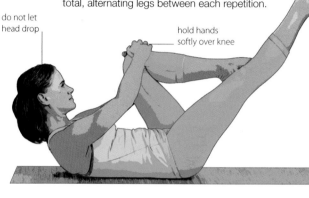

point toes

draw abs inward

press palms firmly into floor

Double Leg Stretch

Try this exercise when you are comfortable with the Single Leg Stretch (see opposite). Imagining a line down the length and center of your body helps to keep you aligned.

1 Lie on your back with your abs drawn in toward your spine. Bring your knees in toward your chest and place your hands on the front of your lower legs, just above your ankles. Lift your head and shoulders off the floor. Inhale to prepare.

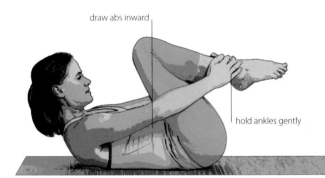

draw abs inward

hold ankles gently

2 As you exhale, let go of your ankles and stretch your arms out straight with your palms facing down. At the same time, extend your legs forward and upward at a diagonal, with your toes pointed. Keep your abs drawn in. As you inhale, tuck your knees back to the start position. Do up to 10 repetitions.

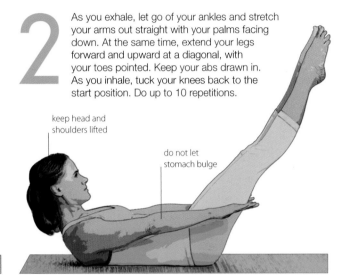

keep head and shoulders lifted

do not let stomach bulge

2 As you exhale, slightly lower both your legs over to one side. Control the movement from your core and do not let the hip farthest from the floor ride up. Keep your arms pressed into the floor. Inhale as you return to center with control, keeping your legs straight. Repeat on the other side. Do up to 10 times in total, alternating sides between each repetition. Then lower your legs and relax into the floor.

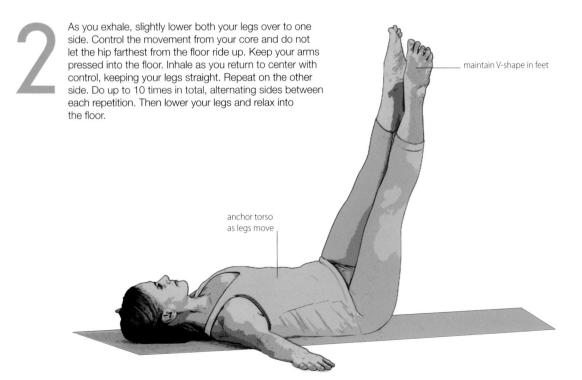

maintain V-shape in feet

anchor torso as legs move

Roll-back

This exercise reveals any weakness in your core abdominals if you try to let your shoulders or neck do the work.

1 Sit balanced on your sit bones, feeling the weight evenly distributed. Pull your belly button toward your spine to flatten your tummy. Place your hands behind your knees. Flex your feet as shown, or keep them flat on the mat. Inhale to prepare.

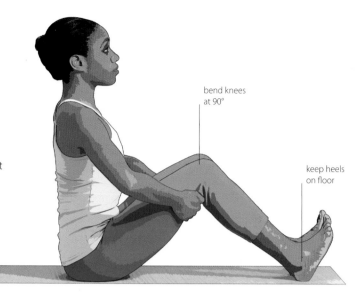

bend knees at 90°

keep heels on floor

2 As you exhale, slowly curl your back toward the floor. Keep lifting and pulling back your abs as you lengthen out through your spine. Take 3 deep breaths, exhaling more deeply as you go farther down.

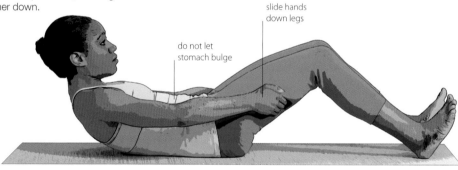

slide hands down legs

do not let stomach bulge

3 After the third exhale, curve your spine up again and tuck your head in, consciously keeping your shoulders down. Keep your mind focused on the imaginary central line of your body and keep your legs parallel throughout the movement. Feel as if your abs are fighting to come back up. Repeat all steps 3–5 times.

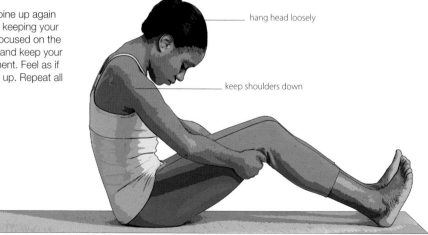

hang head loosely

keep shoulders down

Roll-up

This exercise will strongly work your abdominal muscles. It requires controlled, fluid, and rhythmic movement, and promises great results.

1 Sit with your weight evenly balanced and your legs lengthened out in front of you. Point your toes forward. Scoop in your abs and reach your arms out in front of you at shoulder height. Drop your head between your outstretched arms. Inhale to prepare.

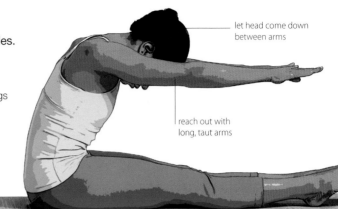

let head come down between arms

reach out with long, taut arms

reach fingers upward

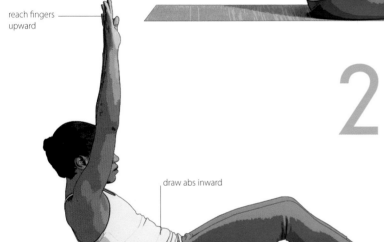

draw abs inward

2 As you exhale, slowly lower yourself down while raising your arms above your head. At the same time, slide your feet up along the mat to bend your knees. Work from your abs to move your body. Hold the position for a couple of seconds, then inhale deeply.

3 As you exhale, lower your arms back to shoulder height and curl your spine up, letting your head come down between your arms again, while gradually lengthening your legs out in front of you to take you back to the start position. Repeat all steps 3–5 times, then come up to sitting.

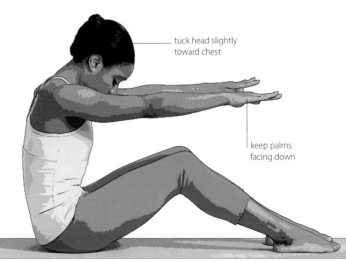

tuck head slightly toward chest

keep palms facing down

Pelvic stability

These exercises strengthen the muscles that support and stabilize your pelvis and hips, and are great for your back muscles, too. They're simple to do and, as you move with purpose and concentration, they will help to reinforce the six principles of Pilates (see pp.198–99). A strong pelvic girdle will improve your performance at any aerobic activity that uses the legs to drive you forward.

Shoulder Bridge

This exercise works both the front and back of your body since it requires a lot of strength from not only your abs, but also your back, buttocks, and the back of your legs.

1 Lie on your back with your knees bent, feet and knees hip-width apart, and your spine in neutral (see p.201) so that your belly doesn't bulge. Keep your arms straight and long by your sides, and palms pressed down into the floor. Inhale to prepare.

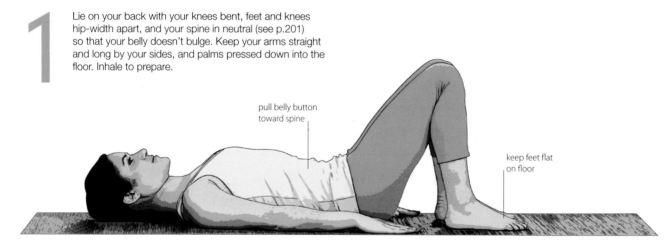

pull belly button toward spine

keep feet flat on floor

2 As you exhale, lift your buttocks off the floor to bring your body into a straight line from your shoulders to your knees, supporting your weight evenly on your shoulders and arms. Inhale to hold, then exhale to lower. Do up to 10 repetitions.

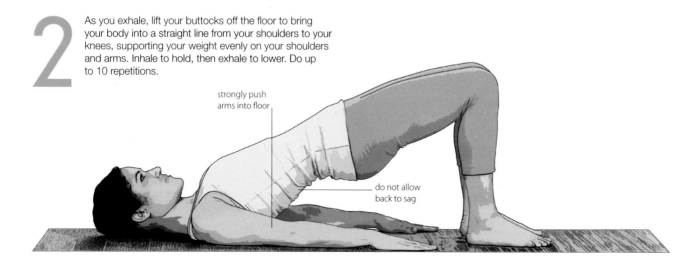

strongly push arms into floor

do not allow back to sag

Focus on stability

Visualizing a central plumb line through your body (from the crown of your head to your toes) helps your mind and body become aware of the imbalances in how the weight of your muscles and bones are distributed. A symmetrical body will perform the exercises with precision. The central point for stability is the pelvis—the place from where imbalances elsewhere often stem.

Leg Circles

Anchoring your core makes a simple movement have impact. This exercise helps to control leg movements from your core.

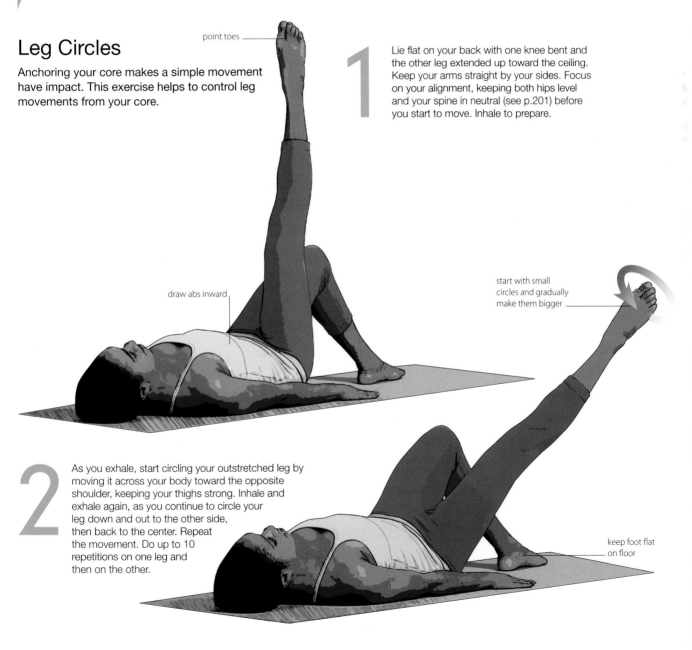

point toes

draw abs inward

start with small circles and gradually make them bigger

keep foot flat on floor

1 Lie flat on your back with one knee bent and the other leg extended up toward the ceiling. Keep your arms straight by your sides. Focus on your alignment, keeping both hips level and your spine in neutral (see p.201) before you start to move. Inhale to prepare.

2 As you exhale, start circling your outstretched leg by moving it across your body toward the opposite shoulder, keeping your thighs strong. Inhale and exhale again, as you continue to circle your leg down and out to the other side, then back to the center. Repeat the movement. Do up to 10 repetitions on one leg and then on the other.

Core glutes

We often forget the rear when we talk about the "core" but, to truly embrace the importance of symmetry and precision, the back of your body cannot be neglected. All of these exercises work in a multi-directional way to activate and strengthen both the front and back of your whole body, with the driving force coming from your core glutes.

Double Leg Lift

The focus here is on precision, working from your core glutes to strengthen the lateral muscles. We don't often work laterally, so this will help to add definition to your legs.

1 Lie on your side. Place one hand on the mat in front of your abs for support. Rest your head in your other hand, elbow on the floor. Angle your legs toward the front of the mat, with your heels touching and toes pointing away from each other. Inhale to prepare.

do not let top hip roll forward

keep heels together, toes apart

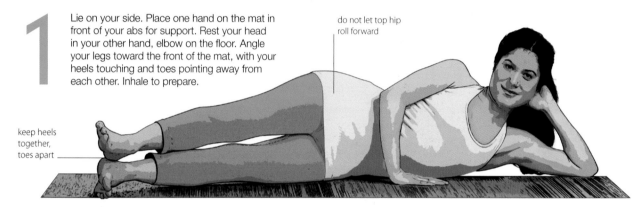

2 As you exhale, slowly lift both your legs off the floor, squeezing them together tightly as you raise them. Inhale to hold them in position, then exhale to gently lower them. As the body gets used to the movement, aim to lift your legs higher so that you work harder. Do up to 10 repetitions on each side.

squeeze legs together

do not sag at waist

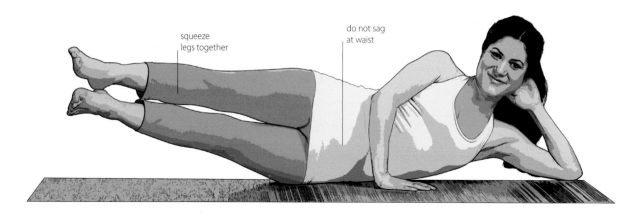

Focus on balance

If you feel that your gluteal muscles aren't working, fire them up by visualizing your sit bones drawing together before moving, and then holding onto them throughout the movement. You can practice using your gluteal muscles in everyday life by drawing your sit bones together as you walk up stairs or uphill since this is when they should be working—but often don't!

Knee Stretch

This exercise uses the strength in your quads and abs and gives your body a really good stretch.

1 Get onto all fours on the floor, keeping your hands in line with your shoulders and your knees in line with your hips. Visualize a line from your tailbone through to the crown of your head, which maintains a solid natural curve of the spine. Inhale to prepare.

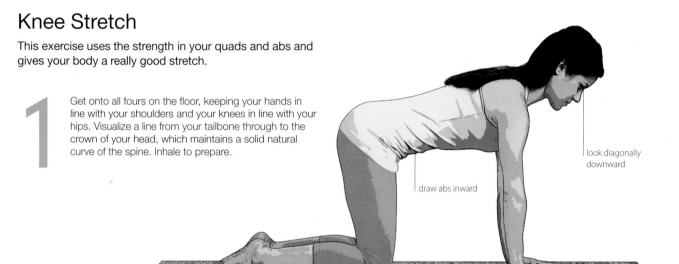

look diagonally downward

draw abs inward

2 As you exhale, extend one leg behind you, lifting your head slightly. Keep your abs working, your hips square, and don't let the hip of your raised leg ride up. Inhale to lower your leg back to the start position. Do up to 10 times in total, alternating sides between each repetition before coming back to sitting.

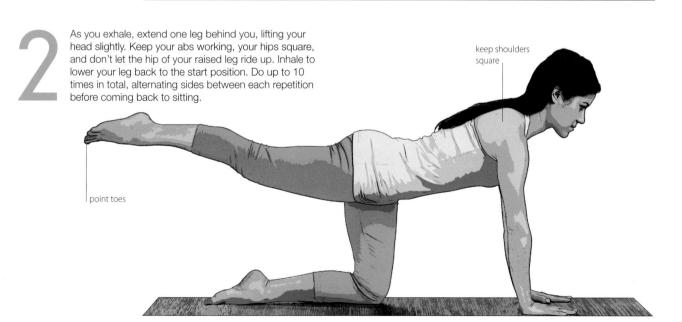

keep shoulders square

point toes

Side-lying Front Kick

Activating your glutes to perform dynamic leg movements needs extra control, so make sure you're working from a strong core. Avoid jerky movements.

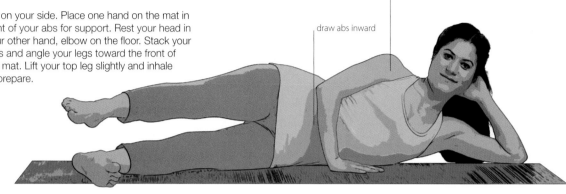

1 Lie on your side. Place one hand on the mat in front of your abs for support. Rest your head in your other hand, elbow on the floor. Stack your hips and angle your legs toward the front of the mat. Lift your top leg slightly and inhale to prepare.

do not let shoulder roll forward

draw abs inward

2 As you exhale, drive your top leg forward as far as you can, keeping it more or less level with your hip. Control the movement by making sure that your core is doing the work by scooping in your abs and contracting your glutes to rotate your leg slightly inward. Do not let the position of your back change. Inhale as you return to center.

keep leg firmly on floor

point toes

3 As you exhale, extend your top leg powerfully behind you by kicking it back, without leaning or rolling forward and keeping your hips as level as you can. Inhale as you return to center. Repeat all steps up to 10 times on each side.

keep leg straight

feel lower back lengthen

Lower Leg Side Kick

This exercise tones your hips and outer legs. The focus is on concentration—you'll need a strong core, good balance, and coordination to perform this exercise effectively.

1 Lie on your side. Place one hand on the mat in front of your abs for support. Rest your head in your other hand, elbow on the floor. Stack your hips, angle your legs toward the front of the mat, and pull your belly button toward your spine. Inhale to prepare.

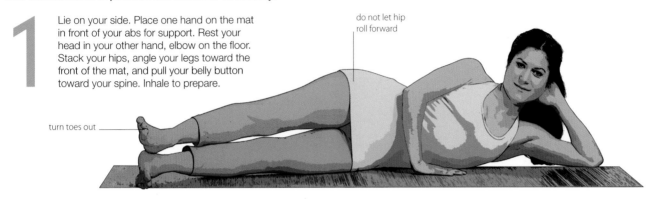

do not let hip roll forward

turn toes out

2 As you exhale, lift both legs off the floor, keeping them angled forward and squeezing them tightly together, with your toes splayed out. Make sure your abs and glutes are fully engaged during the movement so that you remain balanced.

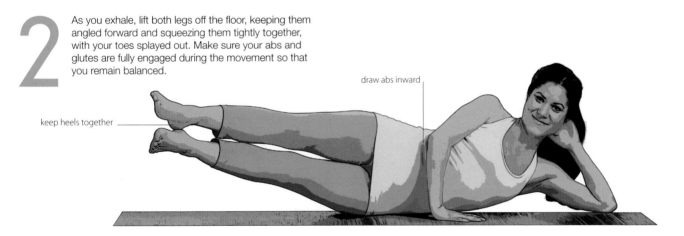

draw abs inward

keep heels together

3 As you inhale, lower your bottom leg to just above the floor, keeping the top leg where it was, then exhale as you lift it back up to meet your top leg. Repeat this movement, working your inner thighs but controlling from your abs and glutes. Repeat all steps up to 10 times before switching sides.

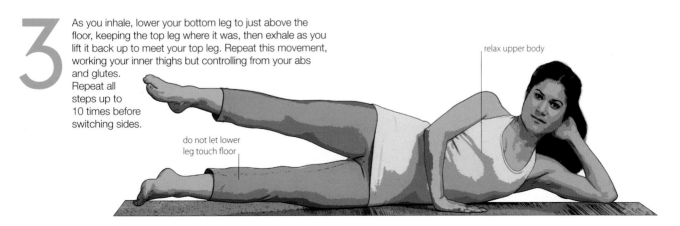

relax upper body

do not let lower leg touch floor

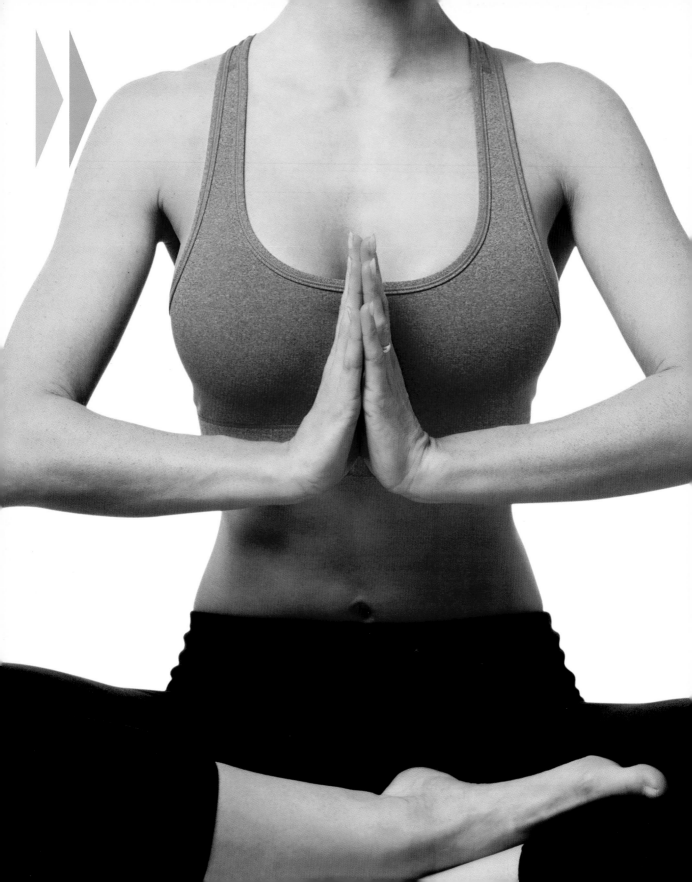

Yoga

Yoga is an ancient Indian approach to health and well-being. By dipping into the physical side of this vast wealth of respected knowledge we can draw on many of its far-reaching health and fitness benefits—both for the body and the mind. The postures, or asanas, that yogic teachings recommend provide a low-impact way to work your body, and will help to develop focus and stillness in both body and mind, strengthening you from the inside out. Yoga can be practiced by anyone and will:

- restore your optimal flexibility and strength

- help to create a leaner, more toned body

- enhance your overall body alignment and posture

- help to deepen your breathing

- encourage you to relax and de-stress

- restore your sense of balance—both physical and emotional

- heighten your performance in both other sports and everyday activities

What is yoga?

Yoga is an ancient Indian system of well-being that dates back 5,000 years. There are many variations, each with a slightly different emphasis. However, underlying all types of yoga is the belief that good health depends on a holistic approach to life—recognizing and working to enhance the mind-body-spirit connection. It is this that sets yoga apart from other forms of exercise.

History of yoga

Traditionally, there are four "paths" of yoga, all of which have the ultimate aim of reaching a higher plane of consciousness and therefore attaining a more balanced, calm state of being:

- jnana yoga involves the pursuit of knowledge
- bhakti yoga is the path of devotion and compassion
- karma yoga involves mindfulness and selfless action
- raja yoga (and its later adaptation hatha yoga) is the form most widely known and practiced in the West. This was codified by Indian sage Patanjali in the *Yoga Sutras* some time between 200BC and 200AD into a system called "ashtanga" yoga, meaning "eight limbs" (see box right).

Practicing yoga involves focusing your energy in an inward direction to help to still your mind.

It's important to note that the postures, called asanas, that many people today view of as "yoga" in its entirety are, in fact, just one part of the overall picture.

Yoga in the West

Yoga was brought to the West in the late 19th century, but it was only in the 1960s that it became popular due to masters like Swami Vishnudevananda, devoted pupil of Swami Sivananda, who presented yogic ideas in easy-to-understand terms. He proposed five principles of yoga: proper exercise, breathing, diet, relaxation, and positive thinking and meditation (see box right).

The "eight limbs" of yoga

The eight-fold path of yoga that Indian sage Patanjali put forward in his now renowned *Yoga Sutras* text offers guidelines for a well-rounded, healthy life:

- **Yama:** positive, ethical, external actions, such as non-violence, no stealing, and truthfulness
- **Niyama:** positive, self-disciplined, internal "actions," such as cleanliness and self-study
- **Asanas:** development of discipline through physical postures in preparation for meditation
- **Pranayama:** breath control exercises to gain mastery over our internal energy, known as prana
- **Pratyahara:** sensory transcendence
- **Dharana:** concentration
- **Dhyana:** meditation
- **Samadhi:** spiritual enlightenment

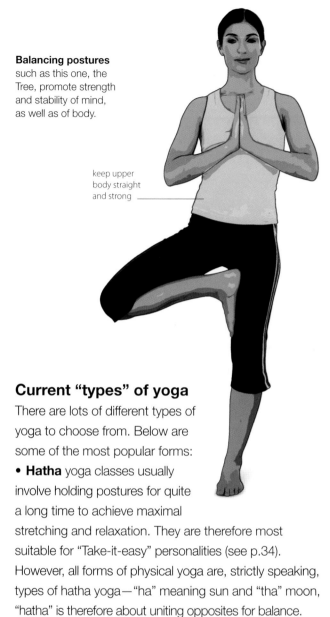

Balancing postures such as this one, the Tree, promote strength and stability of mind, as well as of body.

keep upper body straight and strong

Current "types" of yoga

There are lots of different types of yoga to choose from. Below are some of the most popular forms:
• **Hatha** yoga classes usually involve holding postures for quite a long time to achieve maximal stretching and relaxation. They are therefore most suitable for "Take-it-easy" personalities (see p.34). However, all forms of physical yoga are, strictly speaking, types of hatha yoga—"ha" meaning sun and "tha" moon, "hatha" is therefore about uniting opposites for balance.
• **Iyengar** focuses on accurate body alignment and may use props, such as blocks or straps, to help you into the positions. It's ideal for "Get-up-and-go" personalities.
• **Ashtanga vinyasa** (or power) yoga involves moving into each posture in rhythm with the breath. This flowing, dynamic yoga is perfect for "Let's-do-it!" personalities.
• **Bikram** (or hot) yoga involves doing a series of 26 postures in rooms heated to between 95–105°F (35–40°C), chiefly to promote flexibility. This yoga is also perfect for "Let's-do-it!" personalities.

Five principles of yoga

Yoga guru Swami Vishnudevananda condensed the essence of yoga into the five principles below—for physical and mental health as well as spiritual growth:

Proper exercise: Yoga postures, known as asanas, are believed to build flexibility, keeping the spinal area strong, the nervous system healthy, the body young and supple, the mind focused, and the soul nourished on its journey to perfection (samadhi—see box left).

Proper breathing: Deep, rhythmical breathing (see p.226) not only provides the body with energy, but also clears harmful toxins, thereby purifying both the body and mind. Specific breathing exercises known as pranayama (see box left) are particularly useful.

Proper diet: A diet of fresh, healthy, easy-to-digest food is recommended to supply the body with the vital energy that it needs to function optimally. Dedicated yogis are often vegetarian.

Proper relaxation: Regular and complete relaxation—both physical and mental—are considered an essential way to restore energetic balance.

Positive thinking and meditation: With a balanced, strong, and relaxed body comes increased clarity and peace of mind. Meditation declutters the mind and leads to awareness of what is really of value to you.

• **Kundalini** yoga focuses on doing exercises to awaken the subtle energy within the body, known as "kundalini," which travels up through energy centers known as chakras. It's ideal for "Get-up-and go" personalities.
• **Sivananda** yoga focuses on the five principles of yoga (see above) and particularly on getting the most from twelve key postures by holding them for quite a long time to relax into them. It's ideal for "Take-it-easy" personalities.
• **Jivamukti** yoga, meaning "liberation while living" combines intense exercise with music, meditation, and chanting—perfect for "Get-up-and-go" personalities.

Principles of yoga

The physical element of yoga, known as the postures or asanas, can be used as part of your regular fitness program to increase your strength, enhance your flexibility, and tone up your body, as well as boost your capacity for concentration. Before you do this, it's useful to understand a little more about their benefits, the type of movement they involve, and when and how to do them, so read on.

What are the benefits?

The yoga exercises in the pages that follow will work all the muscles and joints in your body, increasing not only your overall strength and flexibility, but also grounding you, nourishing you, rebalancing you, relaxing you, and re-energizing you. Gently stretching with mindfulness in each posture will restore your full range of movement. It will also allow areas of tightness and compression to unfurl and release, causing a sense of increased lightness and length throughout the body, as well as improved posture. Some body areas that may have looked a little bulky might, in fact, have been the result of muscular compression, rather than diet, which means there's even a chance of you appearing leaner, too.

Types of movement

It's important that any yoga session involves a range of movement types in order to ensure a balanced, all-over body workout. Below are the main types of movement involved in yoga asanas:

• **Forward bends:** Postures such as the Standing Forward Bend (see p.229) and the Wide-legged Forward Bend (right), stretch your hamstrings, lengthen your spine, and massage your internal organs, especially the digestive ones. The forward-bending also helps to boost your concentration, calm your mind, and encourage a sense of surrender.

• **Back bends:** Postures such as the Cobra (see p.232) both strengthen your spine and increase its mobility. The backward-bending also stretches out the front of your body, opening your chest, encouraging deep breathing, and leaving you feeling re-energized and reinvigorated.

• **Lateral bends:** Postures such as the Triangle (see p.246) increase the sideways mobility of your spine, as well as opening up the sides of your body, which can easily become compressed in everyday life.

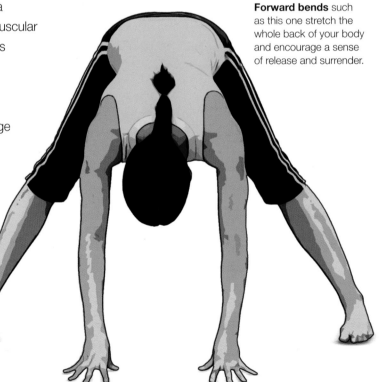

Forward bends such as this one stretch the whole back of your body and encourage a sense of release and surrender.

The importance of focus

All yoga postures should be done with a sense of gentle focus. In astanga yoga, a technique called "drishti" is recommended to cultivate this concentration. This involves directing your gaze at a particular point, the idea being that if you focus your eyes, you will focus your attention and therefore your mind. Drishti brings all the senses into one place and creates stillness of both the senses and the mind so that you are no longer distracted by the external world as you do your postures.

• **Twists:** In postures such as the Seated Twist, (see p.236), the corkscrew movement of your spine and torso releases tension throughout your back and gives your abdomen a nice massage, energizing your digestive system. Twisting movements are uncommon in daily life, so exploring this new way of moving can also help to open up your mind, making it more adaptable.

• **Balances:** Maintaining your balance in one-legged postures such as the Tree (see p.245) and also in postures that involve balancing on your hands helps to develop a strong core (see p.199) and teaches you to really focus your mind (see box above).

• **Inversions:** Upside-down poses, such as the Shoulderstand (see p.235) increase upper body strength, bring more blood to your heart, which improves your circulation, and also bring more blood to your brain, which boosts your ability to concentrate.

When should I practice?

Yoga can be done at any time. Different combinations of postures can be used to various effects, such as to energize you when you feel tired or sluggish or to help you to unwind when you're stressed. But traditionally, a vigorous practice would be done in the morning to get the body fired up for the day, while a gentle, restorative practice would be done in the evening to encourage the body to come into balance. You should always wait 2–3 hours after eating before practicing.

How long should I hold each posture?

Poses can be held for different lengths of time depending on the "type" of yoga you're doing (see p.223) and how you're feeling at the time. Specific guidance is given for each posture within the pages that follow. However, if you want to achieve a deeper stretch or relaxation than the time recommended allows, feel free to hold a pose for a little longer, as long as it's causing you no discomfort.

Do I need props?

A yoga block can be useful to support you and help with posture, alignment, and comfort; a yoga belt can be used as an extension of your arms if you can't quite achieve a desired position or to deepen a pose; and a bolster is ideal under your spine or knees to deepen relaxation.

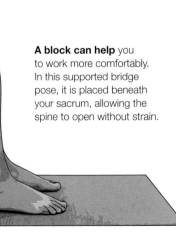

A block can help you to work more comfortably. In this supported bridge pose, it is placed beneath your sacrum, allowing the spine to open without strain.

Breathing and relaxation

Learning to become aware of and deepen your breathing is a key aspect of yoga, since only by breathing fully and deeply can you provide your body with the energy it needs to function optimally. Relaxation is another integral aspect—equally as important as the more physically challenging postures. The exercises below will enable you to get to grips with the fundamentals of both these things.

Yogic Breathing

This exercise encourages full, deep breathing, boosting energy and reducing stress and toxins in your body. It will also rebalance your nervous system and improve concentration.

1 Sit tall with your legs crossed. Place one hand on your abdomen and the other on your chest. As you inhale, feel your abdomen expand and rise like a balloon filling with air. As you continue to draw in air, feel your chest rise, the back and sides of your rib cage expand, and your collar bones lift.

2 As you start to exhale, first feel your abdomen gradually relax and deflate, then feel your rib cage lower again. Finally, empty the last bit of air from your lungs by actively drawing in your abdomen. Repeat both steps at least 10 times in total, drawing up tall through your head and keeping your sit bones firmly anchored to the floor.

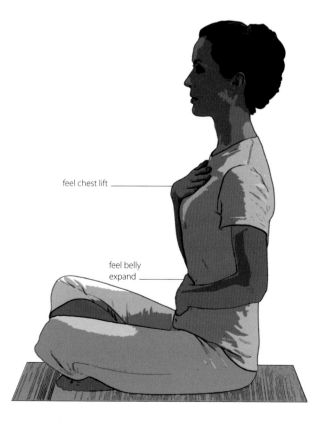

feel chest lift

feel belly expand

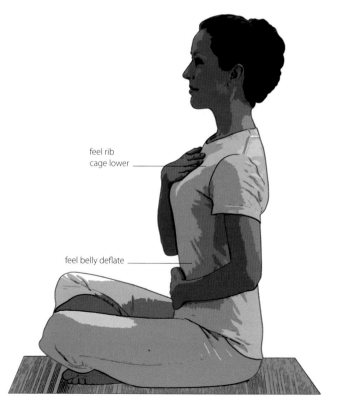

feel rib cage lower

feel belly deflate

The art of pranayama

In yogic terms, our vital energy, or "prana," is gained through our food and our breath. Learning to control our breath through exercises, known as pranayama, is therefore hugely beneficial. The starting point is full, deep, yogic breathing (see below left). To explore pranayama further once you have mastered this, you could consider investing in a yoga—or pranayama-specific book.

Child's Pose

This nourishing posture can be done as a relaxing exercise in itself or as a rest between more active postures to give your body time to absorb their benefits.

Kneel down. Let your big toes touch, keep your knees apart, and sit back on your heels. Lower yourself to rest your head on the floor in front of you. Relax your arms by your sides. Inhale and feel your breath reach your lower back. Exhale and relax. Take at least 10 breaths in this position before returning to seated.

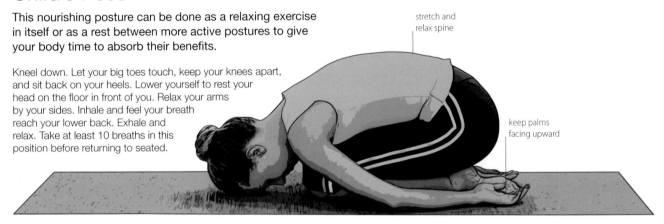

stretch and relax spine

keep palms facing upward

Corpse Pose

This encourages complete relaxation—both physical and mental. It should be done at the end of every yoga practice and can be done any time as a relaxation in its own right.

Lie on your back with your legs apart and your arms diagonally out from your body. Close your eyes. Inhale and tense one leg, exhale and release it. Do the same on the other leg. Move up through your body, tensing each area after inhaling and releasing after exhaling: buttocks, abs, chest, arms, shoulders, neck, and face. Observe the flow of air both in and out through your nose and completely surrender your body into the floor for 25 breaths.

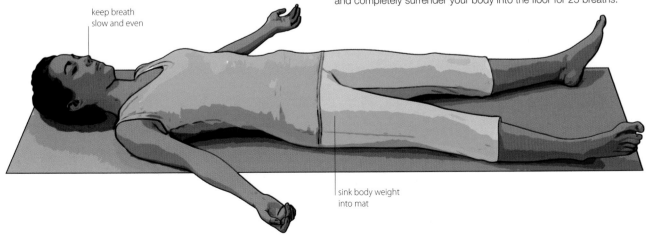

keep breath slow and even

sink body weight into mat

Sun Salutation

A wonderful mainstay of yoga, the flowing Sun Salutation sequence on the pages that follow can be done on its own or as a warm-up to the rest of your yoga practice. If you do nothing else, ten of these a day will start to make a difference to how you look and feel. Aim to move into each new pose on the breath, as indicated, but take an extra breath or two in each pose as required.

Mountain

1 Stand tall with your feet hip-width apart and firmly rooted to the floor and your arms by your sides. Imagine a plumb line through the center of your body to help to keep you in balance. As you inhale through your nose, let your body grow taller. As you exhale through your nose, draw your shoulder blades backward and downward.

relax shoulders

ensure weight is evenly distributed between both feet

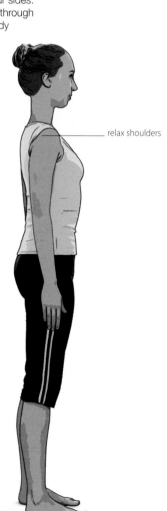

Extended Mountain

2 As you inhale, pull your belly button toward your spine and sweep your arms above your head so that they are close to your ears, with your palms facing inward. Feel all the muscles in your body lengthen and ensure that you keep your body in a straight line.

stretch fingertips upward

draw tailbone straight down

The importance of flow

When doing a sequence of yoga poses, such as in the Sun Salutation below, it's important that everything flows smoothly together: the transition between one pose and the next is just as important as each pose in itself. The main way to achieve this is to do each movement either on an inhalation or an exhalation. This creates what is called *vinyasa*—smooth, breath-connected movement.

Standing Forward Bend

3

As you exhale, fold your body forward from your waist, aiming for your torso to touch your thighs and your hands to touch the floor on either sides of your feet—palms down if possible, fingertips if not. Keep your legs straight if you can but if this is too intense, bend them a little to help you to reach farther toward the floor. Allow your head, neck, and shoulders to relax.

keep neck long

keep legs straight
if possible

Lunge

4

As you inhale, extend your right leg behind you and place your knee on the floor, while bending your front leg to 90° so that you are in a deep lunge. Place your hands on the floor on either side of your front foot—palms down if possible, fingertips if not, and let your chest rest gently on your knee. Look downward.

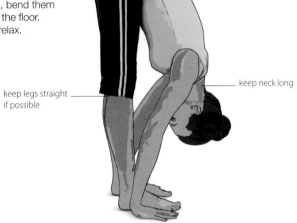

keep knee in
line with ankle

keep back
knee on floor

Plank

5 As you exhale, turn the toes of your right foot under so that you are on the ball of your foot, straighten your leg, and step your left foot back to join your right one, hip-width apart. As you inhale, ensure that your arms are in a straight line with your shoulders, strongly engage your abdominal and leg muscles, and look downward to keep your body in more or less a straight line from your head to your heels.

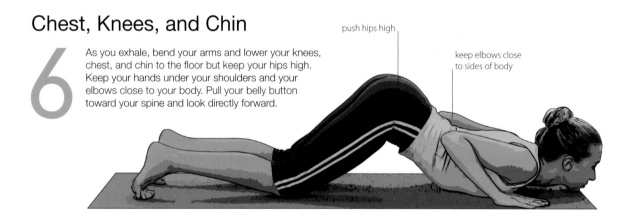

draw abs inward

look directly downward

Chest, Knees, and Chin

6 As you exhale, bend your arms and lower your knees, chest, and chin to the floor but keep your hips high. Keep your hands under your shoulders and your elbows close to your body. Pull your belly button toward your spine and look directly forward.

push hips high

keep elbows close to sides of body

Upward Dog

7 As you inhale, bring your hips down, rest the tops of your feet on the floor, lift your head, shoulders, and chest off the floor, and look forward so that your chest is open. Pull your shoulder blades back and down and your elbows into your sides, while pressing your hands into the floor. An easier option, if required, is to let your forearms support you on the floor, while pulling your shoulders downward.

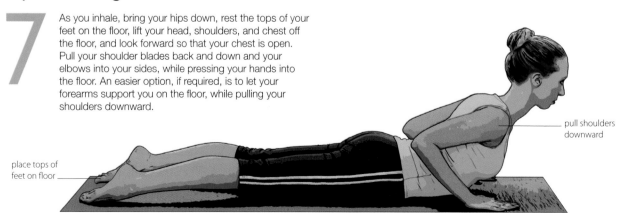

place tops of feet on floor

pull shoulders downward

Downward Dog

8 As you exhale, tuck your toes under, push your hips as high as you can in the air, and aim to press your heels toward the floor, with straight legs. At the same time, straighten your arms and press your palms into the floor, fingers spread wide. Pull your belly button toward your spine and look toward your belly. Bend your knees, if necessary, for comfort. Hold for 5 breaths.

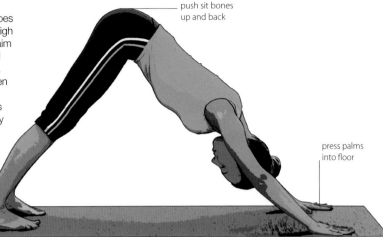

push sit bones up and back

press palms into floor

Standing Forward Bend

9 As you inhale, press your weight into your hands, step your feet up between your hands, then exhale as you straighten your legs so that you come into a forward bend. Relax your head and neck and bend your knees slightly for comfort, if required. Strongly pull in your abdominal muscles and really engage both your front and back thigh muscles.

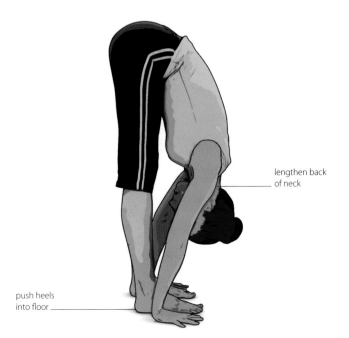

lengthen back of neck

push heels into floor

Extended Mountain

10 As you inhale, come slowly up to standing, sweeping your arms above your head as you do so and extending your fingertips toward the ceiling. Pull your shoulder blades back and down, and reach higher. As you exhale, lower your arms to your sides and stand in Mountain Pose (Step 1), looking straight ahead.

Gradually build up to doing 10 rounds of this 10-step Sun Salutation sequence as you become more confident with it.

keep legs straight but not locked

keep weight even through both feet

Upper body strength and toning

The yoga poses that follow will release tension and create an increased sense of internal space and length throughout your body. At the same time, they'll build a stronger, leaner upper body, allowing you to carry out daily activities with more ease and efficiency, whether carrying groceries or lifting your kids. A strong body means you'll also be more effective at other forms of exercise.

Cobra

This front-lying back bend will not only strengthen your back, but also increase the flexibility of your spine and release any held tension in your upper back.

1 Lie on your front with your forehead resting on the floor, hands placed by the sides of your chest, fingertips in line with your shoulders and pointing forward, and elbows bent in the air. As you exhale, make your legs long and point your toes so that the top of your feet are on the floor.

keep elbows close to body

press top of feet into floor

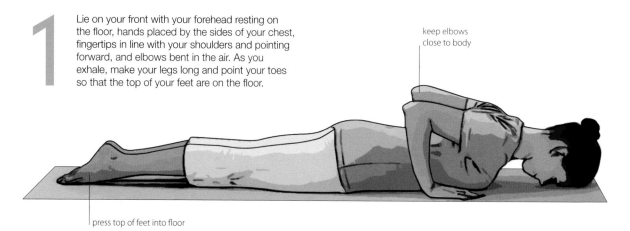

2 As you inhale, press your hands into the floor and lift your head, shoulders, and upper chest off the floor, lengthening your spine. Keep your elbows close to your body and pull your shoulder blades back and down so that your shoulders are away from your ears. Look forward. Hold for at least 5 breaths, breathing smoothly and evenly, then lower your body to the floor as you exhale.

relax buttocks

engage thigh muscles

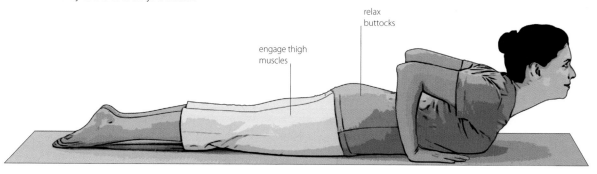

Energetic lightness

In any yoga poses that you do, it's important to aim for a sense of what can be called energetic lightness. This means that as well as being firmly rooted and grounded—whether through the feet when standing, the sit bones when seated, or the head or hands in inversions—you should always draw up through your body also, to achieve an opposing sense of length, openness, and lightness.

Inclined Plane

This challenging exercise stretches the front of your body and strengthens the back of your body. It therefore helps to balance out the work of forward bends.

1 Sit tall with your legs long and your toes pointing forward. Place your hands behind you, fingers pointing away from you, and strongly pull your belly button toward your spine. Open your chest and slowly tilt your head backward, lengthening the front of your neck. Squeeze your shoulder blades together to expand your chest more.

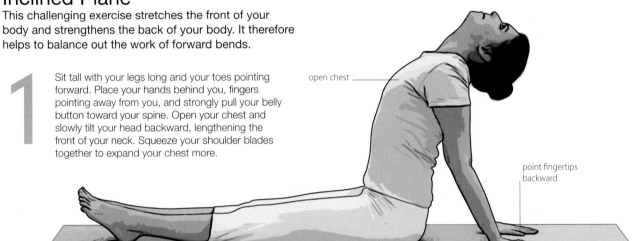

open chest

point fingertips backward

2 As you inhale, press your hands and feet into the floor and lift your hips forward and upward so that your legs form a diagonal line with the floor. Keep your head tilted back, letting go of any tension in your neck and making sure that your shoulders are directly above your hands. Hold for at least 5 breaths. Exhale to return to Step 1 before returning your head to neutral.

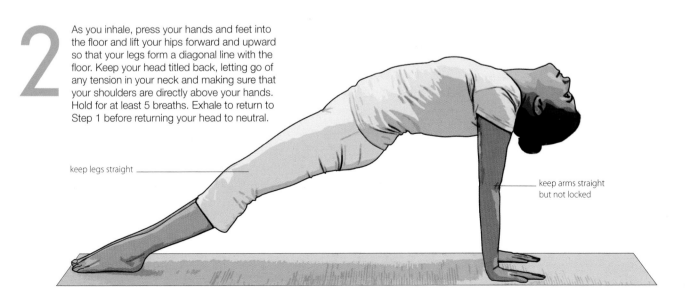

keep legs straight

keep arms straight but not locked

Bow

This exercise stretches the whole front of your body as you take on the shape of a bow, with your arms forming the strings. It also releases tension from your upper back.

1 Lie on your front, with your forehead on the floor. As you inhale, stretch your left arm in front of you and your toes out behind. As you exhale, bend your right leg, using your right hand to draw your ankle toward your bottom. Inhale, then exhale as you release your leg. Repeat on the other side.

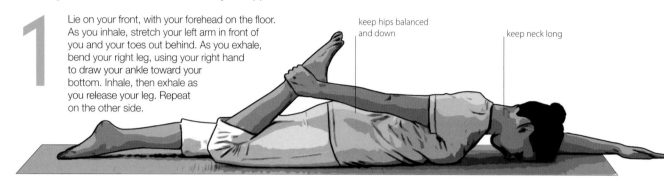

keep hips balanced and down

keep neck long

2 Inhale to prepare. Then as you exhale, bend both legs toward your buttocks holding your ankles with your hands to keep them in place. Keep your arms straight, forehead relaxed on the floor, abs drawn in, and hips balanced.

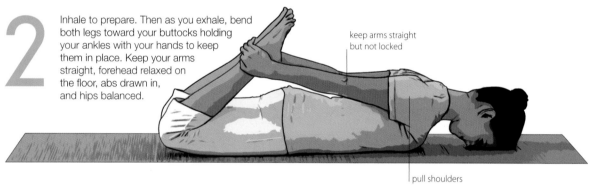

keep arms straight but not locked

pull shoulders back and down

3 As you inhale, push your feet up until your knees come as high off the floor as possible. At the same time, lift your whole upper body as high as you can off the floor, keeping your abs engaged to protect your back, your lower back long, and your arms straight but not locked. Hold for at least 5 breaths. As you exhale, release your feet and slowly lower your knees, upper body, and forehead back onto the floor.

look diagonally upward

strongly engage thighs

Shoulderstand

This challenging inversion really strengthens your shoulders and upper back muscles. Do not move your head throughout the movement.

1 Lie on your back with your abs drawn in, hips level, shoulders relaxed, and neck and head long and centered. Inhale deeply, then exhale and raise your legs to 90°. Keep your legs straight and flex your feet so that your soles face the ceiling. Let your arms lie straight alongside your body, palms down.

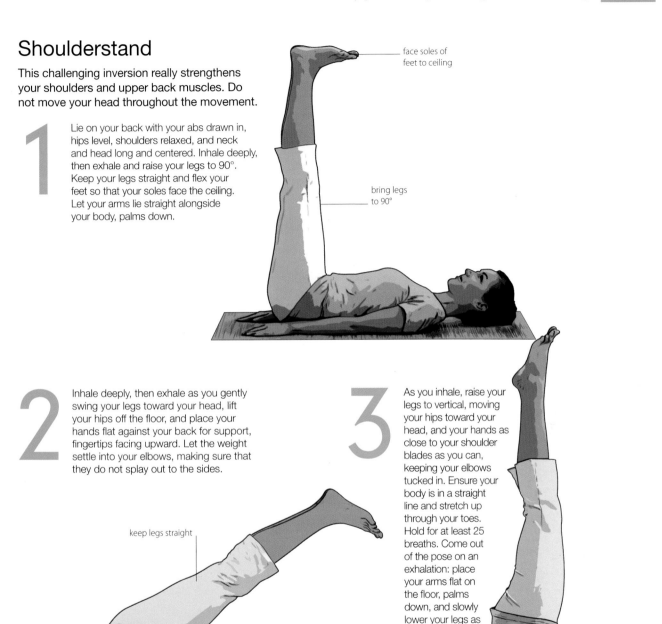

face soles of feet to ceiling

bring legs to 90°

2 Inhale deeply, then exhale as you gently swing your legs toward your head, lift your hips off the floor, and place your hands flat against your back for support, fingertips facing upward. Let the weight settle into your elbows, making sure that they do not splay out to the sides.

keep legs straight

keep back long and strong

3 As you inhale, raise your legs to vertical, moving your hips toward your head, and your hands as close to your shoulder blades as you can, keeping your elbows tucked in. Ensure your body is in a straight line and stretch up through your toes. Hold for at least 25 breaths. Come out of the pose on an exhalation: place your arms flat on the floor, palms down, and slowly lower your legs as you roll your spine down, using your abs for control.

tuck chin in toward chest

keep weight in elbows

Spine fluidity

The spine is a complex mechanism that moves forward and backward (sagittal), side to side (lateral), and also in a rotating motion (axial). The yoga poses on the following pages aim to make the spine more fluid and free to move in all directions, but focus particularly on the movements that we tend to do less in everyday life, mainly twists and back bends, in order to maximize mobility.

Seated Twist

This exercise improves the flexibility and fluidity of your entire spine—from base to neck. It also gives your abdomen a nice massage as you twist it against your leg.

1 Sit tall, with your legs straight in front of you. Bend your right knee and cross it over your left leg, placing your right foot alongside your left calf. As you inhale, place your right hand slightly behind your back with your palm on the floor, fingers pointing away from you, and reach your left arm up toward the ceiling. Keep your spine straight throughout.

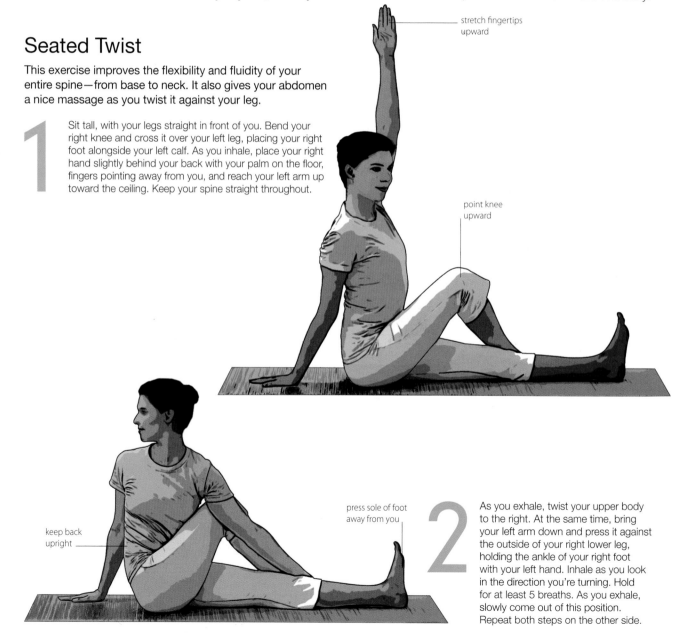

stretch fingertips upward

point knee upward

keep back upright

press sole of foot away from you

2 As you exhale, twist your upper body to the right. At the same time, bring your left arm down and press it against the outside of your right lower leg, holding the ankle of your right foot with your left hand. Inhale as you look in the direction you're turning. Hold for at least 5 breaths. As you exhale, slowly come out of this position. Repeat both steps on the other side.

The importance of the spine

A strong, flexible spine is essential for good posture and effective movement, as well as for a healthy nervous system due to the spinal column housing the spinal cord. In yoga, this superhighway of nerves is conceptualized as the central energy channel known as the *sushumna nadi*, at the base of which lies our kundalini energy (see p.223), coiled like a serpent, waiting to be awakened and rise up through the body.

Lying Twist

A nourishing rotation that opens your rib cage and provides a lovely twist through your waist, this pose will ease stiffness and release tension.

1 Lie on your back. As you inhale, extend your arms out to your sides at shoulder level and pull your belly button toward your spine to engage your abdominal muscles. As you exhale, bend your knees, lift your feet off the floor, and bring your thighs slightly toward your chest. Inhale to prepare.

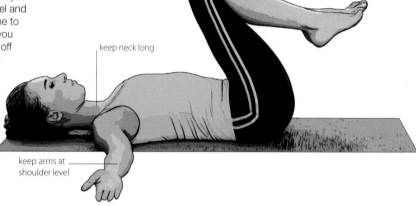

keep neck long

keep arms at shoulder level

2 As you exhale, slowly lower your knees to one side while turning your head to the other, feeling the twisting sensation through your middle. As you twist, feel your rib cage expand and open like a fan. Hold for at least 5 breaths. Then inhale as you come back to the center, as in Step 1. Repeat on the other side, your knees now going to the left and your head to the right.

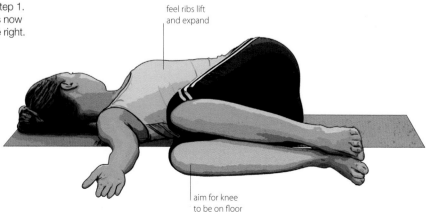

feel ribs lift and expand

aim for knee to be on floor

Wheel

This intense exercise stretches out the whole front of your body, works your back muscles, increases the flexibility of your spine, and boosts energy levels.

1 Lie on your back and bend your legs so that your knees point upward and your feet face forward, hip-width apart. Slowly move your feet in toward your buttocks and take hold of your ankles with your hands, keeping your arms straight.

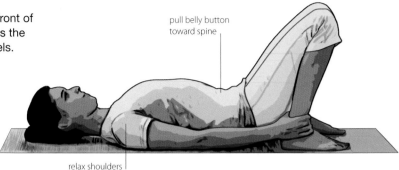

pull belly button toward spine

relax shoulders

2 Keeping your head, neck, and shoulders on the floor, inhale as you energetically lift your hips and bottom off the floor as far as you can, pushing them upward and arching your spine. Press your shoulders and feet firmly into the floor so that your weight is distributed between the two. Hold this position for at least 5 breaths.

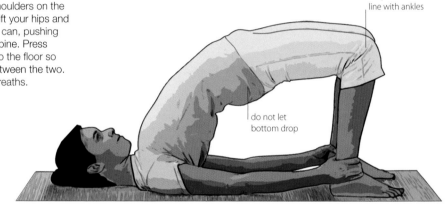

keep knees in line with ankles

do not let bottom drop

Fish

This back bend, the counterpose to the Shoulderstand (see p.235), releases tension in your neck and throat, corrects round shoulders, and opens up your chest area.

1 Lie on your back with your legs and feet together and place your hands beside each other under your buttocks, palms facing downward. Keep your arms straight and tuck them under your upper body so that they raise it slightly off the floor.

pull belly button toward spine

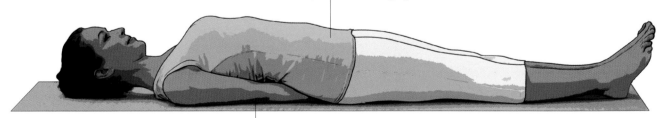

tuck elbows under body

3 If you feel comfortable with Step 2, remove your hands from your ankles and place them, palms down, by your ears, with your fingers pointing toward your shoulders and your elbows in the air. Keep your feet flat on the floor and do not let your back or hips drop.

keep bent arms close to head

strongly engage thigh muscles

4 As you inhale, push on your hands to lift your shoulders off the floor. At the same time, lift your head and gently place the top of it on the floor. Keep your elbows bent and pointing away from your body. Contract your glutes to maintain a good lift of your hips and keep your thighs strong. Aim to hold this extremely challenging pose for at least 5 breaths if you can, but do not force it. To come out of the pose, exhale as you bend your arms and reverse Steps 3, 2, and 1.

do not let knees bend beyond toes

rest crown of head lightly on floor

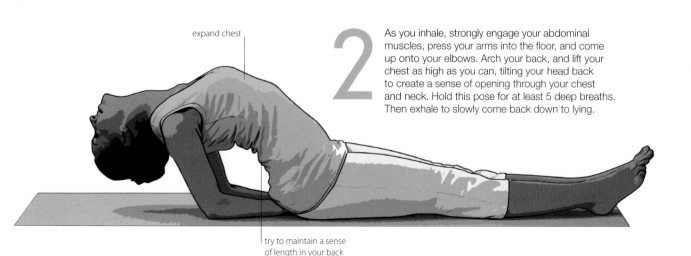

expand chest

2 As you inhale, strongly engage your abdominal muscles, press your arms into the floor, and come up onto your elbows. Arch your back, and lift your chest as high as you can, tilting your head back to create a sense of opening through your chest and neck. Hold this pose for at least 5 deep breaths. Then exhale to slowly come back down to lying.

try to maintain a sense of length in your back

Deep hip release

The yoga poses that follow will help to make everyday sitting, standing, and walking easier by releasing any tension within your hip joints, an area that often becomes tight as we spend so much time sitting during our daily lives—whether at desks, in cars, on trains, or on the sofa. Doing these exercises regularly will help to keep your hips open and mobile into old age.

Horse

Like the animal it is named after, this pose is strong and energetic. It will create powerful legs and glutes as well as giving your inner thighs a fantastic stretch.

1 Stand with your feet wider than hip-width apart, abs drawn in, back long, shoulders down, and feet and knees turned out at 45°. As you inhale, sweep your arms out to the sides and then above your head, with your palms together.

2 As you exhale, bend your knees as low as you can go without your knees moving beyond the line of your toes. At the same time, bring your arms down through your center line into what is called "prayer position": your palms pressed together vertically at chest height. Hold for at least 5 breaths. Inhale as you come up to standing.

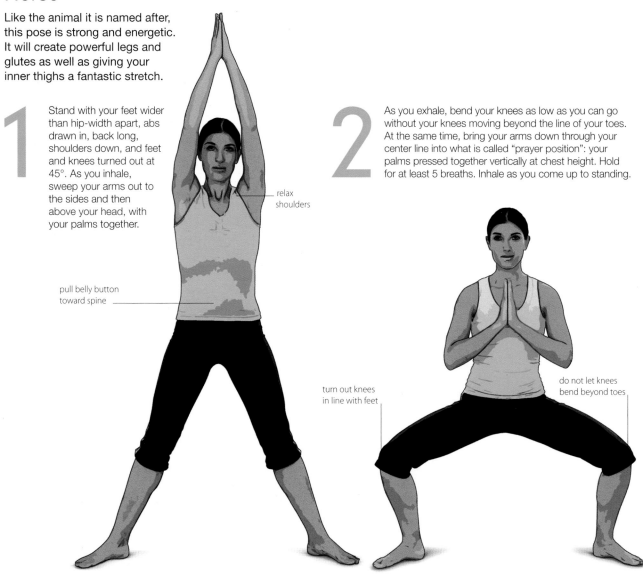

relax shoulders

pull belly button toward spine

turn out knees in line with feet

do not let knees bend beyond toes

Encouraging deep release

One of the many benefits of yoga is that different poses create a sense of release and decompression in different areas of the body. Deep, rhythmical breathing can help with this: imagine each full breath you take reaching deep into your joints, like an invisible, flowing key that unlocks the tension in the surrounding muscles, enabling them to function optimally again.

Sitting Squat

This deep squat works all your leg muscles and is quite a challenge for the hip flexors. It requires real strength and flexibility to get into and maintain the lowest position.

1 Stand tall with your feet hip-width apart and bend your knees into a half squat. As you inhale, bend your arms up in front of you at chest height, palms facing each other, and place them in what is called the "eagle position" by wrapping your right upper arm over your left and aiming to place the fingers of your left hand on your right palm. Bring your thumbs in line with your nose.

relax shoulders

do not over-arch back

2 As you exhale, slowly bend your knees and lower your buttocks with the aim of getting them between your heels just above the floor. If your heels start to rise off the floor, go back to the point at which you could still keep your feet flat. Aim to hold for at least 5 breaths, then slowly come back to standing as you inhale. However, if you feel any discomfort or start to topple over before this, come up earlier. Exhale as you release your arms to your sides. Then repeat both steps with your arms wrapped in the other direction—left over right.

keep back flat

keep heels down if possible

Single-leg Forward Bend

This pose works deeply through each hip and stretches all the muscles of the back of your body. Follow it with its counterpose, the Inclined Plane (see p.233).

1 Sit up tall with your legs straight out in front of you. Bend your right leg so that the sole of your right foot sits against the inside of your left thigh and your right knee points out to the side. Flex your left foot so that your sole presses away from you. As you inhale, reach your arms up above your head.

stretch fingertips upward

pull belly button toward spine

2 As you exhale, bend foward over your left leg and reach your hands toward your toes and your chest toward your thigh. If they don't reach, just stretch your hands as far as they'll reach keeping your back straight and your shoulders down. Take at least 5 breaths in this pose, lengthening out your spine with each exhalation. Release and repeat on the other side.

relax neck

keep foot flexed

Cross-legged Forward Bend

This seated forward bend helps to calm the mind as well as giving the inner thighs a good stretch and the hip flexors a nice challenge. Let gravity do most of the work.

1 Sit cross-legged on the floor. As you inhale, draw up tall through the top of your head. As you exhale, slowly hinge forward from your hips and place your hands on the floor in front of you, fingertips facing forward, without rounding your back. Inhale here, keeping your sit bones firmly rooted and looking diagonally downward.

keep back straight

keep hips grounded

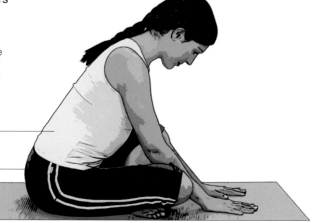

Seated Wide-legged Forward Bend

This forward bend is a wonderful way to open up your hip joints and stretch your entire spine and legs. It is also a useful way to release built-up tension at the end of a day.

1 Sit with your legs opened as wide as you can, flex your feet, and press your heels away from you. Pull your belly button toward your spine, and inhale as you sweep your arms above your head, palms facing forward and fingertips reaching upward. Make sure your body is balanced on both sides.

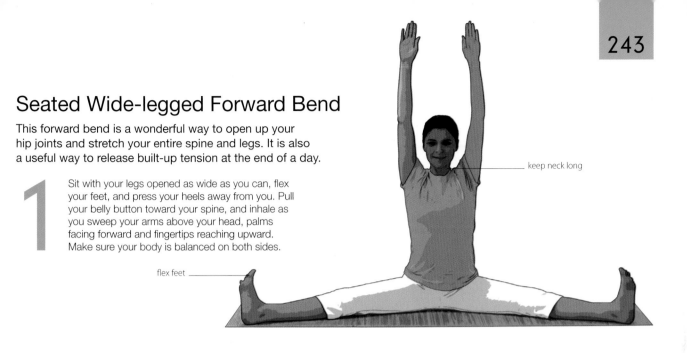

keep neck long

flex feet

2 As you exhale, bend forward from your waist, reaching each arm toward its corresponding leg so that your fingers touch the toes of your outstretched legs. If you can't reach, touch your ankles or calves instead. Keep your sit bones anchored to the floor. Hold for at least 5 breaths, then release. Inhale as you return to upright.

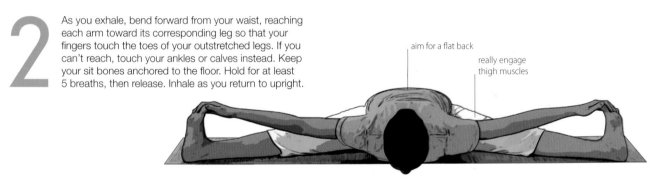

aim for a flat back

really engage thigh muscles

2 As you exhale, reach your hands farther forward on the floor, feeling your hips open wider as you do so. Hold for at least 5 breaths, extending the stretch on each exhalation. However, if there's any discomfort, gradually come back up to sitting. Then do both steps again with the opposite leg on top in the cross-legged position.

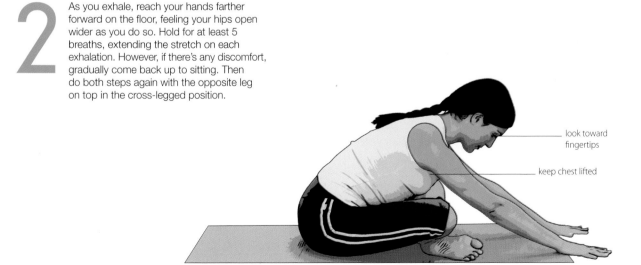

look toward fingertips

keep chest lifted

Lower body strength and toning

The yoga poses that follow have been specially chosen to both strengthen and tone your legs, which will not only make you look and feel better, but will also boost your metabolism since a strong, lean body burns more calories. Regularly doing these exercises will also encourage your lower body joints to open more fully, which will mean less stress on your spine when sitting.

Chair

This classic pose, where you essentially sit down without a chair, stretches and releases your shoulders and chest as well as working your legs.

1 Stand tall with your feet hip-width apart. As you inhale, extend your arms forward and then up above your head, so that your fingers point upward, with your palms together if you can. Otherwise keep them parallel and facing one another. At the same time, raise yourself up onto your toes keeping your legs straight. Hold for at least 5 breaths.

2 As you exhale, place your heels back on the floor and bend your knees as if you are sitting down on a chair, aiming for your thighs to be as close to horizontal as possible. Create length through your spine by drawing your tailbone toward the floor as you lift your chestbone. Hold for at least 5 breaths, then come up to standing as you inhale.

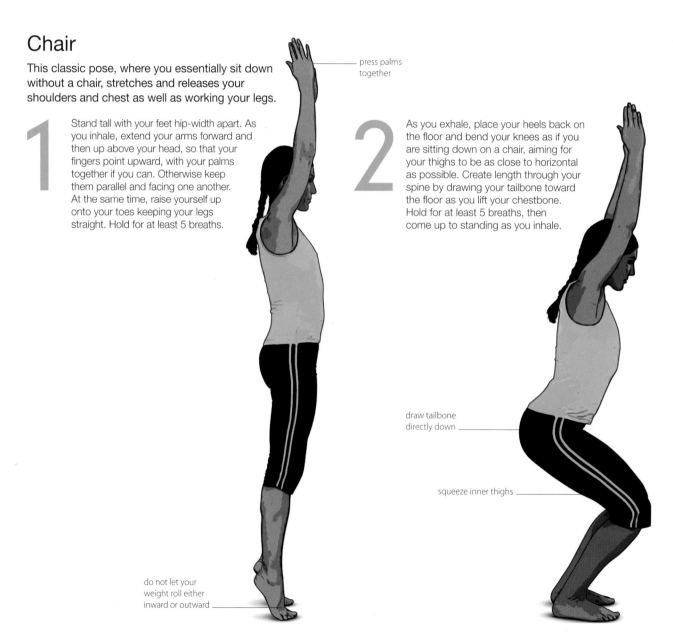

press palms together

draw tailbone directly down

squeeze inner thighs

do not let your weight roll either inward or outward

The importance of pelvic stability

Keeping your pelvis strong is vital to the health of your whole body since it acts as a basin for your spine to sit in and so is a link between your upper and lower body. Many people, especially those who spend a lot of time sitting, underuse this area, which means it can become somewhat collapsed. The lower body exercises below and opposite will help to both strengthen and stabilize it.

Tree

This nature-inspired pose really challenges both your lower body and your abs as you try to maintain balance on just one leg. It also cultivates a strong sense of focus.

1 Stand tall with your feet hip-width apart. As you inhale, raise your right foot and place the sole of it as high as you can on your inner left thigh, with your right knee pointing out to the side. As you exhale, bring your hands into the prayer position: palms pressed together at chest height. Ensure that you remain absolutely upright—do not let your left hip jut out to the side.

keep hips level

strongly root foot into floor

2 As you inhale, sweep your arms up above your head, extending them upward like the branches of a tree. If you're struggling with balance, support yourself against a wall with one hand. Hold for at least 5 breaths. Exhale as you bring your arms and leg down. Then repeat both steps with the other leg raised.

pull belly button toward spine

keep knee out to side

Triangle

This pose helps to develop strength in your feet, legs, and hips, and aids flexibility in your spine. It also helps to bring all your lower joints into correct alignment for better support.

Turn out your right foot by 90° so that it points toward the side, and slightly turn in your left foot. As you inhale, relax your left arm down by your side and extend your right arm up in the air, leaning slightly over your left leg and looking up at the raised arm.

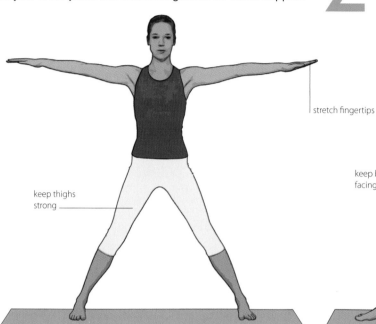

stretch fingertips

lift and open chest

keep both hips facing forward

keep thighs strong

Stand tall, with your feet together and hands by your sides. As you exhale, step your feet wide apart, toes facing forward, and raise your arms to shoulder height out to the sides. Adjust your feet so that they are roughly under your elbows. Keep your abs pulled in and strong.

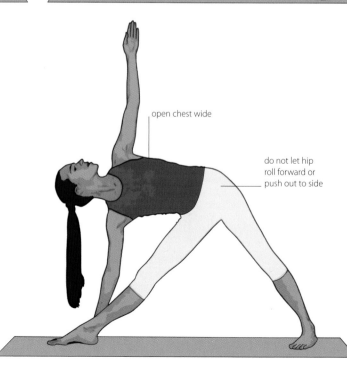

open chest wide

do not let hip roll forward or push out to side

As you exhale, bring your right arm down toward your right foot, bending your body to the side to do so and extending your left arm up in the air with your palm facing forward. Finish by looking toward your raised hand. Hold for at least 5 breaths. Come back up as you inhale. Repeat all three steps on the other side.

Warrior 2 and Side Angle Stretch

The poses in this sequence are all about lower limb strength and stability, and upper body length—a perfect balance between grounding and lightness.

1 Stand with your legs wide. As you inhale, take your arms out to shoulder height, turn your right foot out by 90°, and the toes of the other foot in slightly. As you exhale, bend your right knee at a right angle and pull back your left hip. Inhale as you look down your right arm and stretch out the fingertips of both hands. Hold for at least 5 breaths.

2 Keeping your legs in the same position and not letting your right knee bend past your toes, exhale as you rest your right elbow on your right thigh and place your left arm down your left side. Then inhale as you turn to look over your left shoulder. Hold for at least 5 breaths, then exhale. If you find this difficult, stop here, but if you feel comfortable, go on to Step 3.

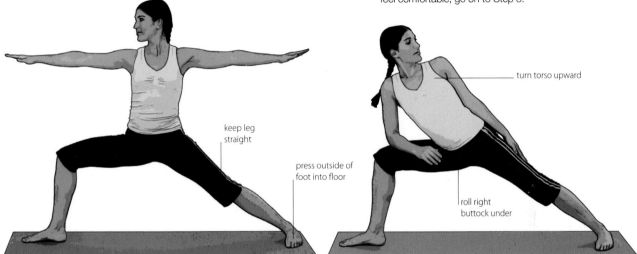

keep leg straight

press outside of foot into floor

turn torso upward

roll right buttock under

3 Still keeping your legs in the same position, inhale as you sweep your left arm up over your head, so that it is in line with your left leg. At the same time, bring your right hand to the floor, if possible, alongside your right foot so that your fingers point the same direction as your toes. Exhale as you look up at the underside of your outstretched arm. Hold for at least 5 breaths, then inhale as you come back up to standing position with wide legs. Repeat all three steps on the other side.

strongly engage thigh muscles

use right elbow to ease back right knee

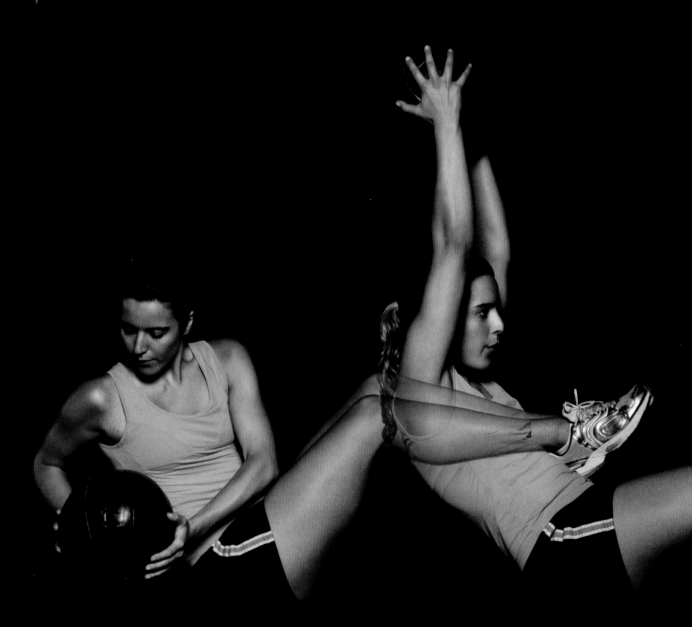

Workouts

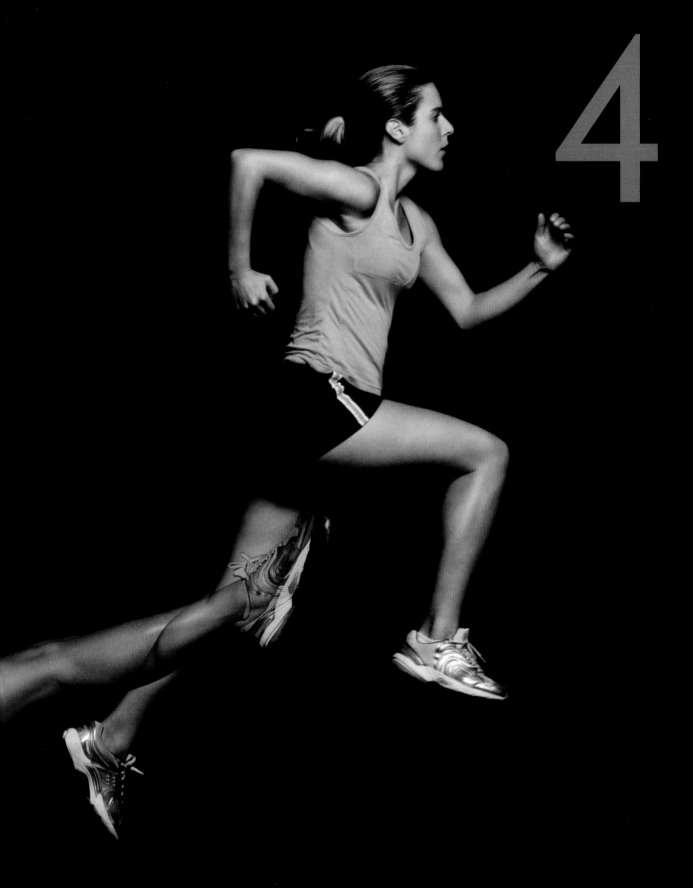

4

How to use this section

This section is your ready-to-use fitness toolkit, providing a range of specially designed Cardio, Sculpting, and Quick-fix workouts for you to mix and match according to your needs and goals. The Cardio and Sculpting workouts are key, since combined in the right balance—3–5 Cardio and 3 Sculpting per week—these will start to get you fitter and in better shape within just 4–6 weeks.

Warming up and cooling down

Firstly, there are three "Universal" workouts:
• Universal warm-up (see pp.252–53)—essential before any of the Cardio or Sculpting workouts; and optional before the Quick-fixes (otherwise do 5 minutes marching in place). See p.17 for more information on the importance of warming up.
• Universal cool-down (see pp.254–55)—essential after any of the workouts in the book, whether Cardio, Sculpting, or Quick-fix. See p.17 for more information on the importance of cooling down.
• Universal relaxation (see pp.256–57)—optional after any cool-down; also useful in its own right at any time.

Cardio workouts

Next up is a choice of nine workouts for each of the five cardio activities covered in the Cardio chapter (see pp.52–97): walking, running, cycling, swimming, and aerobics and dance. That's 45 workouts to choose from in order to get your heart working harder, burn off lots of calories, and therefore both improve cardiovascular fitness and maintain or lose weight. Aim to fit three to five of these into your weekly schedule to see results, choosing each workout based on activity preference, relevant time scale (20, 30, or 60 minutes per session, plus warm-up and cool-down time), and appropriate intensity level (gentle, moderate, or intense).

An easy-to-follow chart offers you a range of nine workouts to choose from for each cardio activity—based on the time you have available and your desired intensity level.

The Cardio workout spreads provide a range of effective workouts for: walking, running, cycling, swimming, and aerobics and dance.

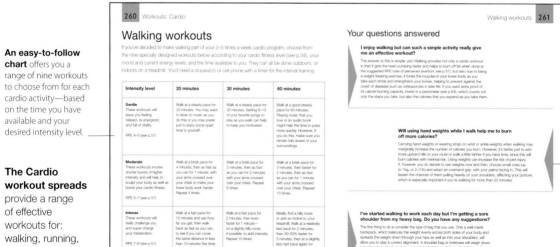

Question and answer features address common issues that people encounter when doing a specific cardio activity.

Sculpting workouts

Now it's time to choose which three out of the 20 sculpting workouts per week will best suit your needs. Look through them to see which ones sound like they'll get you the results you want. For example, if you're eager to tone up your thighs, you might choose "Skinny jeans," "Dream legs," and/or "Pear." If you want to look great for your vacation, you might choose "Bikini body," "Fabulous abs," and/or "Ultimate butt." Or if you want to firm up all over, you might choose "Body blast," "Total body yoga," and/or "Little black dress." It's up to you whether you do the same workout three times a week or a different one each time, but be sure to do your workouts on alternate days for maximal sculpting effect (see p.104).

Each workout consists of a sequence of eight exercises from the Sculpting section (see pp.98–247), which means a healthy combination of resistance, stretching, Pilates, and yoga moves. A summary of each exercise is given, but for step-by-step guidance on how to do each one safely and effectively, you'll need to turn to the page number listed in the blue bar beneath. Guidance on how long to hold each position for or how many reps (repetitions) and sets (the number of times to do the reps) to do on each side of the body is also given within this blue bar (see below for further explanation).

Quick-fix workouts

The seven Quick-fix workouts are presented in the same way as the Sculpting ones; the only difference is that these are "added extras"—workouts for you to fit in when you have a little spare time. So just dip into these when you can, rather than making them weekly fixtures in your diary.

How much time do I need?

Leave 5–10 minutes for your warm-up and the same for your cool-down. The time needed for Sculpting and Quick-fix workouts depends on the level of intensity you choose for the resistance exercises since this will affect the number of sets you do. You'll need about 10 minutes for a "gentle" workout, 15–20 minutes for a "moderate" one, and 25–30 minutes for an "intense" one. Give yourself plenty of time so that there's no need to rush. If you do run out of time, do fewer sets of each exercise rather than leave out certain exercises altogether.

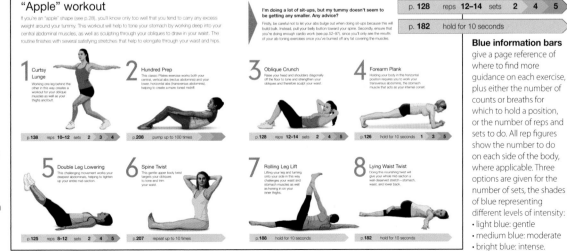

The Sculpting and Quick-fix workouts each recommend a sequence of eight exercises specially chosen to help you to achieve a particular goal.

Blue information bars give a page reference of where to find more guidance on each exercise, plus either the number of counts or breaths for which to hold a position, or the number of reps and sets to do. All rep figures show the number to do on each side of the body, where applicable. Three options are given for the number of sets to do, the shades of blue representing different levels of intensity:
• light blue: gentle
• medium blue: moderate
• bright blue: intense.

Universal warm-up

It's essential to do this warm-up before doing any of the cardio or sculpting workouts in this book in order to gradually raise your core body temperature and prepare both your muscles and your heart for the more challenging activity to come. Before you begin the specially selected range of stretching exercises, spend two minutes marching on the spot to get you moving.

1 Elbow Circling

This exercise will mobilize your upper body, opening your chest as you circle your elbows backward, and stretching your upper back as you circle them forward.

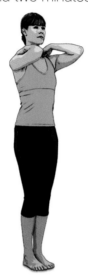

p.**164**   circle 8 times each way

2 Quad Stretch

Warm up your front thighs one at a time with this strong balancing exercise.

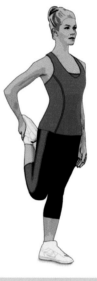

p.**186**   hold for 10 seconds

5 Standing Waist Twist

Further mobilize your shoulders and arms, and stretch out through your waist, with this combined rotation and arm extension.

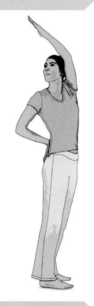

p.**182**   hold for 10 seconds

6 Triceps Overhead

Apply gentle pressure to your elbow with one hand to move the other hand down your back as far as possible. This will warm up the back of your upper arms.

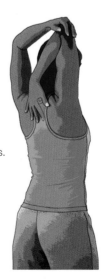

p.**180**   hold for 10 seconds

I understand that I need to warm up before cardio exercise, but why do I need to do it before sculpting workouts too?

Most sculpting workouts in this book include a range of resistance exercises, which can really challenge your muscles to the max, giving you a mini cardio workout in many cases (due to engaging large muscles, such as your quads). It's therefore essential that you are fully warmed up in preparation for them.

3 Calf Lunge

Now warm up your lower legs with this simple lunge, keeping your back heel on the floor.

p.**190**   hold for 10 seconds

4 Standing Hamstring Stretch

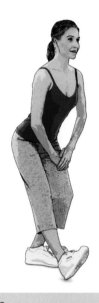

Next warm up the back of your thighs one at a time by leaning your weight into your back bent leg in this classic stretch position.

p.**187**   hold for 10 seconds

7 Backward Arm Raise

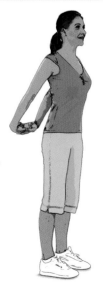

Lift your clasped hands behind you to really open up through your chest and release any tightness.

p.**174**   hold for 10 seconds

8 Front Hip Stretch

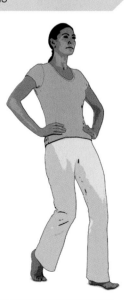

Finally warm up through your hips with this forward step and pelvic tilt, your back heel raised off the floor.

p.**184**   hold for 10 seconds

Universal cool-down

It's essential to do this cool-down after any other workout in this book to give your body a chance to gradually return to a state of "normality" after working so hard. It will also help to prevent post-exercise stiffness and further enhance your flexibility. Follow it with the Universal relaxation (see pp.256–57) if you have time but if not, simply do Child's Pose (see p.227) to give your back a final stretch.

1 Quad Stretch

Stretch out the large muscles in the front of your thigh, keeping your pelvis tilted forward in this balancing position.

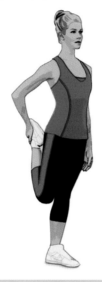

p.**186**   hold for 10 seconds

2 Calf Lunge

Stretch not only the gastrocnemius and soleus muscles that form your calves, but also your Achilles tendons which attach your calves to your heels.

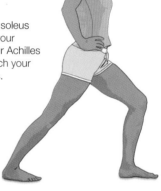

p.**190**   hold for 10 seconds

5 Triceps Overhead

Stretch out the back of each upper arm by applying gentle pressure on your raised elbow in this position.

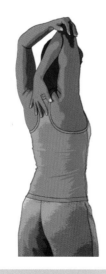

p.**180**   hold for 10 seconds

6 Straddle Side Bend

Stretch the inside of your thighs and open down each side of your upper body as you bend in this way.

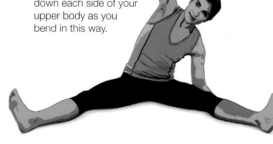

p.**189**   hold for 10 seconds

Sometimes when I exercise it's not until two days later that my muscles begin to feel sore. Why is this?

This is what is known as DOMS—delayed onset muscle soreness—which is normally felt between 24 hours and 48 hours after exercising. Caused by muscles having been challenged particularly intensely, it can be reduced by always doing the cool-down below after you do a workout of any kind.

3 Deep Lunge

A further stretch for the front of your thighs, this deep lunge also targets your hip flexors, improving mobility throughout your lower body.

p.**186**   hold for 10 seconds

4 Corner Press

Using two walls for resistance in this way gives you a fantastic stretch through your chest and shoulders.

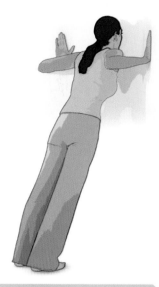

p.**174**   hold for 10 seconds

7 Lying Hamstring Stretch

Give the back of your thighs and your calves an intense stretch, being sure to keep your lower leg flat on the floor.

p.**187**   hold for 10 seconds

8 Lying Waist Twist

Stretch through your chest, waist, hips, and buttocks, as you twist your lower body first to one side, then to the other, keeping your shoulders firmly on the floor.

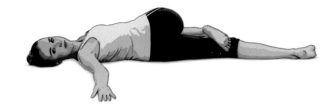

p.**182**   hold for 10 seconds

Universal relaxation

It's just as important for your health and fitness to make time to relax as well as to exercise. This workout, made up of stretching, Pilates, and yoga movements, will give your whole body a chance to do exactly this. Do it after your cool-down if you have time. Otherwise, do it any time you feel stressed, wound up, tired, or sore. Dim the lights and get ready to unwind and feel super-relaxed.

1 Roll-down

Curl your body down and up again, one vertebra at a time, to relieve tension in your back and shoulders.

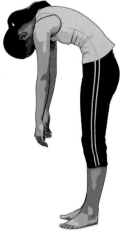

p.**206**　　repeat 3–5 times

2 Straddle Side Bend

Give both your upper and lower body a nice stretch as you bend to the side in this wide-legged position.

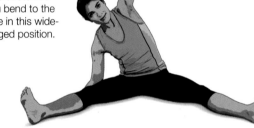

p.**189**　　hold for 10 seconds

5 Child's Pose

Stretch out your neck, shoulders, back, buttocks, and thighs as you curl into this lovely introspective yoga pose.

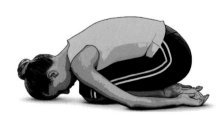

p.**227**　　hold for at least 10 breaths

6 Knees to Chest

Give your entire spine a nourishing stretch as you curl your legs in toward your chest. This will also release any tension in your buttocks.

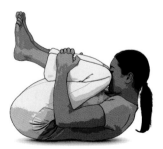

p.**168**　　hold for 10 seconds

I find it really hard to switch off and relax even when I do manage to fit exercise into my hectic schedule. Any advice?

Try to establish regular slots for your exercise, even if only 20 minutes at a time. That way, your body will know when it's going to have time dedicated to it, which can help it to unwind. Also explore different types of exercise—a flowing yoga sequence or the workout below might do the trick if an intense run or swim doesn't.

3 Cross-legged Forward Bend

Relax and let gravity do the work as you bend forward in this cross-legged yoga pose.

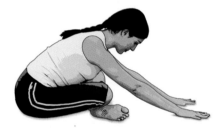

p.**242**　hold for at least 5 breaths

4 Front-lying Back Bend

Stretch through your chest and stomach as you come up into this back bend. Then enjoy relaxing down into a front-lying position.

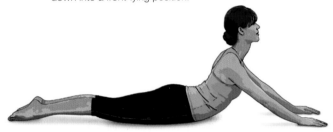

p.**172**　hold for 10 seconds

7 Lying Twist

Ease out any remaining tightness in your body with this slow, controlled rotation of both legs first to one side, then to the other.

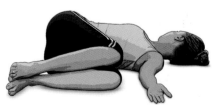

p.**237**　hold for at least 5 breaths

8 Corpse Pose

Simply lie on your back, with your legs and arms slightly wide, and relax all your muscles into the floor in this classic yoga relaxation pose.

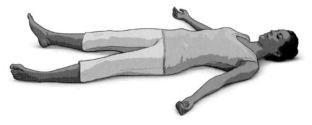

p.**227**　hold for 25 breaths

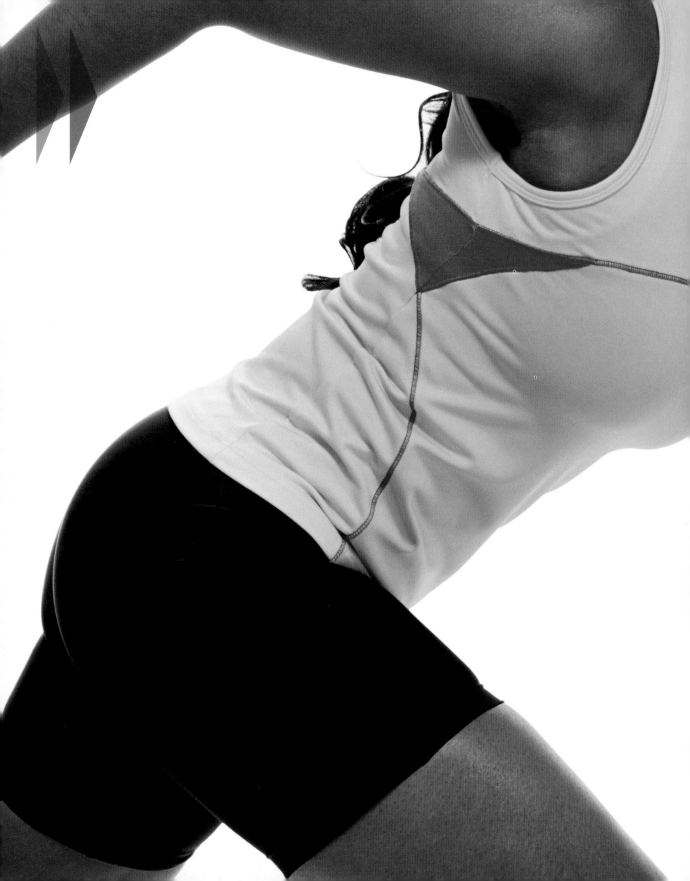

Cardio workouts

As the main calorie-burning form of exercise, cardio training should form the backbone of your fitness routine if you want to slim down and get in better shape. The workouts that follow have been specially created to give you a good range of heart-pumping, fat-burning options across five main activities: walking, running, cycling, swimming, and aerobics and dance. All you need to do is:

- decide which of the cardio activities appeal to you the most—you might want to stick to the same activity for 4–6 weeks, or you may prefer to mix it up

- schedule three to five cardio workouts into your weekly diary

- establish how long you can afford to devote to each workout —20, 30, or 60 minutes

- consider which intensity level matches your current fitness level needs —gentle, moderate, or intense

- keep at it—remember that any new fitness regimen can feel difficult at times, but it will be worth it in the end!

Walking workouts

If you've decided to make walking part of your 3–5 times a week cardio program, choose from the nine specially designed workouts below according to your cardio fitness level (see p.34), your mood and current energy levels, and the time available to you. They can all be done outdoors, or indoors on a treadmill. You'll need a stopwatch or cell phone with a timer for the interval training.

Intensity level	20 minutes	30 minutes	60 minutes
Gentle These workouts will leave you feeling relaxed, re-energized, and full of vitality. RPE 4–5 (see p.57)	Walk at a steady pace for 20 minutes. You may want to listen to music as you do this or you may prefer just to enjoy some quiet time to yourself.	Walk at a steady pace for 30 minutes. Setting 6–10 of your favorite songs to play as you walk can help to keep you motivated.	Walk at a good steady pace for 60 minutes. Playing music that you love or an audio book might help the time to pass more quickly. However, if you do this, make sure you remain fully aware of your surroundings.
Moderate These workouts involve shorter bursts of higher intensity and will help to sculpt your body as well as boost your cardio fitness. RPE 5–7 (see p.57)	Walk at a brisk pace for 4 minutes, then as fast as you can for 1 minute, with your arms crossed over your chest to make your lower body work harder. Repeat 4 times.	Walk at a brisk pace for 3 minutes, then as fast as you can for 2 minutes with your arms crossed over your chest. Repeat 6 times.	Walk at a brisk pace for 3 minutes, then faster for 2 minutes, then as fast as you can for 1 minute, with your arms crossed over your chest. Repeat 10 times.
Intense These workouts will really challenge you and super-charge your metabolism. RPE 7–8 (see p.57)	Walk at a fast pace for 10 minutes and see how far you get, then walk back as fast as you can, to see if you can cover the same distance in less than 10 minutes this time. This mini challenge is a great stress buster.	Walk at a fast pace for 2 minutes, then even faster for 1 minute— on a slightly hilly route, if possible, to add intensity. Repeat 10 times.	Ideally, find a hilly route or add an incline to your treadmill. Walk at a relatively fast pace for 2 minutes, then 30–50% faster for 3 minutes, then at a slightly less fast pace again for 1 minute, pumping your arms up and down above your head during this last minute. Repeat 10 times.

Your questions answered

I enjoy walking but can such a simple activity really give me an effective workout?

The answer to this is simple: yes! Walking provides not only a cardio workout in that it gets the heart pumping faster and helps to burn off fat when done at the suggested RPE (rate of perceived exertion; see p.57), but also due to being a weight-bearing exercise, it tones the muscles in your lower body as you take each stride and strengthens your bones, helping to prevent against the onset of diseases such as osteoporosis in later life. If you want extra proof of its calorie-burning capacity, invest in a pedometer (see p.64), which counts not only the steps you take, but also the calories that you expend as you take them.

Will using hand weights while I walk help me to burn off more calories?

Carrying hand weights or wearing strap-on wrist or ankle weights when walking may marginally increase the number of calories you burn. However, it's better just to add more upward hills to your route or walk a little farther if you have time, since this will burn calories with minimal risk. Using weights can increase the risk of joint injury. If, however, you do decide to use weights now and then, choose small ones (up to 1kg, or 2–3 lb) and adopt an overhand grip, with your palms facing in. This will lessen the chances of them pulling heavily on your shoulders, affecting your posture, which is especially important if you're walking for more than 20 minutes.

I've started walking to work each day but I'm getting a sore shoulder from my heavy bag. Do you have any suggestions?

The first thing to do is consider the type of bag that you use. Only a well-made backpack, which balances the weight evenly across both sides of your body and spreads the weight down through your hips as well as into your shoulders, will allow you to stay in correct alignment. A shoulder bag or briefcase will weigh down one side of your body and cause potential twisting and discomfort. You might therefore want to switch to using a backpack for your walks, even if this means keeping a nicer bag in the office—to transfer your belongings into when you arrive. It's also best to minimize what you carry: only bring what you really need.

Running workouts

If you've decided to make jogging or running part of your 3–5 times a week cardio program, choose from the nine specially designed workouts below according to your cardio fitness level (see p.39), your mood and current energy levels, and the time available to you. They can all be done outdoors, or indoors on a treadmill. You'll need a stopwatch for the interval training.

Intensity level	20 minutes	30 minutes	60 minutes
Gentle These workouts will leave you feeling refreshed, supple, and re-energized. RPE 4–5 (see p.57)	Jog at a mild pace for 3 minutes, then walk at a brisk pace for 2 minutes. Repeat 4 times.	Jog at a steady pace for 30 minutes. Setting 6–10 of your favorite songs to play as you run can help to keep you motivated.	Jog at a steady pace for 60 minutes. Listening to the radio or setting your MP3 player to "shuffle" can help to add an element of interest and surprise to your run. Music of 135–140 bpm is ideal if you want to run to the beat.
Moderate These workouts use simple interval training to increase your cardio fitness and really boost your calorie burn. RPE 5–7 (see p.57)	Jog at a reasonable pace for 4 minutes, then pick up speed and run for 1 minute. Repeat 4 times.	Jog at a reasonable pace for 3 minutes, then pick up speed and run for 2 minutes. Repeat 6 times.	Jog at a reasonable pace for 4 minutes, then pick up speed and run for 2 minutes. Repeat 10 times.
Intense These workouts provide a high-impact, high-energy workout that will help you to de-stress and get fitter all round. RPE 7–8 (see p.57)	Jog at a reasonable pace for 3 minutes, then run at a reasonable pace for 1 minute 30 seconds, then sprint for 30 seconds. Repeat 4 times.	Run at a reasonable pace for 4 minutes, then sprint for 1 minute. Repeat 6 times.	Ideally, find a hilly route or change your treadmill to an incline setting for at least part of the journey. Run at a reasonable pace for 30 minutes and see how far you get. Then run back as fast as you can to see if you can cover the same distance in less than 30 minutes this time.

Your questions answered

I find running hard and keep wanting to stop. How can I make it easier?

Try focusing on the 2 R's—rhythm and relaxation. To get into a natural "rhythm," breathe in time with your feet as they hit the floor: inhale deeply as you take two strides, then exhale fully as you take the next two strides. Aim to "relax" into this rhythm by actively letting go of all the tension in your body—"unscrunch" your face, drop your shoulders back and down, shake out your arms, unclench your hands, and focus your mind entirely on your breathing. This should allow you to reduce any wasted effort, move with a greater sense of freedom, and therefore enjoy your run more.

How can I stop myself from getting pain in my shins when I run?

This is most likely the injury known as shin splints—a common problem among runners and people who take part in activities that involve a lot of sudden stops and starts, such as soccer and tennis. Caused by too much force or impact being exerted on your tibia bones when your heels strike a hard surface, it can be prevented to some extent by running on softer surfaces, such as grass, and also by being aware of how heavy each step you take is: if you thud on each landing, try to change your running style to make it lighter. It's also vital to ensure that your sneakers are well enough cushioned and in good condition; consider changing them if not. If, however, the shin pain persists, make an appointment with your doctor.

Am I better off running on a treadmill or outdoors?

Outdoor running is fantastic because it gets you out in the fresh air, gives you a sense of real movement, and provides you with a set of natural challenges through different surfaces, different inclines, and elements such as wind resistance, all of which will help to improve your running. However it's often more convenient to run indoors, especially during periods of bad weather or on dark mornings or nights if you run alone—both for comfort and safety. The main benefits of a treadmill are that it's specially designed for impact so tends to be easier on your joints than tarmac, plus progress is easier to monitor due to the computerized readings. You can also create tailor-made programs on it.

Cycling workouts

If you've decided to make cycling part of your 3–5 times a week cardio program, choose from the nine specially designed workouts below according to your cardio fitness level (see p.39), your mood and current energy levels, and the time available to you. They can all be done either outdoors, or indoors on an exercise bike. You'll need a stopwatch for the interval training.

Intensity level	20 minutes	30 minutes	60 minutes
Gentle These workouts will leave you feeling refreshed, revitalized, and brimming with renewed energy. RPE 4–5 (see p.57)	Cycle at a mild pace for 20 minutes on a mainly flat surface. You may want to listen to music as you do so or you may prefer simply to relax and enjoy your surroundings.	Cycle at a mild pace for 30 minutes on a mainly flat surface. You may want to listen to music as you do so to help keep you motivated, but if you are cycling outdoors, make sure you are still fully aware of your surroundings in order to remain safe.	Cycle at a mild to moderate pace for 60 minutes on a mainly flat surface. This can be a good chance to go cross-country—planning a route through nice parks or countryside could help to rejuvenate your mind as well as your body.
Moderate These interval workouts will tone your buttocks, hips, thighs, and abs while burning off calories and enhancing your cardio fitness. RPE 5–7 (see p.57)	Cycle at a moderate pace for 3 minutes, then 50% faster for 2 minutes. Repeat 4 times. Include some small inclines in your route, if possible, to really tone your legs and buttocks.	Cycle at a moderate pace for 3 minutes, then faster for 2 minutes. Repeat 6 times. Include some small inclines in your route, if possible, to increase the calorie burn.	Cycle at a moderate pace for 6 minutes, then faster for 4 minutes. Repeat this 6 times. Go cross-country if you want—planning a scenic route with small to moderate inclines will provide an extra challenge.
Intense These high-energy workouts will give you a really good physical challenge, enhancing all-around fitness. RPE 7–8 (see p.57)	Cycle at a reasonable pace for 10 minutes and see how far you get. Then cycle back as fast as you can to see if you can cover the same distance in slightly less than 10 minutes this time.	Cycle at a moderate pace for 2 minutes, then faster for 4 minutes, aiming to include some cross-country or small inclines throughout, if possible. Repeat 5 times.	Cycle at a moderate speed for 2 minutes, then faster for 2 minutes, then faster still for 2 minutes. Repeat 10 times. Aim to cover as much distance as you can in this hour, including hills and cross-country terrain, if possible.

Your questions answered

Sometimes when I cycle for a long time the muscles across my chest start to feel tight? Why might this be?

Although cycling strongly works your legs, you are, of course, using your upper body muscles, too—to hold you in position and provide core strength to drive you forward. Slight tightness in the chest is not uncommon in cyclists as a result of the slightly rounded upper body position sometimes adopted, which causes the upper back to overstretch and the opposing chest muscles to contract. Try to stay aware of this and only round your shoulders when really required as you ride. After every bike ride add a few extra chest stretches (see pp.174–77) to your cool-down (see pp.254–55). If, however, the tightness persists, consult your doctor.

Will cycling bulk up my thighs?

This is a question that lots of women ask since they tend to want long, lean legs, with toned thighs, rather than overly muscular ones, with bulky thighs. But there's no need to worry. Although cycling provides a strong workout for your legs due to all the pedaling, you'd have to do extreme hill training for your thigh muscles to start to shorten and bulk up in this way, for example, cycling on steep inclines for hours at a time several times a week. Doing the level of cycling suggested in the workouts opposite, on the other hand—for between 20 and 60 minutes at a time on mainly flat surfaces with some hills—will just burn off calories, sculpt your body, and give your legs a lovely athletic but feminine shape.

I often feel sore a while after I've been for a bike ride. Is this ok? And why does this happen?

Well, it depends what you mean by "sore." If your muscles are just aching a little, it might be a healthy post-exercise "burn." Pain in the knees, however, can be the result of your seat being at the wrong height, and back and arm pain can be as a result of you leaning too far forward when you ride. Ensure that the saddle of your bike is at hip-height when you're standing. Also make sure that when your leg is extended on the pedal, there is still a slight bend at your knee: if it's too straight, your seat is too high; if it's too bent, your seat is too low (see p.78). Adjust it accordingly and make sure you find a comfortable riding position.

Swimming workouts

If you've decided to make swimming part of your 3–5 times a week cardio program, choose from the nine specially designed workouts below according to your cardio fitness level (see p.39), your mood and current energy levels, and the time available to you. It's a good idea to have a copy of your local pool's timetable to ensure that your desired workout times tie in with pool availability.

Intensity level	20 minutes	30 minutes	60 minutes
Gentle These workouts will give you an overall sense of increased fitness and well-being. RPE 4–5 (see p.57)	Swim at a gentle pace for 20 minutes—preferably doing the breaststroke. Focus on making big movements to improve your mobility and flexibility.	Swim for 30 minutes, alternating between 1 length at a moderate pace and 1 at a faster pace—preferably both breaststroke. Focus on keeping your abdominals pulled in as you swim.	Spend 60 minutes in the water, alternating between swimming 10 lengths at a good pace (preferably breaststroke) and then walking the width of the shallow end of the pool 10 times to improve core strength and balance.
Moderate These interval workouts involve switching between strokes to give you an all-over body sculpt, to burn fat, and to increase your cardio fitness. RPE 5–7 (see p.57)	Swim at a moderate pace for 20 minutes, alternating lengths between breaststroke and backstroke. Focus on moving as smoothly as possible with each movement.	Swim for 30 minutes, alternating between 2 lengths of the pool at a moderate pace (preferably breaststroke) and 1 length of the pool at a faster rate (preferably backstroke).	Swim for 60 minutes, alternating between three different strokes: preferably breaststroke for one length, backstroke for the next, and the style of your choice for the next.
Intense These workouts offer not only an intense, fat-burning approach to training in the water, but also help you to release stress. RPE 7–8 (see p.57)	Swim at a fast pace using any stroke you want for 20 minutes. Note how many lengths you complete. Each time you do this, see if you can complete more lengths within the same time frame.	Swim at a good pace for 30 minutes, alternating between strokes—something along the lines of 2 breaststroke lengths, 2 front crawl lengths, 1 backstroke length, 1 butterfly length, and 1 length in the stroke of your choice.	Swim 10 lengths at a fast pace, changing stroke on each length, then tread water for 2 minutes. Repeat but doing only 8 lengths, using varied strokes before you tread water again. Do the same with just 6 lengths, then 4, and finally 2. Use any time left to swim freestyle.

Your questions answered

I feel so self-conscious about wearing a bathing suit that it stops me going to the pool. Do you have any suggestions?

It's worth investing in a bathing suit that flatters your body shape (see pp.28–29). If you're an "apple," look for one with tummy control; piping under your bust will also help to accentuate your narrowest point. If you're a "pear," detailing on your chest will move the attention away from your hips. If you're a "ruler" (straight up and down), colored panels down the sides will create the illusion of curves. And if you're an "hourglass," cup support and control panels are good. It's only by doing activities such as swimming that you'll enhance your body shape and feel more confident, so try to get to that pool despite your worries if you possibly can.

I find myself getting exhausted really quickly when I go swimming. Is there anything I can do about this?

On one level it's good if your workout is tiring you out—it means it's challenging your body. And hopefully the more often you go, the less exhausting you'll find it. However, it's important to establish that you're not getting tired for the wrong reasons, so make sure that you're being efficient in the water. Learning to float will encourage you to trust that the water will support you to a certain extent and allow you to make less effort when appropriate. Becoming fully comfortable with putting your head under the water will also help since it will make your movements much smoother and more streamlined than if you're constantly having to hold your head at an uncomfortable angle.

I swim three times a week. Is this a good way for me to protect my bones against osteoporosis in later life?

Swimming is a great all-around exercise. However, unlike a lot of other cardio activities, it is what is known as a non-weight bearing exercise, which means that although it's good for cardio, strength, and also flexibility, unfortunately it won't specifically help to build stronger bones. This needs to be done through weight-bearing activities, such as walking, running, aerobics, and resistance training, which involve applying weight to your bones. If, however, you already have any kind of problem with your bones or joints, you should consult a medical expert before doing any such activities.

Aerobics and dance workouts

If you've decided to make aerobics part of your 3–5 times a week cardio program, choose from the nine specially designed workouts below according to your cardio fitness level (see p.39), your mood and current energy levels, and the time available to you. Whichever workout you choose, you'll need a music system to play your chosen songs and a watch to keep track of the time.

Intensity level	20 minutes	30 minutes	60 minutes
Gentle These workouts are low impact with a focus on coordination, balance, and flexibility. RPE 4–5 (see p.57)	Select 20 minutes of music and do non-jumping aerobics moves in sets of 16, such as: • step touches • heel digs • knee lifts • alternate kicks	Select 30 minutes' worth of your favorite music (6–10 songs) and dance to it, including low-impact moves such as those on the left. Do each move in sets of 16.	Put on the music of your choice and combine moves such as those on the left for 5 minutes, doing each move in sets of 8. Then march in place for about 1 minute. Repeat until your 60 minutes are up.
Moderate These workouts will boost your energy and give you a full-body tone as well as increase your cardio fitness. RPE 5–7 (see p.57)	Do 20 minutes of high- and low-impact moves, with arms, in sets of 16, such as: • step touches or jumps with lateral arm swings • heel digs with biceps curls • knee lifts with hands in air • kicks with alternate forward arm swings	Dance for about 6 minutes, doing moves such as those on the left, in sets of 8. Then: • do 16 Salsa Swing (see p.97) • skip on spot for 1 minute • do 16 more Salsa Swing • skip for 1 more minute Repeat for 30 minutes total.	Dance for about 10 minutes, doing moves such as those far left, in sets of 8. Then: • do 16 Salsa Swing (see p.97) • skip on spot for 1 minute • do 16 more Salsa Swing • skip for 1 more minute Repeat for 60 minutes total.
Intense These high-energy workouts include a combination of low- and high-impact moves that will really boost both your metabolic rate and cardio fitness. RPE 7–8 (see p.57)	Dance for about 2 minutes to fast music, combining low- and high-impact moves such as those listed directly above in sets of 8. Then: • jump from side to side for about 1 minute • do 16 Salsa Swing, then 16 Twist and Shift (see p.97) Repeat for 20 minutes total.	Dance for about 2 minutes to fast music, combining moves such as those listed above left. Then: • jump from side to side for about 1 minute • do 16 Salsa Swing, then 16 Twist and Shift (see p.97) • skip on spot for 1 minute Repeat for 30 minutes total.	Dance for about 5 minutes to fast music, using a combination of any moves you like. Then: • jump from side to side for about 1 minute • do 16 Salsa Swing, then 16 Twist and Shift (see p.97) • skip on spot for 1 minute Repeat for 60 minutes total.

Your questions answered

I love dancing but I find it hard to keep in time to the music. Is there anything I can do to improve this?

Try sitting down and listening to music, focusing only on the beat (not the lyrics) by tapping it out with your feet or drumming it out wth your hands on something. Ask a friend to help you if you can't hear it at first. With practice you will start to feel the rhythm more instinctively and can feed it into your dancing. Bear in mind, however, that you have to anticipate each beat ever so slightly when dancing in order to stay in time—if you only start to move on each beat, you'll end up behind. It's also important to move with control in order to stay in sync with the music: dance is a fine balance between freedom and control of movement.

I wear all my fitness gear when I go to dance classes, but is this necessary when I do these workouts at home?

It's crucial to wear high quality, good-fitting sneakers for adequate ankle support and under-foot cushioning, and a sports bra to support your bust during high-impact moves. But other than that, it's up to you what you wear. Having said that, you're more likely to put 100 percent into what you're doing if you look and feel the part, so it's best to make some kind of effort with what you look like. Also, more practically speaking, fitness clothes are specially designed to allow your body to move freely and your skin to breathe so you'll probably be more comfortable in them as well as more confident, whether it's shorts and a T-shirt or leggings and a short top.

I really struggle with my coordination, so I find aerobics and dance classes hard. Is this something that I can build on?

It's true that dancing and aerobics require good coordination, which some people seem to have more of than others. But it's also a matter of practice—the more you move your body in certain ways, the more accustomed it will get to sending the right messages between your brain and muscles. This is called motor skills fitness, which originates in your motor cortex, a region of the cerebral cortex in your brain that controls voluntary muscle groups. The more complex a move, the more motor skills are required, so if something is too challenging at first, try just one element of it to start, then add other aspects once you feel comfortable.

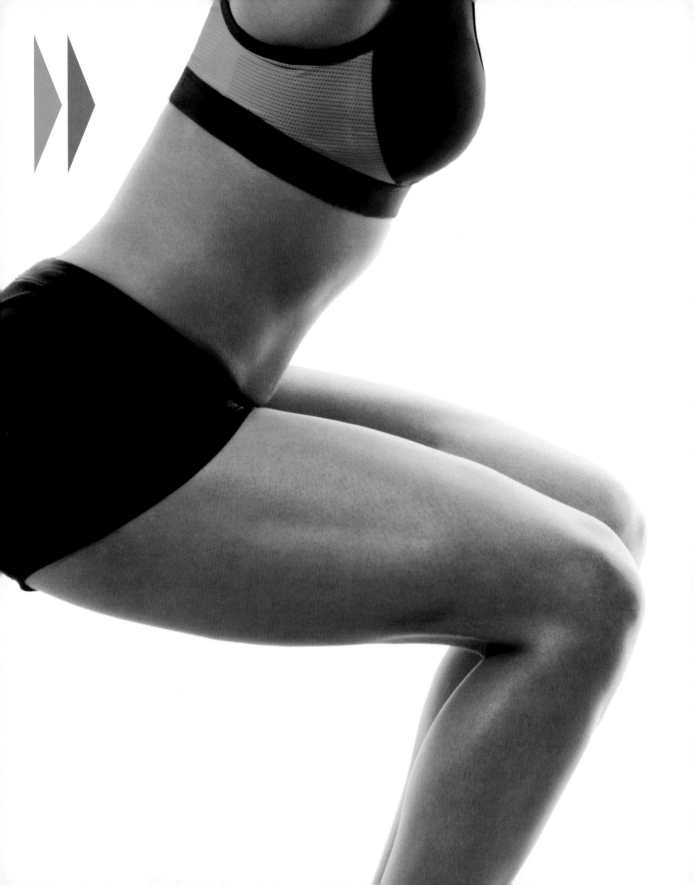

Sculpting workouts

To get the toned body you've always wanted, you need to complement cardio training with a healthy dose of body sculpting. The workouts in the pages that follow, which have been specially created from the wide range of resistance, stretching, Pilates, and yoga exercises on pp.108–247, will start to change your body shape in just 4–6 weeks if done three times a week, with a day of rest between each one:

- Body blast, Core Pilates, and Total body yoga will give you an all-over workout

- Little black dress, Bride-to-be, Skinny jeans, and Bikini body will have you looking fantastic in your LBD, wedding dress, favorite jeans, or on the beach!

- Beautiful back, Ultimate bust, Amazing arms, Fabulous abs, Ultimate butt, and Dream legs will enhance specific body zones

- "Apple," "Pear," "Ruler," and "Hourglass" will enable you to make the most of your natural body shape

- Better-in-bed, Postpartum, and Ten-years-younger will empower you in the bedroom, post-pregnancy, or if you're starting to feel older than your years

Body blast workout

If you want to get fitter and in all-around better shape fast, whether in time for a special event or your upcoming beach vacation, then this is the workout for you. Targeting all the major muscle groups, it will tone your whole body, give you a fantastic calorie-burning boost, and increase both strength and flexibility. Doing it three times a week will increase your fitness level in no time.

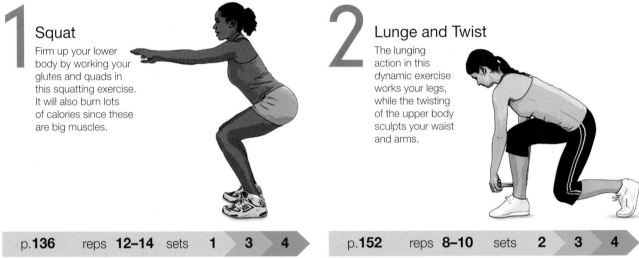

1 Squat
Firm up your lower body by working your glutes and quads in this squatting exercise. It will also burn lots of calories since these are big muscles.

p.**136**   reps **12–14**   sets   **1**   **3**   **4**

2 Lunge and Twist
The lunging action in this dynamic exercise works your legs, while the twisting of the upper body sculpts your waist and arms.

p.**152**   reps **8–10**   sets   **2**   **3**   **4**

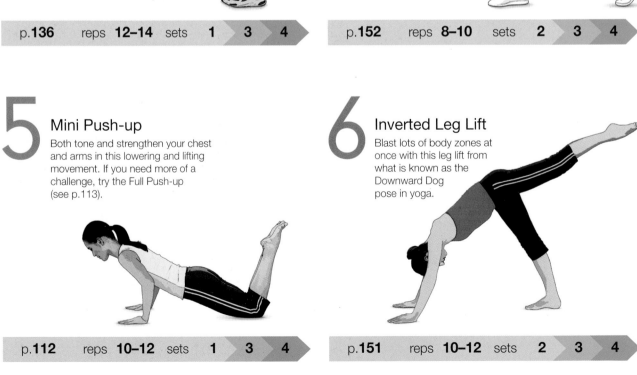

5 Mini Push-up
Both tone and strengthen your chest and arms in this lowering and lifting movement. If you need more of a challenge, try the Full Push-up (see p.113).

p.**112**   reps **10–12**   sets   **1**   **3**   **4**

6 Inverted Leg Lift
Blast lots of body zones at once with this leg lift from what is known as the Downward Dog pose in yoga.

p.**151**   reps **10–12**   sets   **2**   **3**   **4**

I'm worried about resistance exercises making me look like a body builder. If I do them, will I build bulky muscles?

There's no need to worry—you would have to lift very heavy weights to build bulk, and all the exercises in this book work by challenging your muscles through endurance (reps and sets), rather than power (heavy weights). This means that they will give you a lean, defined body, rather than a bulky one.

3 Lateral Lift

This sideways leg lift targets your thighs and core, while the double arm lift boosts your arm and shoulder strength.

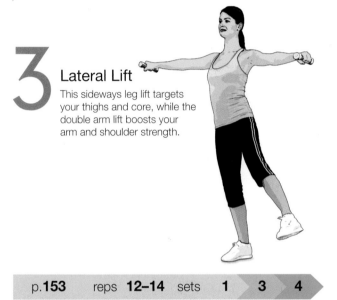

| p.**153** | reps **12–14** | sets | **1** | **3** | **4** |

4 Hamstring Curl

Get those buttocks and thighs in great shape with this bending and straightening leg exercise.

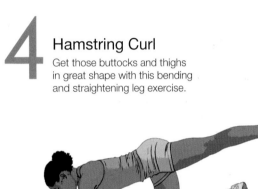

| p.**142** | reps **14–16** | sets | **2** | **3** | **4** |

7 Corkscrew

Tone and sculpt your stomach and waist as you strongly engage your abs in this challenging leg-circling exercise.

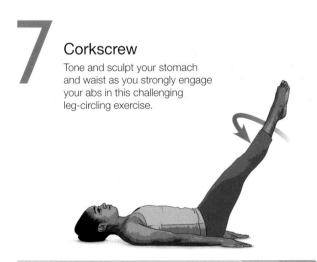

| p.**127** | reps **12–14** | sets | **1** | **2** | **3** |

8 Lunge with Extended Arms

This nice stretch targets both your upper and lower body and will release any tension after your workout.

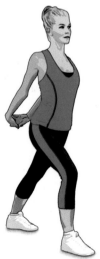

| p.**192** | hold for 10 seconds |

Core Pilates workout

If you're a Pilates fan, particularly enjoyed the Pilates section of this book (see pp.194–219), or are specifically eager to strengthen the core muscles in your stomach, back, and buttocks, then you'll love this workout. With its combination of stretching and strength exercises, regular practice will have you feeling fitter, stronger, and more flexible from the inside out within just three to four weeks.

1 Hundred Prep

Deeply engage your abdominal muscles as you pump your arms in this classic Pilates position. Be sure not to strain your neck as you do so.

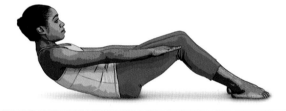

p.**208**   pump up to 100 times

2 Roll-back

Continue to challenge your abdominals, and also mobilize your spine, as you curl firstly back toward the floor and then up toward your knees.

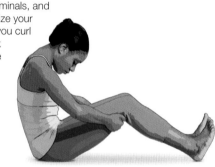

p.**212**   repeat 3–5 times

5 Side-lying Front Kick

The kicking motion in this exercise will really tone up your buttocks and thighs, while the abdominal effort required to maintain balance lying on your side works your stomach and back.

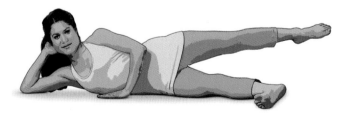

p.**218**   repeat up to 10 times

6 Knee Stretch

This backward leg lift really targets your buttock muscles. It's important to do it slowly and with control so that you don't overarch your spine.

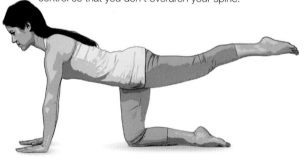

p.**217**   repeat up to 10 times

I thought Pilates involved exercises on specially designed machines. Can I do it without specialist equipment?

In short, yes, you absolutely can! All you need to do most of the Pilates exercises in this book are comfortable fitness clothes and an exercise mat. Although Joseph Pilates, founder of the fitness method, did indeed develop specialist equipment, floor exercises are recognized as the core of his approach.

3 Single Leg Stretch

Extending your legs one at a time with your head and shoulders raised off the floor works your legs as well as your abs.

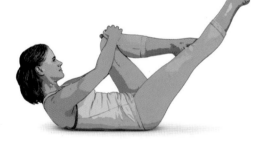

p.**210**   repeat up to 10 times

4 Shoulder Bridge

This movement mobilizes your spine while strengthening the glutes and deep abdominals.

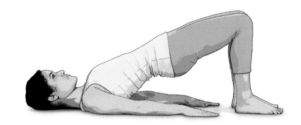

p.**214**   repeat up to 10 times

7 Swan Prep

This movement will help to open and stretch the front of your chest, while strengthening the muscles in your back and shoulders.

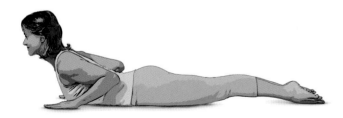

p.**204**   repeat up to 10 times

8 Roll-down

Ease any stiffness and encourage maximal spine mobility with this simple but highly effective curling and uncurling movement.

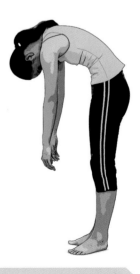

p.**206**   repeat 3–5 times

Total body yoga workout

If you enjoy a less adrenaline-fuelled, more holistic approach to exercise, then you'll appreciate this body-sculpting yoga workout. If you do it at least three times a week, it will not only develop your strength and greatly enhance your flexibility, but it will also put you firmly on the path to a leaner, more toned body, and potentially a calmer frame of mind, within just three to four weeks.

1 Cobra

This front-lying back bend opens your chest and draws back your shoulders, while at the same time mobilizing and strengthening your spine. It is therefore a great posture enhancer for anyone with a tendency to slouch.

p.**232**   hold for at least 5 breaths

2 Downward Dog

Adopting this inverted V-shape creates both strength and length throughout your body.

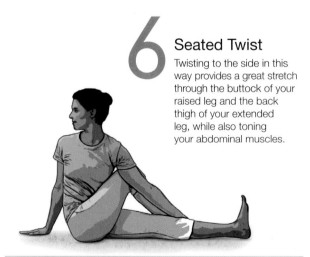

p.**231**   hold for at least 5 breaths

5 Single-leg Forward Bend

This nourishing seated forward bend really stretches out the entire length of your spine at the same time as strengthening your leg muscles.

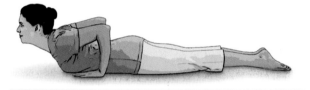

p.**242**   hold for at least 5 breaths

6 Seated Twist

Twisting to the side in this way provides a great stretch through the buttock of your raised leg and the back thigh of your extended leg, while also toning your abdominal muscles.

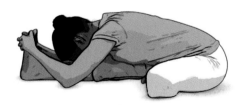

p.**236**   hold for at least 5 breaths

Yoga has a reputation for being mainly a means of relaxation so can it really give me a thorough workout?

Although the underlying focus of yoga is to reach a point of peace and stillness, and some postures, such as Corpse Pose (see p.227), reflect this, most poses are very dynamic and require a great deal of effort to do well, especially in a flowing sequence, so yes—yoga can definitely give you a fantastic all-around workout.

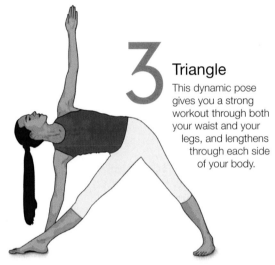

3 Triangle

This dynamic pose gives you a strong workout through both your waist and your legs, and lengthens through each side of your body.

p.**246**　hold for at least 5 breaths

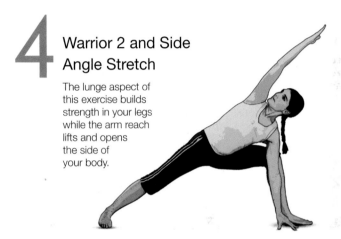

4 Warrior 2 and Side Angle Stretch

The lunge aspect of this exercise builds strength in your legs while the arm reach lifts and opens the side of your body.

p.**247**　hold for at least 5 breaths

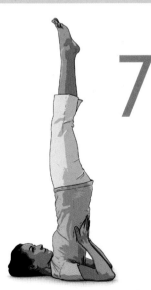

7 Shoulderstand

This classic inverted pose engages the muscles throughout your whole body. It also has a calming effect on the mind. However, it's best to omit it if you're having your period.

p.**235**　hold for at least 25 breaths if possible

8 Fish

An important counter-posture to the Shoulderstand, this exercise can also be done in its own right to lengthen through the front of your body and strengthen through your back, arms, and shoulder.

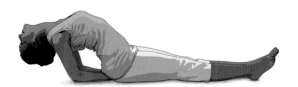

p.**238**　hold for at least 5 breaths

Little black dress workout

Whether you want to look your best for an upcoming special event or you just want to get back into your favorite LBD, this is the workout for you. The first two exercises will firm up your arms, the next two shape your hips and thighs, as well as burn calories, and the final four target your abs for a flat stomach and trim waist. The Mini Bridge will also enhance calf definition for killer legs.

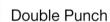

1 Double Punch

Punch forward and draw backward with both arms to firm up the back of your arms, tone your chest and shoulders, and lift your bust.

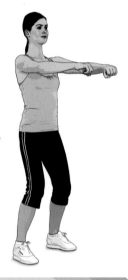

p.**119**   reps **10–12**   sets   **2**   **3**   **4**

2 Front Raise

Lift your arms up and out from your thighs to sculpt your upper arms and shoulders. This will also enhance your posture.

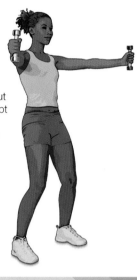

p.**109**   reps **8–10**   sets   **2**   **3**   **4**

5 Twist and Reach

Do this seated twist to target your obliques and define your waist. It will also open up your chest area, enhancing posture.

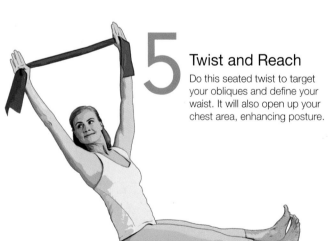

p.**130**   reps **8–10**   sets   **1**   **2**   **3**

6 Mini Bridge

Stretch your front and work your back with this mini back bend for increased length and strength throughout your body. It will particularly tone your abs, thighs, and calves.

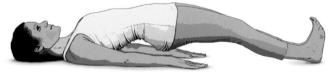

p.**143**   reps **10–12**   sets   **1**   **2**   **3**

I'd love to go down a dress size so I can fit into some of my favorite clothes again. How can I best achieve this?

The workout below is perfect for you to do as a starting point toward this goal. However, you'll only see the benefits of this whole-body toning work if you complement it with both a healthy, balanced diet (see p.48) and five moderate to intense cardio workouts a week (see pp.258–69) to bring on the fat-burning.

3 Lunge with Weights

This deep forward lunge will help to create luscious legs and a lifted bottom. Lunging also burns calories.

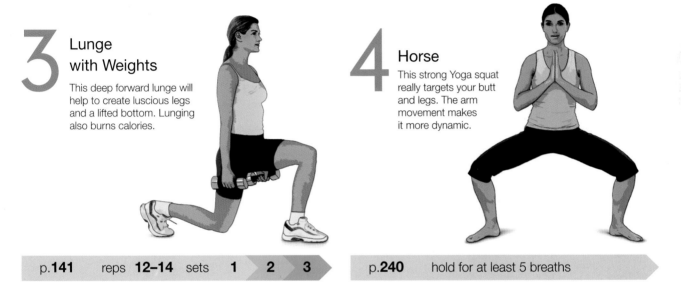

| p.**141** | reps **12–14** | sets | **1** | **2** | **3** |

4 Horse

This strong Yoga squat really targets your butt and legs. The arm movement makes it more dynamic.

| p.**240** | hold for at least 5 breaths |

7 Ab Crunch

Engage your abdominal muscles in this classic sit-up move to strengthen your core and flatten your tummy.

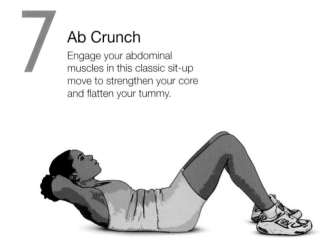

| p.**122** | reps **12–15** | sets | **2** | **3** | **4** |

8 Double Leg Lowering

A more challenging movement, this works your deep abdominal muscles to further tone and flatten your stomach area.

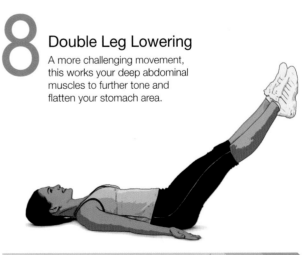

| p.**125** | reps **8–10** | sets | **1** | **2** | **3** |

Bride-to-be workout

If your "big day" is approaching and you want to look and feel fantastic for the happy occasion when all eyes (and cameras) will be on you, then the Bride-to-be workout can help. Although designed to tone your whole body, it particularly targets your chest, shoulders, arms, back, stomach, and waist so that you will be sure to look your very best in your dream dress.

1 Pull-up

The inward turn of your arms during this exercise means that you really blast the back of your arms, eliminating bat wings for good.

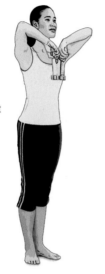

| p.**118** | reps **10–12** | sets | **2** | **3** | **4** |

2 Plié with Lateral Raise

This squat with out-turned toes particularly targets your inner thighs, while the sideways arm raise blasts your chest, shoulders, and arms.

| p.**152** | reps **10–12** | sets | **2** | **3** | **4** |

5 Twist and Bend

This seated rotation beautifully targets your obliques, helping to trim your waist. It will also lengthen your back and legs.

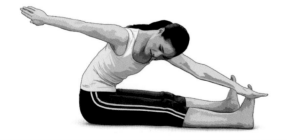

| p.**131** | reps **12–16** | sets | **1** | **2** | **3** |

6 Alternating Kicks

Continue to sculpt your stomach and waist by alternately bending and extending your legs while lying on your back.

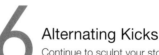
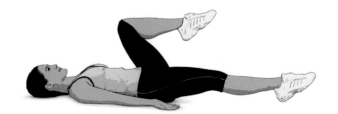

| p.**124** | reps **12–15** | sets | **2** | **3** | **4** |

> ## What exercises would you advise me to do the night before my wedding so that I look my absolute best?
>
> The workout below is perfect for you to do in the weeks or months leading up to your wedding. However, the night before the big event it's best not to overstrain yourself. Save your energy for the celebrations and just do the Universal relaxation workout (see pp.256–57) to encourage a good night's sleep.

3 Shoulder Extension

This dynamic reaching and twisting exercise tones your arms and shoulders, while at the same time strengthening your back and abdominals.

4 Chest Expansion

Lifting your arms forward and backward in the way that this exercise requires sculpts your shoulders and arms, and is a great posture enhancer.

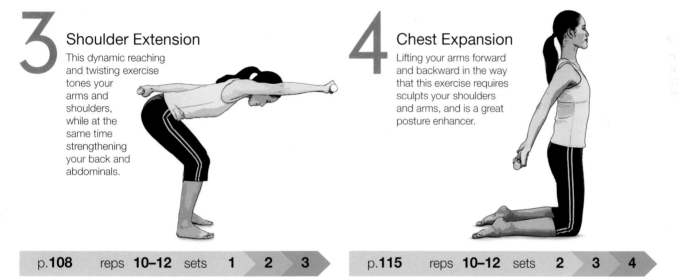

| p.**108** | reps **10–12** | sets | **1** | **2** | **3** |

| p.**115** | reps **10–12** | sets | **2** | **3** | **4** |

7 Oblique Crunch

This diagonal sit-up will help to firm and tone your stomach and waist. Strong abdominals also help to improve posture.

8 Extended Heel Taps

Lifting both your legs and upper body off the floor, then opening and closing your legs, enhances length through your front body and sculpts your back and glutes.

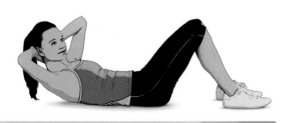

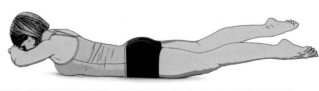

| p.**128** | reps **14–16** | sets | **2** | **3** | **4** |

| p.**133** | reps **10–12** | sets | **2** | **3** | **4** |

Skinny jeans workout

Whether you want to get back into your favorite jeans after an over-indulgent vacation or you want to wear skinny jeans for the first time, this workout will give you both the shape and confidence to do so. Masterfully blasting your lower body from every angle, it sculpts not only your hips, thighs, and butt, but also your abs and waist so that you can do up that zip without a care in the world.

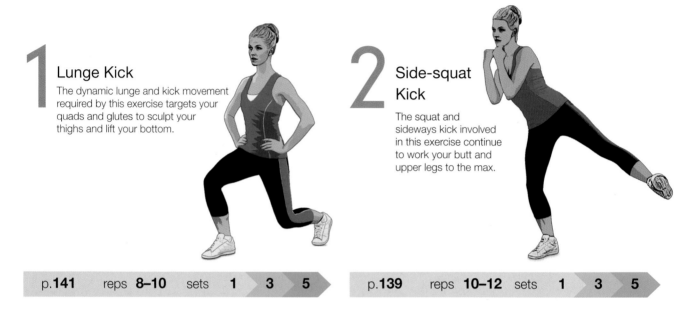

1 Lunge Kick
The dynamic lunge and kick movement required by this exercise targets your quads and glutes to sculpt your thighs and lift your bottom.

| p.141 | reps **8–10** | sets | **1** | **3** | **5** |

2 Side-squat Kick
The squat and sideways kick involved in this exercise continue to work your butt and upper legs to the max.

| p.139 | reps **10–12** | sets | **1** | **3** | **5** |

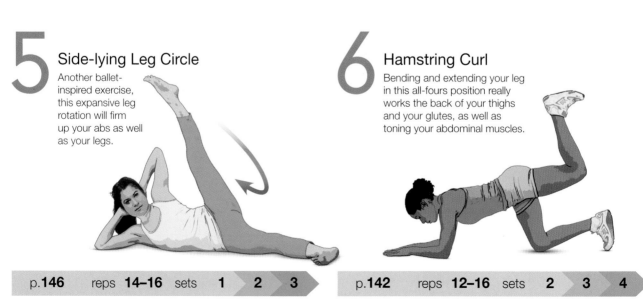

5 Side-lying Leg Circle
Another ballet-inspired exercise, this expansive leg rotation will firm up your abs as well as your legs.

| p.146 | reps **14–16** | sets | **1** | **2** | **3** |

6 Hamstring Curl
Bending and extending your leg in this all-fours position really works the back of your thighs and your glutes, as well as toning your abdominal muscles.

| p.142 | reps **12–16** | sets | **2** | **3** | **4** |

> **I have a roll of tummy that sticks over the top of my jeans, especially at the sides. What can I do to get rid of it?**
>
> The workout below is the perfect starting point for you to work towards getting rid of this overhang. However, this will only tone up the muscles in the offending area. To actually reduce the size of the area, you'll need to up your cardio workouts (see pp.258–69) to burn off the fat currently covering the muscles.

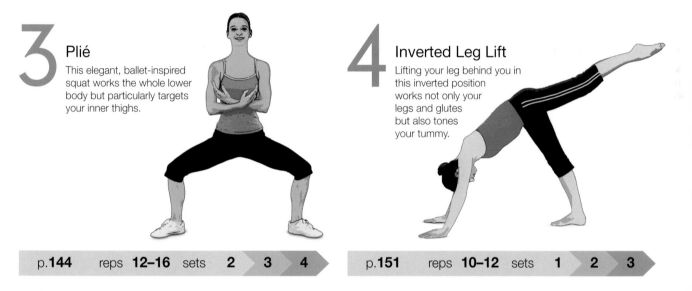

3 Plié

This elegant, ballet-inspired squat works the whole lower body but particularly targets your inner thighs.

p.**144**   reps **12–16**   sets   **2**   **3**   **4**

4 Inverted Leg Lift

Lifting your leg behind you in this inverted position works not only your legs and glutes but also tones your tummy.

p.**151**   reps **10–12**   sets   **1**   **2**   **3**

7 Plank with Leg Lift

Challenge your abs and glutes with alternate leg lifts from the already-tough plank position for a toned midriff and enhanced core strength.

8 Criss-cross Leg Extension

Give not only your legs, but also your stomach and waist a great workout in this diagonal sit-up with alternate leg extensions.

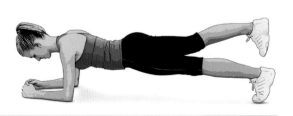

p.**126**   reps **8–10**   sets   **1**   **2**   **3**

p.**129**   reps **12–14**   sets   **2**   **3**   **4**

Bikini body workout

So you've booked your vacation and want to look your best in your bikini or one-piece? The Bikini body workout can help. Starting with a total body exercise, it goes on to sculpt your buttocks and thighs, firm up your arms (getting rid of those "bat wings"), define your abs and back, tone your chest and shoulders, trim down your waist, and finally give your whole body a blast from the core.

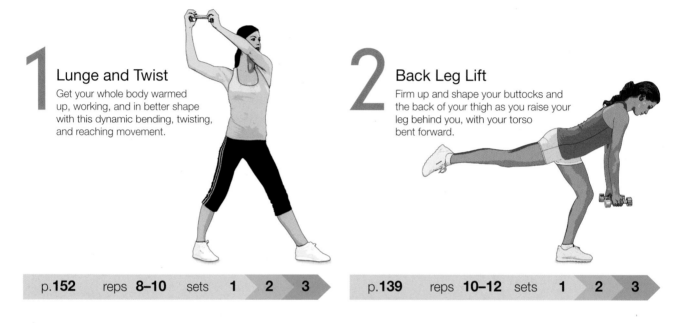

1 Lunge and Twist

Get your whole body warmed up, working, and in better shape with this dynamic bending, twisting, and reaching movement.

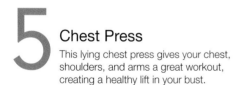

p.152   reps **8–10**   sets   **1**   **2**   **3**

2 Back Leg Lift

Firm up and shape your buttocks and the back of your thigh as you raise your leg behind you, with your torso bent forward.

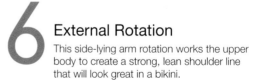

p.139   reps **10–12**   sets   **1**   **2**   **3**

5 Chest Press

This lying chest press gives your chest, shoulders, and arms a great workout, creating a healthy lift in your bust.

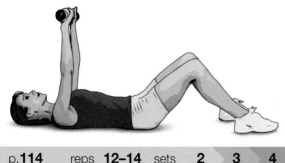

p.114   reps **12–14**   sets   **2**   **3**   **4**

6 External Rotation

This side-lying arm rotation works the upper body to create a strong, lean shoulder line that will look great in a bikini.

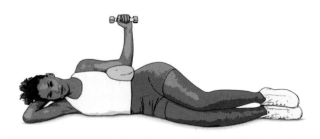

p.110   reps **12–14**   sets   **2**   **3**   **4**

I'd love to feel confident enough to wear a bikini rather than a one-piece this summer. Have you got any advice on this?

Presuming that your main worry is exposing what you view as your "flabby" tummy, try a combination of the below workout and the Fabulous abs workout (see pp.292–93) three times a week, on top of a healthy diet (see pp.48–51) and five moderate to intense cardio workouts (see pp.258–69) a week for six weeks.

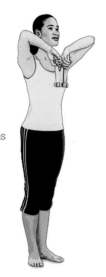

3 Pull-up

Improve your posture and blitz any bat wings by pulling your elbows up and out, and rolling your shoulders back and down, as you lift your inward-turned arms.

p.**118**   reps **12–14**   sets   **2**   **3**   **4**

4 Ab Stretch and Crunch on Ball

This challenging sit-up is a super-sculpting exercise for your abdominals, while the back bend that precedes it lengthens your spine and improves your posture.

p.**123**   reps **10–12**   sets   **2**   **3**   **4**

7 Lying Twist with Weight

Work your oblique muscles and therefore enhance the shape of your waist with this nourishing two-way twist.

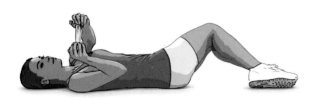

p.**130**   reps **12–14**   sets   **2**   **3**   **4**

8 Single Leg Stretch

The upper body lift in this Pilates exercise works your abdominals while the alternate leg extensions sculpt your legs and butt.

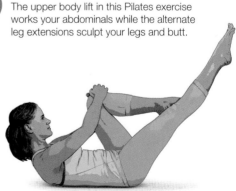

p.**210**   repeat up to 10 times

Beautiful back workout

A healthy spine is vital to our well-being yet we often tend to forget about our back until we have aches or pains there or want to reveal it in summer clothes. This workout will help to prevent such issues from occurring and give you a lovely defined back and shoulder line to show off. It will also dramatically enhance your posture, making you both look and feel more vibrant and confident.

1 Pull-up

Target your upper arms, shoulders, and upper back by doing this central pull-up, with inward-turned arms. It will also open your chest, helping to enhance your posture.

| p.118 | reps **10–12** | sets | **2** | **3** | **4** |

2 Front Raise

Strengthen and define the front and back of your shoulders as you raise your arms diagonally outward from your thighs.

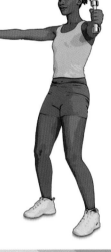

| p.109 | reps **10-12** | sets | **2** | **3** | **4** |

5 Kneeling Back Extension

As well as relieving any tension in your lower back, this satisfying stretch creates a lovely sense of openness through your spine and waist.

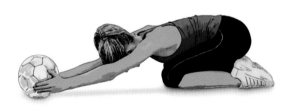

| p.134 | reps **8–10** | sets | **1** | **2** | **3** |

6 External Rotation

Give your upper arms, shoulders, and upper back beautiful definition by doing this side-lying shoulder and arm rotation.

| p.110 | reps **12–14** | sets | **1** | **2** | **3** |

> **I get an achy lower back since I have to sit at a computer all day for work. Will doing exercises like the ones below help with this?**
>
> Many instances of backache are as a result of bad posture (see p.32), so try to be aware of how you stand and take frequent breaks to relieve any pressure on your back throughout each working day. But regularly doing the workout below will also help, since the exercises in it have been specifically chosen to restore beautiful posture for a healthy, pain-free back.

3 Spine Twist

This seated Pilates rotation stretches and strengthens the muscles surrounding your spine, boosting mobility in this area.

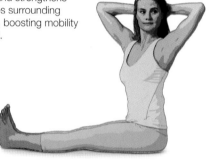

p.**207**   repeat up to 10 times

4 Chest Expansion

This forward and backward arm lift enhances shoulder mobility, as well as toning your upper back, arms, and shoulders.

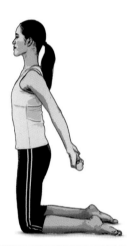

p.**115**   reps **10–12**   sets   **1**   **2**   **3**

7 Letter T

This lying Pilates back bend strongly targets the muscles in your mid and upper back and is wonderful for relieving tension in your shoulders and neck.

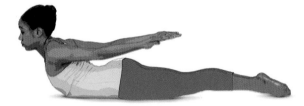

p.**205**   repeat up to 10 times

8 Extended Heel Taps

Engage the whole back of your body to enable this double-whammy lift with heel taps. It will firm up your glutes and thighs as well as strengthening and sculpting your core back and ab muscles.

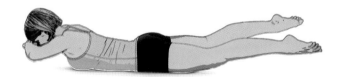

p.**133**   reps **10–12**   sets   **2**   **3**   **4**

Ultimate bust workout

If you feel that your bust area could do with a rejuvenating lift, then try the Ultimate bust workout. The combination of standing and lying exercises will strengthen and open the muscles in your chest and shoulders to encourage not only a pert bust but also healthy overall upper body posture. Regular practice will also result in a smoother and firmer décolletage.

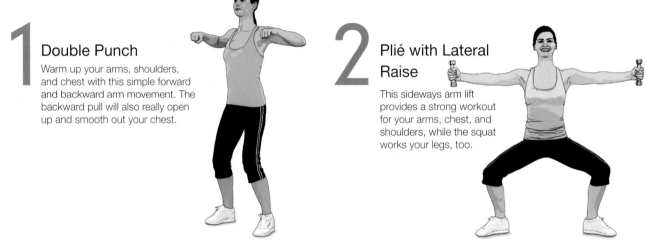

1 Double Punch

Warm up your arms, shoulders, and chest with this simple forward and backward arm movement. The backward pull will also really open up and smooth out your chest.

p.**119**   reps **12–14**   sets   **2**   **3**   **4**

2 Plié with Lateral Raise

This sideways arm lift provides a strong workout for your arms, chest, and shoulders, while the squat works your legs, too.

p.**152**   reps **12–14**   sets   **2**   **3**   **4**

5 Double Arm and Leg Lift

Raising your upper body off the floor in this way lifts and opens your chest, while raising your legs strengthens your lower body.

6 Chest Fly

Blitz the area around your armpits and enhance general lift and definition in the bust area with this inward-pressing arm lift.

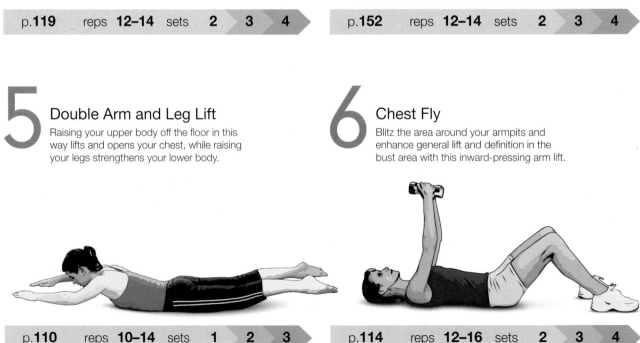

p.**110**   reps **10–14**   sets   **1**   **2**   **3**

p.**114**   reps **12–16**   sets   **2**   **3**   **4**

Do I really need to wear a sports bra when I exercise? Doesn't a normal bra do the same job?

It really is best to wear a sports bra since it provides substantially more support than a normal bra and therefore dramatically reduces the uncomfortable movement and bouncing that can occur during workouts. Sports bras are also made out of fabrics specially designed to cope with increased sweating.

3 Shoulder Extension

This dynamic exercise targets the muscles in your arms, chest, and shoulders, as well as boosting shoulder mobility and toning your abs.

p.**108**   reps **10–12**   sets   **1**   **3**   **4**

4 Full Push-up

Really target your chest with this challenging exercise. If it's too difficult for you at the moment, try the Mini Push-up (see p.112).

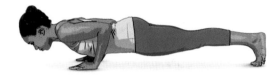

p.**113**   reps **8–10**   sets   **1**   **2**   **3**

7 Chest Press

Further tone your chest, arms, and shoulders as you push upward, and enjoy the sense of opening as you bring your arms down.

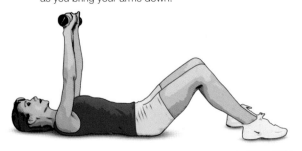

p.**114**   reps **12–16**   sets   **2**   **3**   **4**

8 Opposing Arm Extension

Simultaneously stretching up with one arm and down with the other creates a sense of length throughout your whole body, but particularly through your chest.

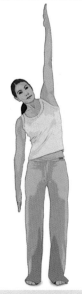

p.**175**   hold for 10 seconds

Amazing arms workout

This workout is the key to banishing "bat wings" for good and getting the lean, sleek upper arms you have always dreamed of. As we get older, muscle strength in our arms is one of the first areas to decrease, so it's important for everyday fitness, as well as for our physical appearance, that we regularly work both the biceps, on the front of our upper arms, and the triceps, on the back.

1 Twisting Punch

Warm up your entire upper body with this dynamic exercise. As you punch first to one side and then upward, you will tone and strengthen your shoulders as well as both sides of your arms.

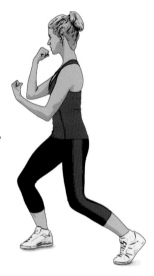

| p.**150** | reps **12–14** | sets | **2** | **3** | **4** |

2 Sitting Side Curl

Hone in on the front of your upper arms with this strengthening biceps curl to give you lovely definition.

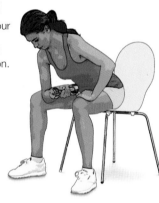

| p.**117** | reps **8–12** | sets | **1** | **3** | **4** |

5 Triceps Dip

Lowering and raising your body in this way further works your upper arms, in particular your triceps.

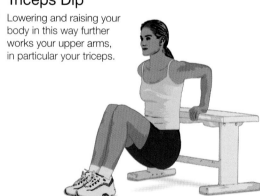

| p.**120** | reps **8–10** | sets | **1** | **2** | **3** |

6 Letter T

The double arm lift in this Pilates back bend means that it stretches and strengthens your arms, as well as your chest and shoulders.

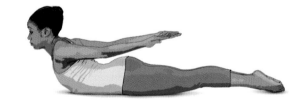

| p.**205** | repeat up to 10 times |

As I get older, the undersides of my upper arms are getting more and more flabby. Is there anything I can do about this?

This a common phenomenon as we age but, fortunately, one that can be addressed with regular arm and shoulder exercises. It is particularly the muscles on the back of the arms (the triceps) and front of the shoulders (the deltoids) that need firming up, so focus on exercises that target these zones. Swimming is also an effective way to tone these areas.

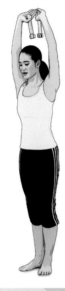

3 Triceps Lift

Target your triceps with this overhead arm extension to firm and sculpt the back of your arms and the areas around your armpits.

p.**118**　reps **10–14**　sets　**1**　**2**　**3**

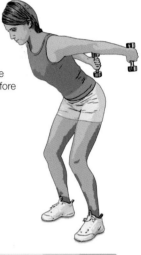

4 Triceps Kickback

Continue to firm and sculpt the back of your arms—and therefore blast any bat wings—with this backward arm raise.

p.**121**　reps **10–12**　sets　**1**　**2**　**3**

7 Side-lying Triceps Push-up

Challenge your triceps and shoulder muscles as you do this tricky side-lying push-up. It also works your abdominals.

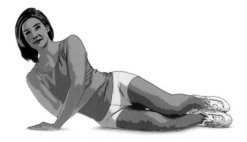

p.**120**　reps **8–10**　sets　**1**　**2**　**3**

8 Mini Push-up

Give your arms and chest a final boost with this classic push-up exercise. If you want more of a challenge, try the Full Push-up (see p.113).

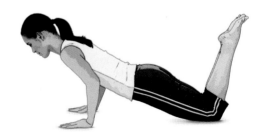

p.**112**　reps **10–14**　sets　**1**　**2**　**3**

Fabulous abs workout

The tummy area is a key worry for many women, especially those with "apple"-shaped bodies (see p.28). Targeting all your abdominal muscles at once, this workout will help you to achieve both a flatter stomach and a slimmer waistline in no time. However, it's essential that you complement it with regular cardio workouts to ensure that you burn off any fat currently covering your muscles!

1 Lunge and Twist

Warm up your whole middle and lower body as you reach first up high to one diagonal, then down low to the other.

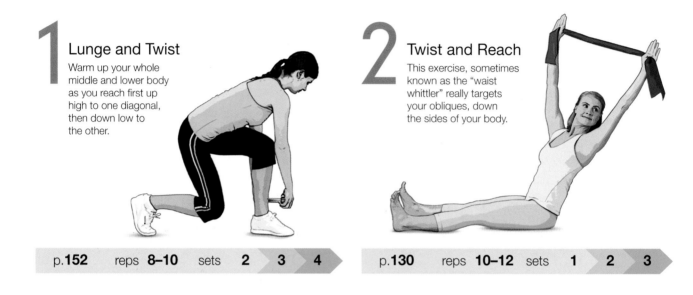

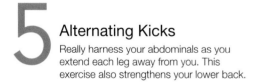
p.152   reps **8–10**   sets   **2**   **3**   **4**

2 Twist and Reach

This exercise, sometimes known as the "waist whittler" really targets your obliques, down the sides of your body.

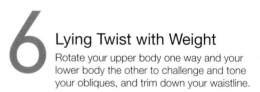
p.130   reps **10–12**   sets   **1**   **2**   **3**

5 Alternating Kicks

Really harness your abdominals as you extend each leg away from you. This exercise also strengthens your lower back.

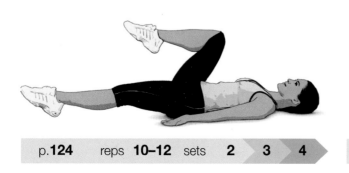
p.124   reps **10–12**   sets   **2**   **3**   **4**

6 Lying Twist with Weight

Rotate your upper body one way and your lower body the other to challenge and tone your obliques, and trim down your waistline.

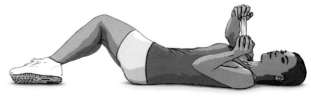
p.130   reps **10–12**   sets   **2**   **3**   **4**

I often get a sore neck when I'm doing sit-ups. Is there anything I can do about this?

The main reason that people tend to get a sore neck when doing sit-ups is that they are bringing their upper body up by pulling their hands on their neck and head, rather than by engaging and moving from their abs. To help to avoid this, only ever place your hands lightly behind your ears or head—do not clasp them.

3 Tick-tock

Hone your deepest abdominal muscle, called your transversus abdominis, with this side-to-side Pilates leg movement.

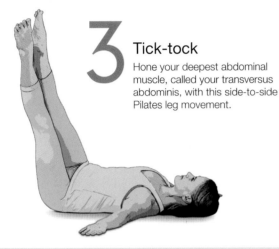

p.**210**   repeat up to 10 times

4 Ab Crunch

Challenge and tone your central abdominal muscles as you raise your head and shoulders in this classic sit-up.

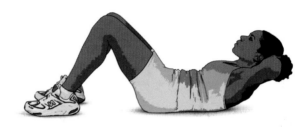

p.**122**   reps **12–14**   sets   **2**   **4**   **5**

7 Kneeling Back Extension

This exercise tones one side of your waist while stretching the other and also provides a nice release for your lower back, which supports your ab work.

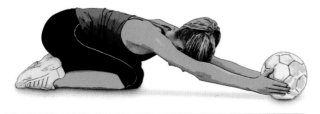

p.**134**   reps **10–12**   sets   **2**   **3**   **4**

8 Forearm Plank

Challenge your corset-style transversus abdominis muscle by pulling your belly button toward your spine in this tough horizontal position.

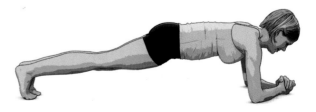

p.**126**   hold for 10 seconds   **1**   **3**   **5**

Ultimate butt workout

For a super-toned and pert butt, look no further than this amazing workout. It targets your glutes (see p.137) through every direction and ensures that the muscles around your thighs and hips are lifted and sculpted, too. In addition to looking good, a well-conditioned butt and thighs can help you to stay slim, because the more healthy these large muscles are, the more calories they burn.

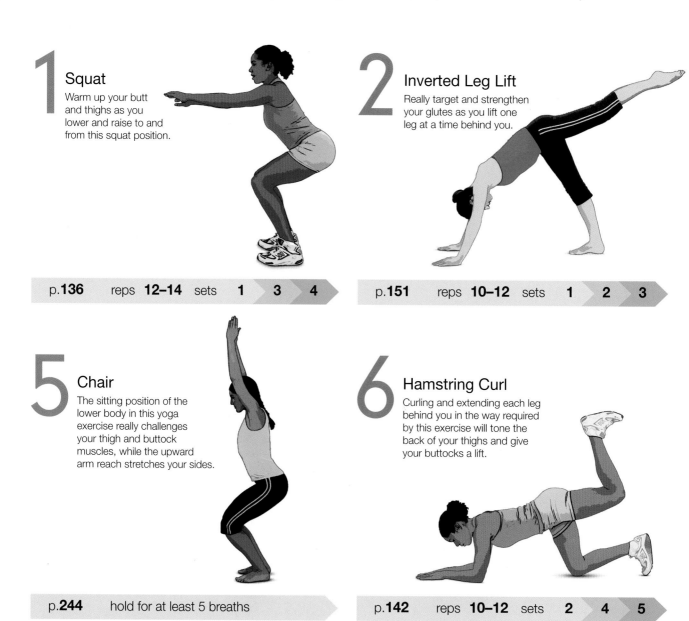

1 Squat

Warm up your butt and thighs as you lower and raise to and from this squat position.

p.136   reps **12–14**   sets   **1**   **3**   **4**

2 Inverted Leg Lift

Really target and strengthen your glutes as you lift one leg at a time behind you.

p.151   reps **10–12**   sets   **1**   **2**   **3**

5 Chair

The sitting position of the lower body in this yoga exercise really challenges your thigh and buttock muscles, while the upward arm reach stretches your sides.

p.244   hold for at least 5 breaths

6 Hamstring Curl

Curling and extending each leg behind you in the way required by this exercise will tone the back of your thighs and give your buttocks a lift.

p.142   reps **10–12**   sets   **2**   **4**   **5**

I do lots of buttock- and thigh-toning exercises but my rear end is still larger than I would like. What else can I do?

Some people naturally have a larger butt and thigh area than others—see p.28 for information on being "pear" shaped. However, doing the workout below and the "Pear" workout on pp.300–01, as well as regular cardio workouts such as running and dancing, will help to keep your lower body as trim and toned as possible.

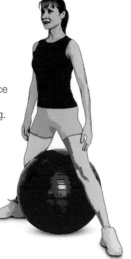

3 Ball Squeeze

Use the ball as resistance each time you come up from a squat to standing. This will really tone your inner thighs as well as your buttocks.

p.**145**   reps **10–12**   sets   **2**   **3**   **4**

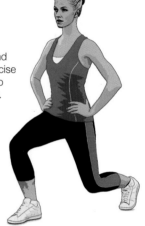

4 Lunge Kick

This alternate lunge and kick is a dynamic exercise that will work deep into your thighs and glutes.

p.**141**   reps **10–12**   sets   **2**   **3**   **4**

7 Plank with Leg Lift

Keep your hips level as you lift each leg to work your glutes. This exercise is also fantastic for your abdominals.

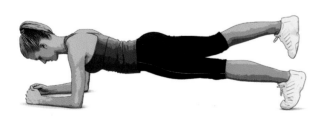

p.**126**   reps **6–10**   sets   **1**   **2**   **3**

8 Kneeling Lean

This exercise will further tone your glutes and abs while also giving the front of your thighs a well-deserved stretch.

p.**140**   reps **8–12**   sets   **2**   **3**   **4**

Dream legs workout

Have you always dreamed of having toned legs that you can show off with confidence? Then the Dream legs workout is for you. Moving your legs through their full range of motion, from bending and extending, forward and backward lifts, to rocks, sideways lifts, and rotations, it sculpts both your thighs and calves to give beautiful all-over definition. Bring on those high hemlines!

1 Plié

Target your inner thighs in particular as you bend and straighten with your feet turned diagonally outward.

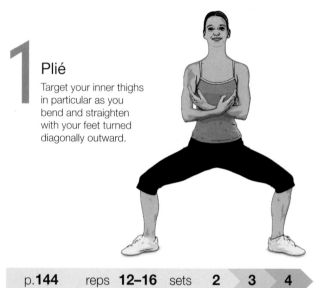

p.**144**   reps **12–16**   sets   **2**   **3**   **4**

2 Heel Raise against Wall

Strengthen and sculpt your calves as you raise and lower your heels. This exercise is also great for balance and foot mobility.

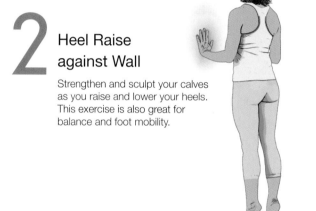

p.**148**   reps **12–14**   sets   **2**   **4**   **5**

5 Lunge with Weights

Strengthen and tone all your leg muscles in this wonderful deep lunge.

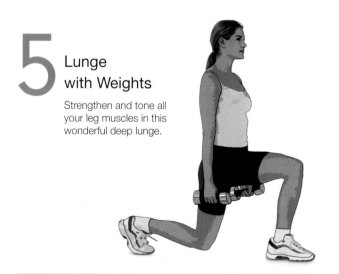

p.**141**   reps **12–16**   sets   **1**   **2**   **3**

6 Leg Circles

This challenging Pilates exercise gives a great workout for not only your legs but also your abs.

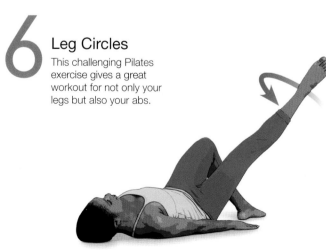

p.**215**   repeat up to 10 times

> **When I'm doing side leg lifts, I start to feel challenged more quickly than with a lot of other leg exercises. Is this okay?**
>
> Sideways leg lifts work the muscles on the inside and outside of your thighs (adductors and abductors, see p.145), which get much less use in everyday movements than the front and back thigh muscles. It's therefore only natural that they tire more easily, so go with this—stop when they "tell" you that you need to.

3 Back Leg Lift

Get the back of your thighs in tip-top shape with this backward leg extension.

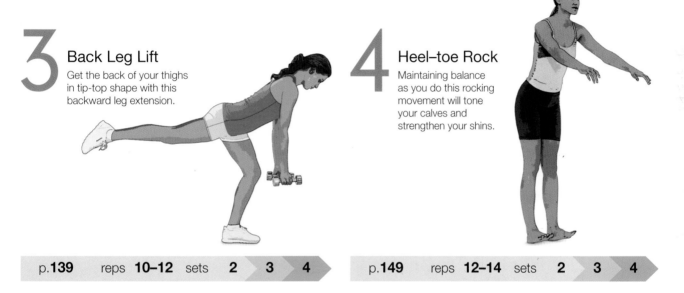

| p.**139** | reps **10–12** | sets | **2** | **3** | **4** |

4 Heel–toe Rock

Maintaining balance as you do this rocking movement will tone your calves and strengthen your shins.

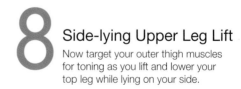

| p.**149** | reps **12–14** | sets | **2** | **3** | **4** |

7 Side-lying Lower Leg Lift

Firm up your hard-to-reach inner thigh muscles as you lift and lower your bottom leg while lying on your side.

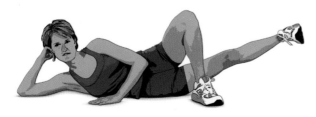

| p.**146** | reps **12–16** | sets | **2** | **3** | **4** |

8 Side-lying Upper Leg Lift

Now target your outer thigh muscles for toning as you lift and lower your top leg while lying on your side.

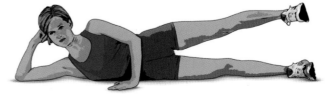

| p.**147** | reps **12–16** | sets | **2** | **3** | **4** |

"Apple" workout

If you're an "apple" shape (see p.28), you'll know only too well that you tend to carry any excess weight around your tummy. This workout will help to tone your stomach by working deep into your central abdominal muscles, as well as sculpting through your obliques to draw in your waist. The routine finishes with several satisfying stretches that help to elongate through your waist and hips.

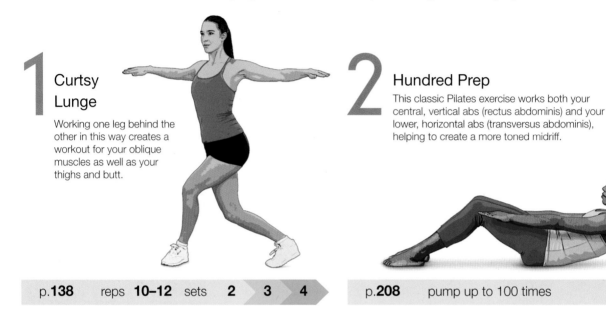

1 Curtsy Lunge

Working one leg behind the other in this way creates a workout for your oblique muscles as well as your thighs and butt.

p.**138**   reps **10–12**   sets   **2**   **3**   **4**

2 Hundred Prep

This classic Pilates exercise works both your central, vertical abs (rectus abdominis) and your lower, horizontal abs (transversus abdominis), helping to create a more toned midriff.

p.**208**   pump up to 100 times

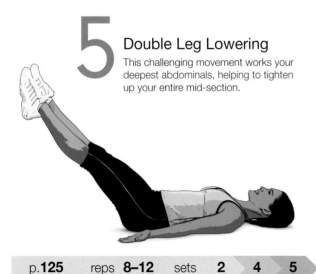

5 Double Leg Lowering

This challenging movement works your deepest abdominals, helping to tighten up your entire mid-section.

p.**125**   reps **8–12**   sets   **2**   **4**   **5**

6 Spine Twist

This gentle upper body twist targets your obliques to tone and trim your waist.

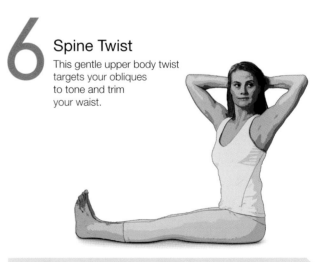

p.**207**   repeat up to 10 times

I'm doing a lot of sit-ups, but my tummy doesn't seem to be getting any smaller. Any advice?

Firstly, be careful not to let your abs bulge out when doing sit-ups because this will build bulk. Instead, pull your belly button toward your spine. Secondly, ensure that you're doing enough cardio work (see pp.52–97), since you'll only see the results of your ab-toning exercises once you've burned off any fat covering the muscles.

3 Oblique Crunch

Raise your head and shoulders diagonally off the floor to tone and strengthen your obliques and therefore sculpt your waist.

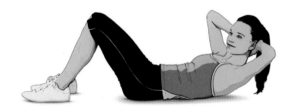

p.**128**   reps **12–14**   sets   **2**   **4**   **5**

4 Forearm Plank

Holding your body in this horizontal position requires you to work your transversus abdominis, the stomach muscle that acts as your internal corset.

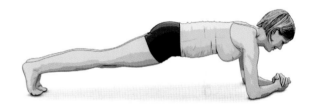

p.**126**   hold for 10 seconds   **1**   **3**   **5**

7 Rolling Leg Lift

Lifting your leg and turning onto your side in this way challenges your waist and stomach muscles as well as honing in on your inner thighs.

p.**188**   hold for 10 seconds

8 Lying Waist Twist

Doing this nourishing twist will give your whole mid-section a well-deserved stretch—stomach, waist, and lower back.

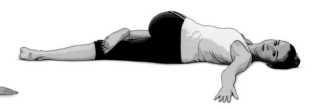

p.**182**   hold for 10 seconds

"Pear" workout

If you're a "pear" shape (see p.28), you'll know only too well that you tend to carry any excess weight around your thighs, hips, and bottom. If this bothers you in any way, then the "Pear" workout can help. Targeting your lower body from all angles, it will enable you to keep your thighs and butt area as streamlined as possible within the parameters of your natural body shape.

1 Chair

Warm up your whole lower body with this powerful yoga move: your thigh and buttock muscles will work hard to keep you in the sitting position required.

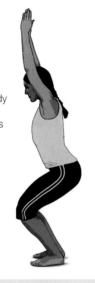

| p.**244** | hold for at least 5 breaths |

2 Side-squat Kick

Tone and sculpt your front and outer thighs as you firstly squat, and then kick to the side.

| p.**139** | reps **10–12** | sets | **2** | **3** | **4** |

5 Leg Circles

This challenging Pilates movement works not only your entire lower body but also deep into your abdominal muscles.

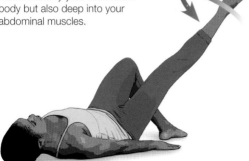

| p.**215** | repeat up to 10 times |

6 Shoulder Bridge

Your thighs and abs work hard to keep you stable in this position, which will both strengthen and tone them. Meanwhile, your front body gets a nice stretch.

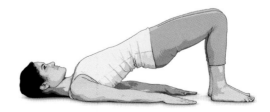

| p.**214** | repeat up to 10 times |

**I have quite bad cellulite around the back of my thighs.
Is there anything I can do about this?**

Cellulite is an accumulation of toxins and fatty deposits that get trapped in the
cells beneath the skin. The key to reducing this is eating a healthy, balanced diet
(see pp.48–51), drinking lots of water to flush it out, and doing regular exercise
(both cardio and sculpting) to stimulate blood flow and lymph drainage.

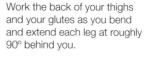

3 Ball Squeeze

Enhance your thigh and butt
definition by squeezing your
inner thighs against the ball
each time you come up to
standing from the Plié position.

p.**145**   reps **10–12**   sets   **2**   **4**   **5**

4 Hamstring Curl

Work the back of your thighs
and your glutes as you bend
and extend each leg at roughly
90° behind you.

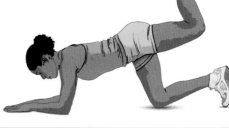

p.**142**   reps **10–12**   sets   **2**   **3**   **4**

7 Criss-cross Leg Extension

While the diagonal sit-up movement works
your abs to tone your waist and stomach,
the alternate leg extensions sculpt your leg
muscles—for a more streamlined silhouette.

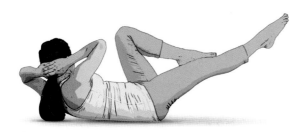

p.**129**   reps **14–16**   sets   **2**   **4**   **5**

8 Cross-knee Forward Bend

Finally, give your butt and thighs
a well-deserved stretch with this
challenging seated forward bend.

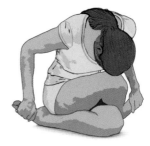

p.**188**   hold for 10 seconds

"Ruler" workout

If you're a "ruler" shape (see p.29), you are the envy of many women in that you're both tall and slim. But if, like many "rulers," you long for a more shapely body, then this workout is just what you need. By toning your waist and stomach, strengthening your shoulder and chest area, and sculpting your butt and thighs, it will maximize your capacity for curves, as well as enhancing healthy posture.

1 Wall Squat with Weights

Doing this squat against a wall will develop your lower body strength, while lifting your arms out in front of you enhances your upper body strength.

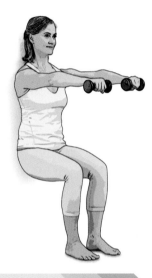

p.**137**   reps **10–12**   sets   **2**   **3**   **4**

2 Knee Squeeze

Restore the natural alignment of your spine and your rightful sense of length throughout your body with this elegant balancing exercise.

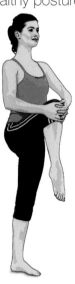

p.**134**   reps **10–12**   sets   **2**   **3**   **4**

5 Twist and Reach

Alternatively called the "waist whittler," this seated twist will help to define your waist as well as pull you up tall to boost your posture.

p.**130**   reps **10–12**   sets   **1**   **2**   **3**

6 Lying Twist with Weight

This rotation to one side with your upper body and to the other side with your lower body further defines your waist and boosts healthy posture through your mid-section.

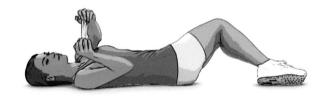

p.**130**   reps **12–14**   sets   **2**   **3**   **4**

I'm ultra-aware of my height (5'10") and often find myself inadvertently slouching. Can any exercises help with this?

Slouching is common among "ruler" shapes. Since it causes the upper back to become overstretched and the chest to tighten, exercises that open your chest will really help. Each time you become aware that you are slouching, try the Knee Squeeze below or Shoulder Circling (see p.164) in a backward direction.

3 Kneeling Lean

Challenge both your upper and lower body with this backward lean, with forward raised arms, while at the same time toning your abs.

p.**140**   reps **10–12**   sets   **1**   **2**   **3**

4 Knee Stretch

This Pilates movement will define your central and side abs, while shaping your glutes and the back of your thighs.

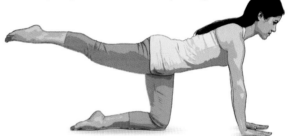

p.**217**   repeat up to 10 times

7 Mini Push-up

Doing this challenging exercise will help to build upper body definition to increase the sense of shapeliness throughout your body.

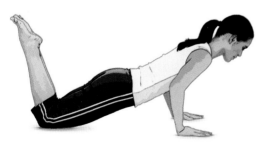

p.**112**   reps **10–12**   sets   **2**   **3**   **5**

8 Roll-up

This Pilates exercise really focuses on building spinal awareness and abdominal strength to further enhance good posture.

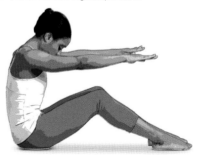

p.**213**   repeat 3–5 times

"Hourglass" workout

If you have a balanced, feminine shape with a substantial bust, slim waist, and curvy hips and thighs, you're lucky enough to have an "hourglass" figure (see p.29). This workout will help you to maintain this much-desired shape via total body toning. The exercises involved will also help you to manage your weight since they'll keep your main muscle groups active, which boosts your metabolism.

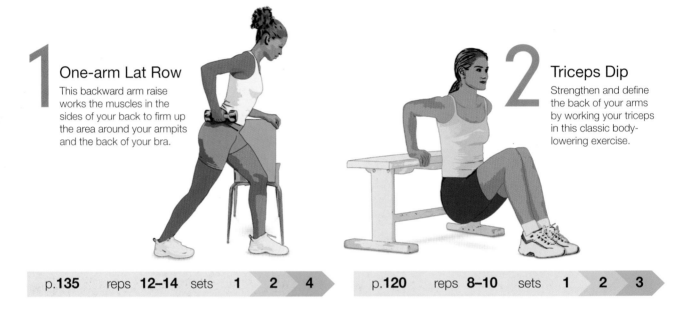

1 One-arm Lat Row

This backward arm raise works the muscles in the sides of your back to firm up the area around your armpits and the back of your bra.

p.**135**   reps **12–14**   sets   **1**   **2**   **4**

2 Triceps Dip

Strengthen and define the back of your arms by working your triceps in this classic body-lowering exercise.

p.**120**   reps **8–10**   sets   **1**   **2**   **3**

5 Ab Stretch and Crunch on Ball

The backward stretch element of this exercise opens your chest, encouraging good posture, and the sit-up aspect then strongly works and sculpts your abs.

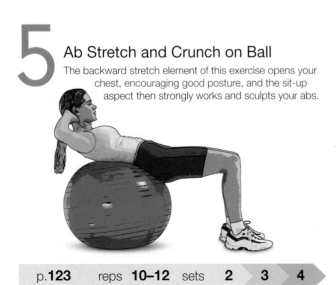

p.**123**   reps **10–12**   sets   **2**   **3**   **4**

6 Mini Push-up

Tone and strengthen your chest muscles and the back of your arms as you push up. Doing this exerise correctly will also open out your shoulders to improve posture.

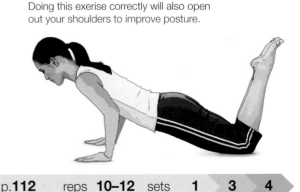

p.**112**   reps **10–12**   sets   **1**   **3**   **4**

As I get older, I'm starting to get thicker around my mid-section. Is there anything I can do about this?

Many women, especially "hourglass" and "apple" shapes, have this problem. Ensure that you are eating a balanced, healthy diet (see pp.48–51) and doing enough cardio exercise (see pp.58–97), and commit to a regular combination of the workout below, the Fabulous abs workout (see pp.292–93), and the "Apple" workout (see pp.298–99).

3 Wall Squat with Weight

Tone the front of your thighs as you squat and your glutes as you push back up, as well as sculpting your arms, shoulders, and upper back with the arm raise.

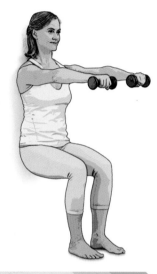

p.**137**   reps **10–12**   sets   **1**   **3**   **4**

4 External Rotation

Strengthen and define your upper arms and the muscles around the back of your shoulders for an elegant, toned shoulder and arm line from behind.

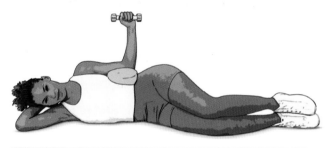

p.**110**   reps **10–12**   sets   **1**   **2**   **3**

7 Tick-tock

This challenging, side-to-side Pilates leg movement targets your waist and abdominal area for excellent toning and sculpting.

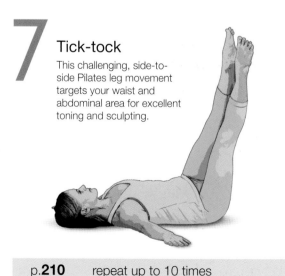

p.**210**   repeat up to 10 times

8 Side-lying Leg Circle

Making large circles with your legs in this way will really work both your inner and outer thighs, as well as further sculpting your abs.

p.**146**   reps **12–14**   sets   **1**   **2**   **3**

Better-in-bed workout

If you want to look good naked and give yourself a boost of confidence in the bedroom, then try the Better-in-bed workout. The specially chosen exercises will energize and tone your whole body, relieve tiredness and stress, boost motivation, and improve your flexibility. Shoulder Bridge and Pelvic Curl focus on toning through your pelvic floor which will enhance your sexual pleasure.

1 Chair

This dynamic yoga pose gives you a fantastic whole body stretch, makes your muscles work hard, and also gets your blood pumping. It will therefore leave you feeling more vibrant and alert, as well as giving you an all-over tone.

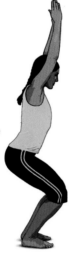

p.**244**   hold for at least 5 breaths

2 Shoulder Bridge

Firm up your abs, your buttocks, and the back of your legs as you lift into this Pilates back bend. It will also strengthen your spine, enhancing both stamina and flexibility. Be sure to engage your pelvic floor as you lift.

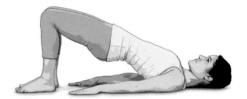

p.**214**   repeat up to 10 times

5 Side-lying Lower Leg Lift

This lateral leg lift will soon firm up and strengthen the inside of your thighs, an area that is notoriously hard to target.

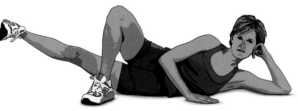

p.**146**   reps **14–16**   sets   **2**   **3**   **4**

6 Side-lying Upper Leg Lift

This lateral lift of your upper leg moves the toning focus to the outside of your thighs so that you can feel more at ease with and confident about this area.

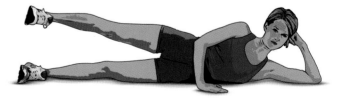

p.**147**   reps **14–16**   sets   **2**   **3**   **4**

My libido has recently been on the decline—I've neither been wanting nor enjoying sex as much. Can exercise help?

If your flagging sex drive feels like it's a result of a general lack of energy, regular exercise may help since, once you get used to doing it, it will give you more get-up-and-go in all areas of your life. Other reasons why exercise can boost your boudoir activities are: increased cardio fitness, endurance, and flexibility, all of which can make things much more active, lengthy, and varied, if desired!

3 Pelvic Curl

This subtle but effective Pilates movement will lengthen the front of your thighs and firm up your abs and buttocks. Be sure to engage your pelvic floor as you lift.

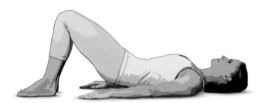

p.**203**   repeat up to 10 times

4 Extended Heel Taps

Strengthen the entire back of your body and lengthen the whole front of your body as you lift into this front-lying back bend. The dynamic heel-tapping further adds to the toning effect, particularly in your legs.

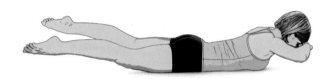

p.**133**   reps **12–14**   sets   **1**   **2**   **3**

7 Ab Crunch

This classic sit-up move will help you on your way to getting the honed abs you've always wanted, boosting your self-image and self-confidence.

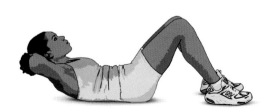

p.**122**   reps **12–14**   sets   **2**   **4**   **6**

8 Rolling Leg Lift

Give your lower body flexibility a dramatic boost with this dynamic, ballet-inspired rolling leg stretch. It will also help to sculpt through your waist and strengthen your back.

p.**188**   hold for 10 seconds

Postpartum workout

This workout is designed to recondition your entire body after pregnancy and help you to feel stronger and more energized again, but it particularly focuses on rebuilding abdominal and pelvic floor strength. However, it's best to consult a medical professional before undertaking any post-pregnancy exercise regimen to ensure that the movements are suitable for you.

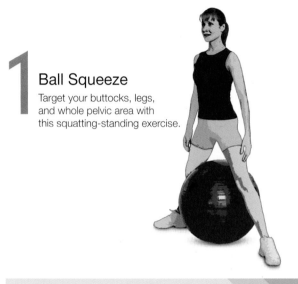

1 Ball Squeeze

Target your buttocks, legs, and whole pelvic area with this squatting-standing exercise.

p.**145**   reps **10–12**   sets   **2**   **3**   **4**

2 Heel Raise against Wall

Boost your lower leg strength with this simple lifting and lowering exercise. It will also help to improve foot mobility if you've had any ankle swelling or other issues during your pregnancy.

p.**148**   reps **12–14**   sets   **2**   **3**   **4**

5 Chest Press

This simple arm exercise helps to lift and support your bust, tone your arms, and boost your upper body strength—useful for carrying your newborn baby.

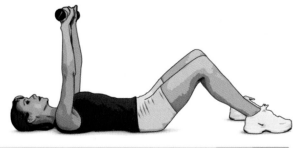

p.**114**   reps **10–12**   sets   **2**   **3**   **4**

6 Pelvic Curl

This subtle Pilates movement is useful for relieving any tension lurking in your lower back as you curl through your spine, one vertebra at a time.

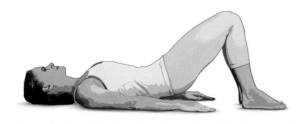

p.**203**   repeat up to 10 times

I've been told to wait six months before doing any high-impact exercise such as running and dancing. Is this right?

This is indeed right because you still have the hormone relaxin in your body for the first six months after your baby's birth. Relaxin is the hormone that causes the loosening of the ligaments in your pelvis and birth canal to facilitate birth, but it also affects other joints. To prevent joint injury, it's therefore best to stick to low-impact cardio exercise such as walking or swimming for this period.

3 Knee Stretch

This Pilates movement requires you to pull your abs in tight toward your spine as you lift and lengthen your leg, toning both your stomach and your legs.

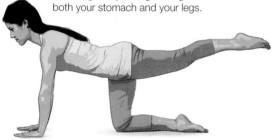

p.**217**   repeat up to 10 times

4 Back Extension

This front-lying back bend helps to strengthen and relieve any tension in your back after the strain of carrying pregnancy weight for nine months.

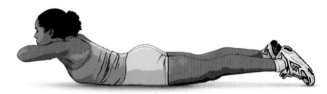

p.**132**   reps **10–12**   sets   **1**   **2**   **3**

7 Shoulder Bridge

Give both the front and back of your body a nice workout with this strong Pilates movement—to boost both length and strength throughout your body.

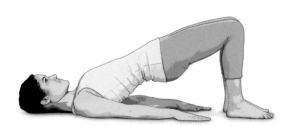

p.**214**   repeat up to 10 times

8 Knee to Shoulder

Give your lower back and buttocks a lovely stretch and your abs a gentle massage as you draw your bent leg toward your chest.

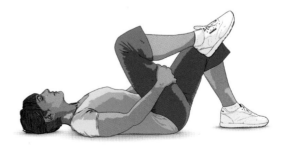

p.**173**   hold for 10 seconds

Ten-years-younger workout

Exercise can keep you looking and feeling fitter, younger, more vibrant, and in better shape than any expensive cream or invasive treatment. So if you want to alleviate stress, increase energy, and maintain or re-establish a firm, strong body, then try the workout below. As we get older, our calorie-burning capacity declines, so it's crucial to complement it with adequate cardio exercise.

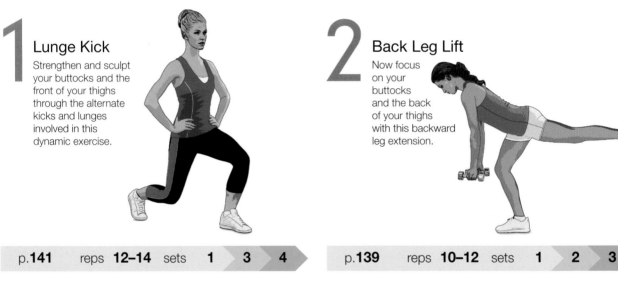

1 Lunge Kick

Strengthen and sculpt your buttocks and the front of your thighs through the alternate kicks and lunges involved in this dynamic exercise.

p.**141**   reps **12–14**   sets   **1**   **3**   **4**

2 Back Leg Lift

Now focus on your buttocks and the back of your thighs with this backward leg extension.

p.**139**   reps **10–12**   sets   **1**   **2**   **3**

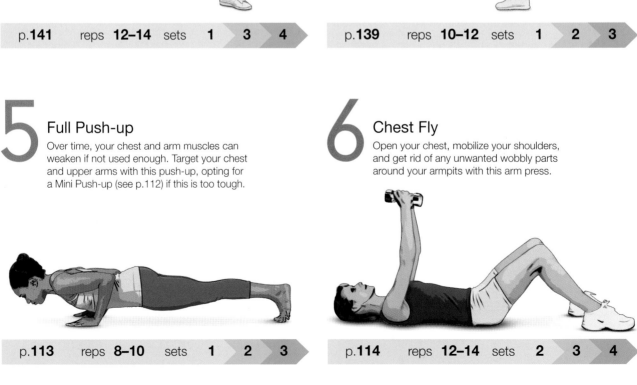

5 Full Push-up

Over time, your chest and arm muscles can weaken if not used enough. Target your chest and upper arms with this push-up, opting for a Mini Push-up (see p.112) if this is too tough.

p.**113**   reps **8–10**   sets   **1**   **2**   **3**

6 Chest Fly

Open your chest, mobilize your shoulders, and get rid of any unwanted wobbly parts around your armpits with this arm press.

p.**114**   reps **12–14**   sets   **2**   **3**   **4**

I am now in my 50s and am increasingly aware of my joints feeling sore when I run. What can I do about this?

As with anything that's causing discomfort or pain, it's best to stop it and try something new. For example, you might want to consider a lower-impact cardio activity, such as walking, cycling, or swimming. Any of these will keep you just as fit and firm without putting the same pressure on your bones: it's intensity, not impact, that counts.

3 Horse

This yoga pose strengthens and sculpts both your lower and upper body due to the combination of the deep squat and the arm movement.

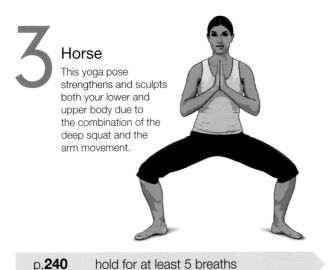

p.**240**	hold for at least 5 breaths

4 Sitting Side Curl

Saggy arms can be very aging. Firm them up and add definition to them with this isolated arm exercise.

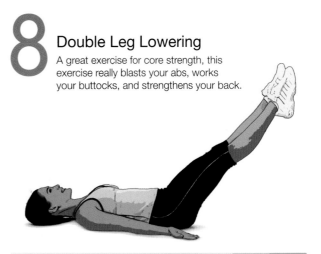

p.**117**	reps **12–14**	sets	2	3	4

7 Criss-cross Leg Extension

Target both your central and side abdominals to tone both your stomach and waist with this twisting bicycle move.

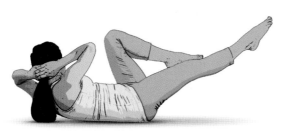

p.**129**	reps **14–16**	sets	2	4	6

8 Double Leg Lowering

A great exercise for core strength, this exercise really blasts your abs, works your buttocks, and strengthens your back.

p.**125**	reps **12–14**	sets	1	3	4

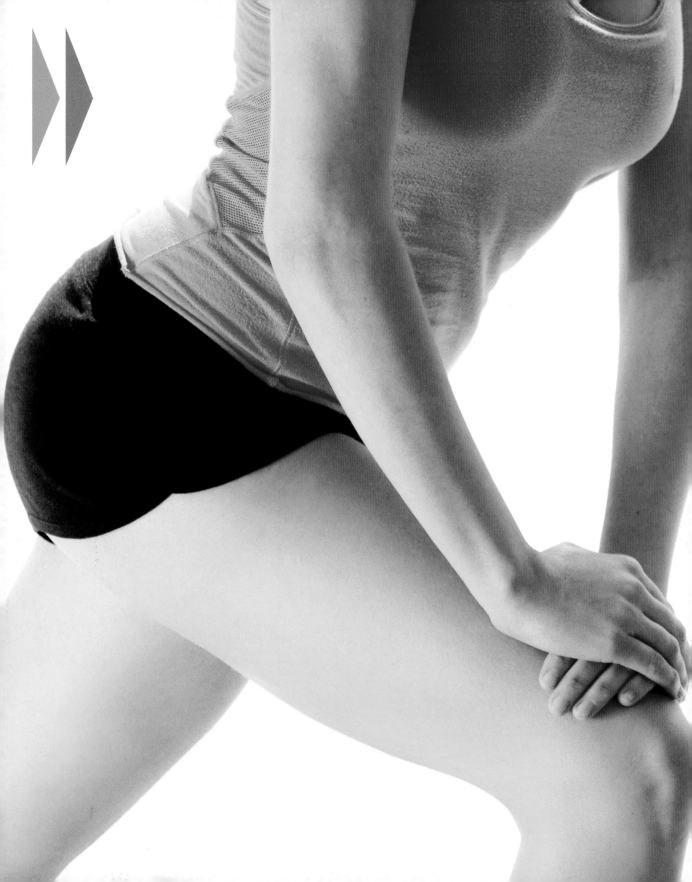

Quick-fix workouts

While it's important to have a regular program of cardio and sculpting workouts built into your weekly schedule in order to work toward your designated goals, it can also be useful to supplement your routine with other exercises from time to time when you find yourself stiff, stressed, flagging in energy, or simply with a bit of time to spare. The seven workouts that follow have been designed to:

- give a kick-start to your morning

- counteract the pressures of hunching over a computer for long periods of time

- provide a welcome mid-day mobilizer

- offer a breath of fresh life to your weary body in times of need

- release any tension or stress that you're carrying

- give your flexibility a welcome boost

- loosen up stiff muscles and make you feel better—any time, anywhere

Morning wake-up workout

If you find it hard to get going in the morning, then try the Morning wake-up workout. A gentle but invigorating energy booster, it includes a combination of easy stretches to shake off stiffness, Elbow Circling to mobilize your upper body, balancing moves to simultaneously ground and uplift you for the day, and arm and leg work to get your limbs warmed up and strengthened.

1 Arm Reach and Palm Press

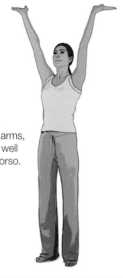

Start the day with this fantastic activating stretch through your arms, shoulders, and upper back, as well as through both sides of your torso.

p.**178**   hold for 10 seconds

2 Elbow Circling

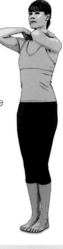

Do this exercise to get your shoulders and arms moving and to open your chest for enhanced posture throughout the day.

p.**164**   circle 8 times each way

5 Double Punch

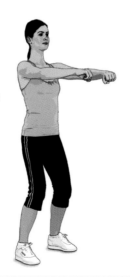

Energize your upper body with this dynamic punching action.

p.**119**   reps **8–10**   sets   **1**   **2**   **3**

6 Heel Raise against Wall

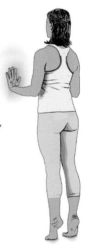

Boost your lower leg strength, tone your calves, enhance your foot mobility, and further challenge your sense of balance, as you rise up onto your toes.

p.**148**   reps **10–12**   sets   **2**   **3**   **4**

Lots of people say that it's best to exercise first thing in the morning. Is this true?

Many people find that a morning workout is a motivating start to the day. However, as with everything, what works "best" for one person may not work at all for another, so experiment with your exercise timings to discover what suits you the best in terms of both your schedule and your energy levels.

3 Opposing Arm Extension

This tilt to the side while stretching your arms in opposing directions relaxes your chest, which can feel tight in the morning, and will stretch out the sides of your body.

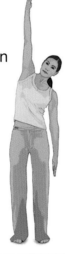

p.**175**   hold for 10 seconds

4 Knee Squeeze

Work both your back and abs with this balancing knee lift. The exercise will also encourage you to approach your day with more of a sense of equilibrium.

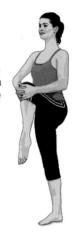

p.**134**   reps **8–10**   sets   **1**   **2**   **3**

7 Warrior 2 and Side Angle Stretch

Gain a sense of length in your upper body and strengthen your lower body in this powerful yoga move.

p.**247**   hold for at least 5 breaths

8 Plié with Lateral Raise

Finally, grab your hand weights or two small bottles of water and do this elegant but invigorating ballet-inspired exercise.

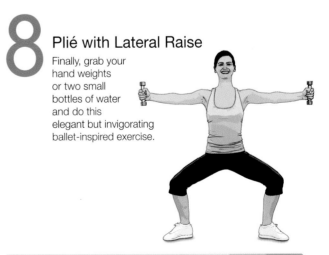

p.**152**   reps **8–10**   sets   **1**   **2**   **3**

Computer workout

Sitting in front of a computer all day, doing repetitive actions such as moving your mouse and typing, can lead to neck and head tension, eye strain, backache, and tightness in your hands, wrists, arms, and shoulders, as well as poor posture due to the hunched position we often adopt. This workout is designed to ease these problems and leave you feeling recharged and revitalized.

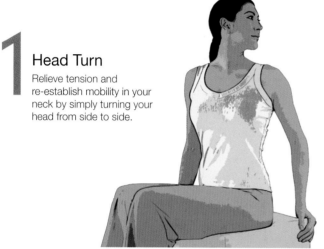

1 Head Turn

Relieve tension and re-establish mobility in your neck by simply turning your head from side to side.

p. **161**   hold for 5 seconds

2 Eye Exercises

Give your eyes a break from their normal position by looking first up and down, then side to side, then from diagonal to diagonal.

p. **160**   hold for 5 seconds

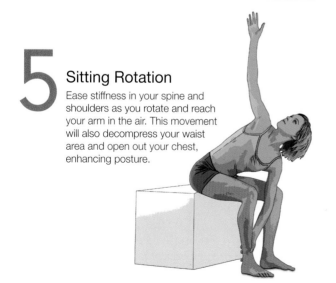

5 Sitting Rotation

Ease stiffness in your spine and shoulders as you rotate and reach your arm in the air. This movement will also decompress your waist area and open out your chest, enhancing posture.

p. **177**   hold for 10 seconds

6 Chest Expansion

Develop mobility through your shoulders and get a good workout for your whole upper body with this arm raise.

p. **115**   reps **8–10**   sets   **1**   **2**   **3**

How can I stop myself slouching when I sit at my desk?

Make sure your chair is at the right height for you: your eyes should be level with your screen, your knees just slightly lower than your hip joints, your feet flat on the floor, and your back nice and upright. Every now and then, do a posture-check: roll your shoulders back and down, pull your head up tall, and draw your belly button toward your spine to engage your abdominal muscles.

3 Hand Rotations

Alleviate any stiffness in your hands, wrists, and forearms with these soothing wrist and arm circling exercises.

p. **181**   repeat 8–10 times each way

4 Press and Twist

Counter slumping and stiffness and increase your range of upper body movement with this twisting motion.

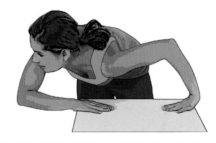

p. **166**   hold for 10 seconds

7 Backward Arm Raise

A strong stretch through your shoulders and into your arms, this will refresh and reinvigorate your upper body.

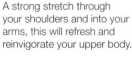
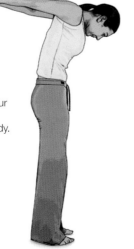

p. **166**   hold for 10 seconds

8 Knee Squeeze

Release tension in your lower back as you lift your knee toward your chest. This also targets your abs as you work to maintain balance.

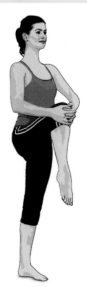

p. **134**   reps **8–10**   sets   **1**   **2**   **3**

Lunch-break workout

Pressed for time to exercise? If you have a busy working life, it can be challenging to fit in regular exercise, but the benefits can really justify the effort. This total body lunchtime workout is therefore just the ticket. As well as offering a nice stretch and sculpt, it will give you a great energy boost for the afternoon, plus it targets lots of big muscle groups, which will enhance your metabolic rate.

1 Lunge and Twist

Mobilize your whole body with this dynamic movement, which moves your arms first up to one diagonal, then down to the other.

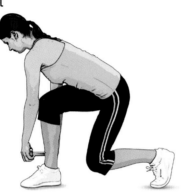

p. **152**   reps **10–12**   sets   **1**   **3**   **4**

2 Biceps Curl

Strengthen the front of your upper arms with this simple double arm curl. Use two small bottles of water if no hand weights are available.

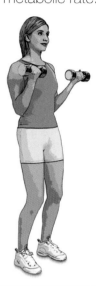

p. **116**   reps **12–14**   sets   **1**   **2**   **3**

5 Lunge Kick

This dynamic exercise targets the back of your legs and your buttocks as you kick and the front of your thighs as you lunge.

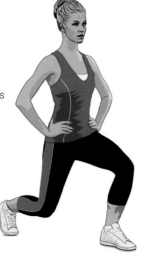

p. **141**   reps **10–12**   sets   **1**   **3**   **4**

6 Front Raise

Work the front of your shoulders and your upper arms with these diagonal arm lifts. Again, use two small bottles of water if no hand weights are available.

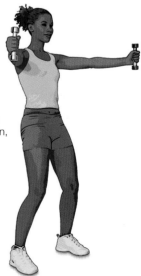

p. **109**   reps **10–12**   sets   **1**   **2**   **3**

I find it hard to fit exercise into my daily life because I've got so much else going on. Do you have any advice?

Our busy, modern lifestyles make it really difficult to fit in everything we want but it's important to remember that regular exercise won't just get you in better shape. It will also enhance your underlying health and fitness, which will make you more able to deal with all the other demands placed on you, so try to make it a priority.

3 Heel–toe Rock

Re-energize your lower legs and feet as you rock forward and backward in this exercise.

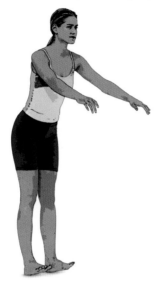

p. **149**   reps **10–12**   sets   **1**   **2**   **3**

4 Triceps Dip

Strengthen and tone the back of your arms using your own body weight for resistance.

p. **120**   reps **8–10**   sets   **1**   **3**   **5**

7 Twist and Bend

Both strengthen and tone your whole mid-section and stretch out your whole back with this diagonal forward bend.

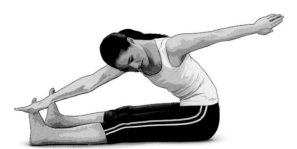

p. **131**   reps **8–10**   sets   **1**   **2**   **3**

8 Oblique Crunch

The diagonal twist in this sit-up variation means that you really work your waist as well as your central abdominal muscles.

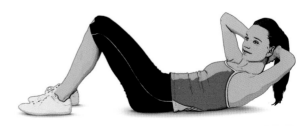

p. **128**   reps **12–14**   sets   **2**   **3**   **4**

Pick-me-up workout

If ever you're feeling tired, sluggish, and in search of an instant energy boost, then this is the workout you need. Designed to blast your body with fresh oxygen and increase the level of adrenaline in your bloodstream, the range of specially selected dynamic exercises will target all your main muscles and enhance your energy levels, leaving you feeling refreshed and invigorated.

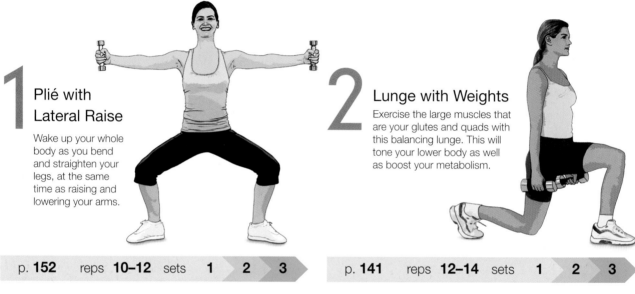

1 Plié with Lateral Raise

Wake up your whole body as you bend and straighten your legs, at the same time as raising and lowering your arms.

p. **152**   reps **10–12**   sets   **1**   **2**   **3**

2 Lunge with Weights

Exercise the large muscles that are your glutes and quads with this balancing lunge. This will tone your lower body as well as boost your metabolism.

p. **141**   reps **12–14**   sets   **1**   **2**   **3**

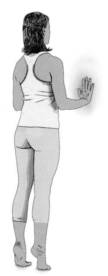

5 Heel Raise against Wall

Reactivate your calves and feet, plus boost lower leg definition, with this simple lift and lower against a wall.

p. **148**   reps **10–12**   sets   **2**   **3**   **4**

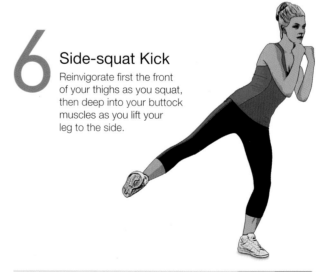

6 Side-squat Kick

Reinvigorate first the front of your thighs as you squat, then deep into your buttock muscles as you lift your leg to the side.

p. **139**   reps **12–14**   sets   **1**   **2**   **3**

The workout below helps to give me a boost when I'm flagging. What else can I do to remain more energized?

The key to feeling as vibrant as possible on an everyday level is a combination of a balanced diet, enough water, regular exercise, and adequate rest. And the most energizing forms of exercise are quite simply the ones you enjoy the most, whether that's walking, swimming, hula hooping, or tennis, so get exploring!

3 Triceps Kickback

Target your triceps to tone and enliven the back of your arms, being sure to keep your abs engaged throughout.

p. **121**   reps **8–10**   sets   **1**   **3**   **4**

4 Shoulder Extension

Work your back, shoulders, arms, abs, and thighs as you do this dynamic opposing arm reach.

p. **108**   reps **8–10**   sets   **1**   **2**   **3**

7 Criss-cross Leg Extension

Challenge and energize all your abdominal muscles, as well as work through your legs, as you twist and kick in this bicycling motion.

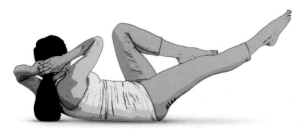

p. **129**   reps **14–16**   sets   **2**   **3**   **5**

8 Hundred Prep

Rolling back into this classic Pilates position, and holding and "pumping" here, will strongly activate your abs and enliven your spine.

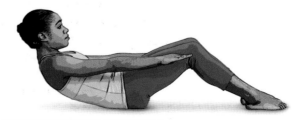

p. **208**   pump up to 100 times

Stress-buster workout

When you feel stressed, exercise is often the last thing you feel like doing, but try to remember that it'll make you feel better in the end because it's a natural mood booster as well as an effective means of releasing tension. Full of dynamic exercises that will give you a new focus, this workout will soon have your mind off your worries and on to getting into the best physical shape possible.

1 Twisting Punch

Alleviate tension in your shoulders and upper back with this dynamic, double-punching exercise.

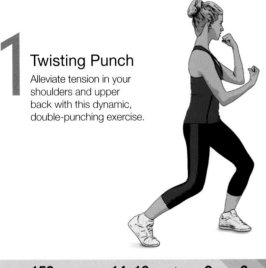

| p. **150** | reps **14–16** | sets | **2** | **3** | **4** |

2 Full Push-up

Doing this super-challenging exercise requires complete focus so will take your mind off any worries. Do the Mini Push-up on p.112 if this is too tough.

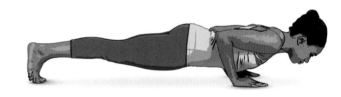

| p. **113** | reps **8–10** | sets | **1** | **2** | **3** |

5 Horse

Doing this powerful yoga pose will boost your body with fresh oxygen, enlivening and empowering your whole being.

| p. **240** | hold for at least 5 breaths |

6 Leg Circles

Focusing on the slow, flowing nature of the leg circling in this Pilates movement will help you to unwind at the same time as seriously working your abs and legs.

| p. **215** | repeat up to 10 times |

The more stressed I get with my work, the harder I find it to get into the frame of mind for exercise. Any advice?

The more stressed you feel, the more you really need a vigorous cardio blast or a relaxing yoga session to release the tensions of your day. So don't give yourself too much time to think about exercise: just finish work as soon as you can and get to it! Advance planning in terms of where, when, and in what clothes also helps.

3 Lunge Kick

This alternate kicking and lunging exercise is a great lower body tension reliever.

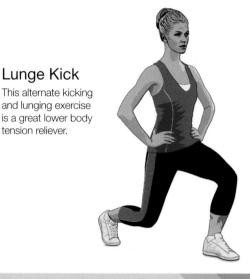

p. **141**   reps **14–16**   sets   **2**   **3**   **4**

4 Pull-up

Keeping your shoulders down as you do this dynamic arm lift will help to ease any tension in your upper body.

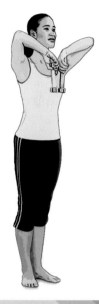

p. **118**   reps **10–12**   sets   **1**   **2**   **3**

7 Double Leg Lift

This strong Pilates movement targets your under-used side muscles, toning your waist and thighs. It will leave you feeling invigorated from the core.

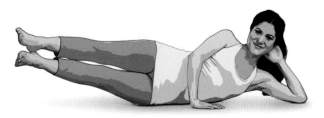

p. **216**   repeat up to 10 times

8 Plank with Leg Lift

This challenging abdominal exercise actually activates your entire body, so is a great way to unload stress—breathe out any tension on each exhalation.

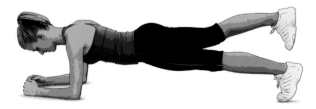

p. **126**   reps **8–10**   sets   **1**   **2**   **3**

Flexibility workout

Any time you're feeling stiff or tense, give this workout a try. Composed of a combination of stretching, Pilates, and yoga movements, it creates a sense of openness and increased mobility throughout your body, which will improve the function of your muscles and enable them to respond more effectively to your everyday needs. It will also relax and re-energize your entire being.

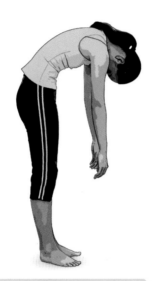

1 Roll-down

Spine flexibility is vital for feeling energized and mobile. Curl and uncurl your spine, one vertebra at a time, with this Pilates roll-down movement.

p. **206**   repeat 3–5 times

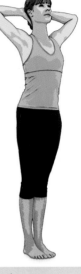

2 Elbow Push Back

Open across your chest and armpits to relieve tension and improve flexibility in your shoulders, as well as smooth the skin across your décolletage.

p. **176**   hold for 10 seconds

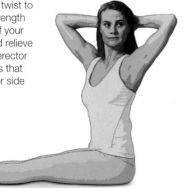

5 Spine Twist

Do this seated twist to improve the strength and flexibility of your lower back and relieve tension in the erector spinae muscles that run down either side of your spine.

p. **207**   repeat up to 10 times

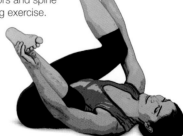

6 Hip Rocking

Stretch through your buttocks and thighs and enhance flexibility in your hip flexors and spine with this rocking exercise.

p. **185**   rock 10 times

When I go to exercise classes, I can't stretch half as far as the people around me. Is there something wrong with me?

Not at all—there's really no need to worry. Some people naturally have a wider range of movement through their joints than others. However, it's also within your own power to enhance your flexibility to the max by working on this particular component of fitness via regular stretching, Pilates, or yoga exercises.

3 Warrior 2 and Side Angle Stretch

Open up through the sides of your body and strengthen your lower body with this dynamic yoga movement.

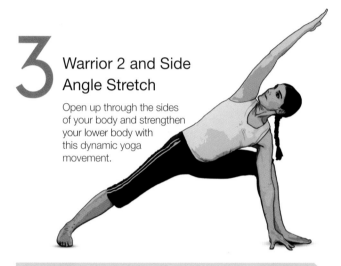

p. **247**   hold for at least 5 breaths

4 Wrist Mobilizer

Stretch your forearms and mobilize your wrists in this yoga-inspired movement. Aim for your forearms to be horizontal.

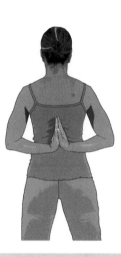

p. **180**   hold for 10 seconds

7 Lying Arm Twist

Open up your chest and shoulders and stretch through each side of your body and into your middle back as you twist.

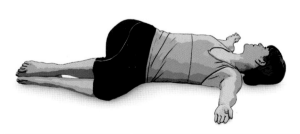

p. **169**   hold for 10 seconds

8 Swan Prep

Challenge your whole body as you lift your chest with control into this front-lying backbend, which will increase backward flexibility through your spine.

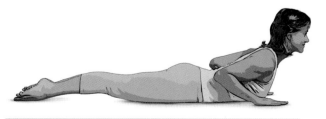

p. **204**   repeat up to 10 times

"Anywhere" workout

Designed to be done pretty much wherever you are, with very little space and minimal equipment, this workout is ideal if you're away from home, whether on a day trip or for longer. It can be easy to lose motivation when you're not in the groove of your home routine, so this set of exercises has been specially selected to help to keep you on track, blasting all your major body zones.

1 Squat

Start by toning and strengthening your front thighs and buttocks with this squatting exercise.

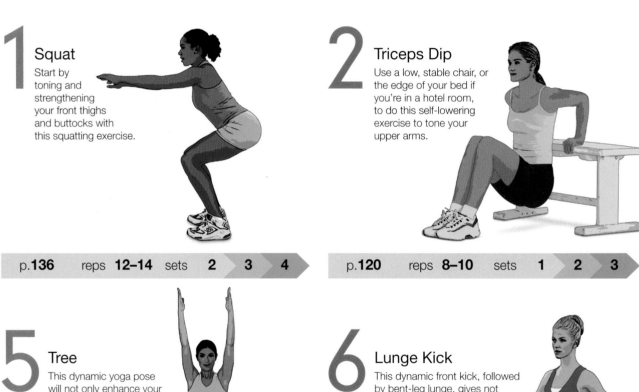

p.**136**   reps **12–14**   sets   **2**   **3**   **4**

2 Triceps Dip

Use a low, stable chair, or the edge of your bed if you're in a hotel room, to do this self-lowering exercise to tone your upper arms.

p.**120**   reps **8–10**   sets   **1**   **2**   **3**

5 Tree

This dynamic yoga pose will not only enhance your sense of balance, but also strengthen and lengthen your entire body.

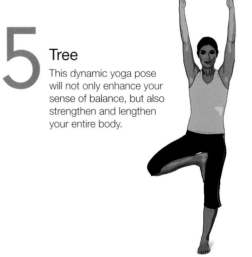

p.**245**   hold for at least 5 breaths

6 Lunge Kick

This dynamic front kick, followed by bent-leg lunge, gives not only your legs but also your abs a nice strong workout as they work to keep your back straight.

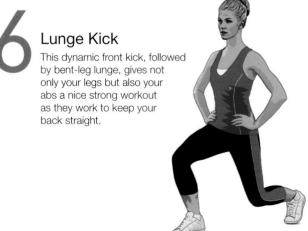

p.**141**   reps **12–14**   sets   **2**   **3**   **5**

Is it okay to have a break from exercise when I go away on business trips and vacations?

It's good to have a couple of days of rest from exercise now and then, but generally it's best never to go for more than 48 hours without doing some form of exercise, whether it's a few stretching moves, a nice walk, or a full workout to remind the body that you're fit and active. That way, you won't lose the momentum of your normal fitness regimen.

3 Heel Raise against Wall

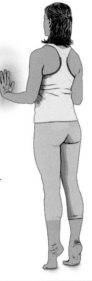

Lean gently against a wall for support, if necessary, and simply raise and lower your heels to boost lower leg strength and tone your calves.

p.**148**   reps **10–12**   sets   **2**   **3**   **4**

4 Biceps Curl

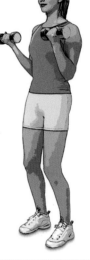

Tone and strengthen the front of your upper arms with these arm curls. Use small bottles of water if no hand weights are available.

p.**116**   reps **12–14**   sets   **1**   **2**   **3**

7 Double Punch

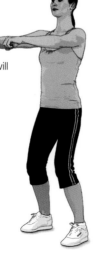

This forward punching exercise will help to keep your upper body in good all-around shape. Feel free to do it holding hand weights, or smalll bottes of water, if you want more of a challenge.

p.**119**   reps **12–14**   sets   **2**   **3**   **5**

8 Knee Squeeze

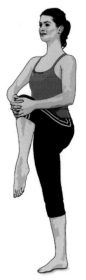

This balancing exercise targets not only your legs, but also your abs and back as you work to stay upright.

p.**134**   reps **10–12**   sets   **1**   **2**   **5**

Index

Useful addresses

America Bikes
(coalition of cycling organizations that advocates for the cycling community)
1612 K Street NW
Suite 802
Washington, DC 20006
Tel: (202) 223-3726
www.americabikes.org

American Dietetic Association
(for information on following a healthy diet)
120 South Riverside Plaza
Suite 2000
Chicago, IL 60606-6995
Tel: (800) 877-1600
www.eatright.org

American Hiking Society
(information on local walking groups, events, and campaigns)
1422 Fenwick Lane
Silver Spring, MD 20910
Tel: (301) 565-6704
www.americanhiking.org

American Running Association
(for information on jogging and running)
www.americanrunning.org

Canadian Diabetes Association
(for information on following a healthy diet)
1400-522 University Ave
Toronto ON M5G 2R5
Tel: (800) 226-8464
www.diabetes.ca

Canadian Volkssport Federation
(walking clubs for fitness and fun)
PO Box 2668, Station D
Ottawa, ON K1P 5W7
Tel: (613) 234-7333
www.walks.ca

Classical Pilates
(to find certified Pilates teachers in your area)
classicalpilates.net

YMCA of the USA
(for locations and services offered at your local YMCA)
101 N Wacker Drive
Chicago, IL 60606
Tel: (800) 872-9622
www.ymca.net

YMCA Canada
(for locations and services offered at your local YMCA)
1867 Yonge Street
Suite 601
Toronto ON M4S 1Y5
Tel: (416) 967-9622
www.ymca.ca

Yoga Alliance
(to find out more about yoga)
1701 Clarendon Boulevard
Suite 110
Arlington, VA 22209
Tel: (888) 921-YOGA (9642)
yogaalliance.org

Author and consultants

Kelly Thompson is a freelance writer and editor with a particular passion for all things health- and fitness-related. Having achieved an Oxford Blue in dance, she went on to become a YMCA-qualified fitness instructor, teaching classes in a variety of London venues. A yoga, dance, walking, and hula hoop enthusiast, she believes in finding and doing what you love to stay fit and has contributed to a wide range of books, covering everything from yoga, massage, and dance to meditation, the power of breathing, and living in the moment. She currently lives in London and has been lucky enough to travel to some of the world's leading health and fitness retreats.

Lucy Wyndham-Read is a leading women's fitness expert, personal trainer, and author of several best-selling books published worldwide. She is a regular on British TV and radio, and also produces her own audio workouts, fitness DVDs, and apps. Lucy also specializes in nutrition and weight loss, and ante- and postnatal exercise. Throughout the years she has helped thousands of women to lose weight and get in shape with her effective but easy-to-follow workouts. For more information, go to www.lwrfitness.com.

Graham Stones started out training and competing in kung fu, which he won a national gold medal for and went on to coach, before becoming interested in yoga, which he has since studied extensively in the UK, Crete, and India. He is regarded as one of London's top holistic health practitioners because he brings together his unique skills in remedial massage treatment and yoga teaching. He specializes in identifying, treating, and educating about areas of restriction and compression in the body so that his clients can achieve optimal health, freedom of movement, and maximal performance. He works for the English National Ballet, as well as for a range of yoga and holistic health centers in London. For more information, go to www.grahamstones.com.

Elisa Withers trained as a classical ballerina in Melbourne before going to college where she gained a BA Honours in physiotherapy. After training as a Pilates instructor, she founded the Australian Physiotherapy and Pilates Institute (APPI), an international Pilates teacher training academy, with her husband, Glenn Withers. They then went on to set up several APPI clinics across London and within leading performing arts and sporting arenas, where they teach their modified Pilates method. For more information, go to www.appihealthgroup.com.

Acknowledgments

Dorling Kindersley would like to thank Susannah Marriott for her involvement in the contents, Kathryn Meeker for editorial assistance, Stephen Bere for design, Susie Peachey for picture research, Steve Crozier and Adam Brackenbury for retouching assistance, Alyson Silverwood and Andrea Bagg for proofreading, and Anna Bennett for indexing.

Picture credits

The publisher would like to thank the following for their kind permission to reproduce their photographs:

(Key: a-above; b-below/bottom; c-centre; f-far; l-left; r-right; t-top)

2 Alamy Images: Chris Rout (c). **8–9 Getty Images:** Dave Nagel (c). **9 Getty Images:** Roman Maerzinger (c). **Dave Nagel:** (cr). **15 Getty Images:** Asia Images (br). **26 Getty Images:** Dominic DiSaia (c). **40 Getty Images:** QxQ IMAGES / Datacraft (c). **43 Alamy Images:** Artostock.com (cl); Mode Images Limited (bl); D. Hurst (clb, cra); Alexander Kalina (tr); Hugh Threlfall (cr). **Corbis:** Adrianna Williams (cla). **Getty Images:** Jamie Grill (crb). **45 Getty Images:** Comstock Images (br). **46 Getty Images:** Wirelmage (crb). **51 Getty Images:** Steve Cole (tr). **52–53 Getty Images:** Dave Nagel (c). **58 Alamy Images:** Chris Rout (c). **66 Alamy Images:** Chris Rout (c). **72 Getty Images:** mediaphotos (br). **74 Getty Images:** Don Bayley (c). **80 Getty Images:** Commercial Eye (br). **82 Getty Images:** Mike Powell (c). **85 Alamy Images:** Niall Edwards (c); macana (cl); Henry Iddon (cr). **Dreamstime. com:** Tombaky (cla). **86 Getty Images:** Erik Isakson (bl, br). **87 Getty Images:** Comstock (bl); Dennis O'Clair (br). **88 Getty Images:** Erik Isakson (bl). **90 Getty Images:** blueduck (c). **98 Getty Images:** PhotosIndia.com (cl). **98–99 Getty Images:** PhotosIndia.com (c). **99 Getty Images:** PhotosIndia. com (cr). **154 Getty Images:** Elke Meitzel (c). **194 Getty Images:** Imagemore Co., Ltd (c). **220 Corbis:** Radius Images (c). **248 Getty Images:** The Image Bank / Matt Henry Gunther (clb). **248-249 Getty Images:** The Image Bank / Matt Henry Gunther (c). **249 Getty Images:** The Image Bank / Matt Henry Gunther (cr). **257 Getty Images:** Image Source (c). **270 Getty Images:** Cavan Images (c). **312 Alamy Images:** Chris Rout (c)

Jacket images: *Front and Back:* **iStockphoto.com:** Tom Fullum, Arthur Kwiatkowski

All other images © Dorling Kindersley
For further information see: www.dkimages.com